SHATTERING
the
CANCER
MYTH

SHATTERING *the* CANCER MYTH

A Unique Positive Guide to Cancer Treatment using Traditional and Natural Therapies

KATRINA ELLIS

HINKLER
BOOKS

Shattering the Cancer Myth
A Unique Positive Guide to Cancer Treatment using Traditional and Natural Therapies

First published in 2003 by Hinkler Books Pty Ltd
Reprinted 2004

17–23 Redwood Drive
Dingley VIC 3172 Australia
www.hinklerbooks.com

ISBN 1 7412 1106 9

Cover designer: Sam Grimmer
Editors: Heather Hammonds and Michelle Hessels
Typesetting: Midland Typesetters, Maryborough, Vic Australia
Printed and bound in Australia by Griffin Press

This book details one woman's journey through illness and recovery from
cancer, and gives general advice about dealing with cancer, including
treatment with herbs and other substances. It records what medications and
natural therapies worked for the author; however, the advice contained in this
book cannot be considered and should not be used as a template for treatment
of cancer. It should not be relied upon as a substitute for proper medical
consultation. The author and publisher cannot be held responsible for any
illness or injury arising from failure to seek medical advice from a doctor.

Information on websites provided in this book was current at the time of
printing and Hinkler Books bears no responsibility for the content of said
websites or their future accessibility.

The author and publisher have made every effort to trace sources of references
used in this book and welcome further information from interested parties on
references that have proved untraceable.

FOREWORD

By Leslie Kenton

Clear, inspiring, and brimming with practical information, this book has been long awaited. Too many people find themselves succumbing to fear, hopelessness, and impotence when they receive a diagnosis of cancer and hear their doctor say: 'you have three months to live'. The pronouncement itself is enough to undermine immunity and trigger rampant proliferation of malignancies. Katrina – whom I affectionately call Katya – refused to succumb to a sense of powerlessness when she heard such pronouncements. Against all odds, despite her sense of helplessness and confusion, she chose to find a way to live and to tell the tale of a courageous journey from disease into wholeness. It is a powerful and life-enriching experience for anyone to read.

A beautiful young woman with sparkling eyes and a passion for her work in health and healing, when I met her six years ago, Katya was a glowing testament to the way in which each of us can take control of our own lives by raising our levels of energy, creativity and joy to the highest order. She ate well, she exercised, she loved her work and was much loved by everyone who was fortunate enough to work with her. Then, through no fault of her own, she found herself exposed to chemical poisoning which had been unearthed near where she lived in Thailand. Almost instantaneously her young radiant body developed cancer.

Katya's story is an all too human one of shock, fear, despondence, helplessness and horror as well as the way all of these can be transmuted into a will to survive, the determination not to accept hopelessness, and a willingness to make the most profound life passage anyone ever makes. Not only a passage out of illness into radiant health, it becomes a passage into meaning – one which demanded that she explore the depths of her own soul in the search for who she is at her core, what she values and how she chooses to live her life. All this by itself would make fascinating reading.

However, *Shattering The Cancer Myth* goes much further. Intrinsic to Katya's nature is a passion to empower others with sound, practical, well-researched tools, techniques and information enabling them to make their own passage out of illness and to live out the fullness of their own being.

Just what *is* cancer? What are its causes? What are the *real* possibilities of clearing it from your body regardless of whatever prognosis has been given? Katya examines all of these things with clarity, compassion and honesty. She looks at what effect a change in diet can exert on cancer. She explains how chemotherapy and radiation therapy work, what they have to offer and what their drawbacks are. She tells you how to make use of plant products and leading-edge neutraceuticals and tells us how simple, yet powerful, elements like flower essences can help change attitudes and lives.

The book is beautifully ordered making it easy to read and easy to use as a reference for specific help when you need it. You will find everything from how to use colour to shift mind and mood to wonderful recipes which can help restore balance while deep cleansing the body.

If you are struggling, as Katya once did, with the diagnosis of cancer and the shock and fear that surrounds the disease, you will find powerful, positive direction on what to do next within these pages. What Katya has written is nothing less than a unique manual for turning one's life around with a very special bonus: this book has *soul*.

CONTENTS

CONTENTS

This book is dedicated to all the brave people in this world fighting cancer and chronic illness, including the practitioners, loved ones, volunteers and family supporting this cause. I know it is God's wish for all of us who develop cancer and the loved ones involved to find a way for our true purity, health, compassion and trust to be reborn.

Initially I wanted to call this book 'Reborn as a Babe' – as in many ways experiencing cancer is like a rebirth and a second chance to us all. Instead I named it 'Shattering the Cancer Myth' as this truly signifies the lack of information available and falsities about cancer out there in today's world. For allowing me this opportunity to express myself and for all of their purest love, patience, support and understanding I wish to thank the following unique beings:

My mother Ann, whose unconditional love is like a flower itself, my father Hedley, whose essence is the pillar of strength, my gentle, nurturing brothers Larry and Brett, and my sisters Naree and Jen; my precious Nan, my eternal soul-mate Clayton, my beautiful mentors and friends (angels in disguise) – Roderick, Justin and Roland, my fantastic and knowledgeable soul sister – Leslie Kenton, the beautiful Clay and Nikki, my Thai family, the talented healer, Norm (God bless his soul), the caring and remarkable souls, Dr Bob Grace and Avenel Grace, Richard Thomas. And finally, my unconditionally loving dogs Keeta, Jarrah, Simo and Lucky.

Thank you all for helping me to re-discover my rainbows of love, laughter and eternal happiness hidden deep within my soul!

Introduction

'Shattering the Cancer Myth' contains an inspirational real life story which documents my courageous fight against cancer. My story signifies a journey of the soul through heartbreak and excitement, sadness and courage, disappointment and hope.

This book is not written by an author who does research on the subject of 'cancer' without actually having the firsthand experience herself. I am writing this book to help other people like myself around the world, of all ages, who face this confusing and mysterious disease.

In today's modern world, very little practical and useful information is available to cancer sufferers and our loved ones. Knowledge of a disease such as cancer creates power and self-empowerment makes us feel more confident in our ability to overcome this condition. Without any knowledge or information we can feel helpless and at the mercy of other people's decisions.

I hope to help provide you, the reader, with a greater scope of information on cancer, including feelings and emotions experienced, useful questions and answers, and alternative therapies available to avoid and reduce the side effects of orthodox cancer treatment. Through my own experience, I hope to offer inspiration to the lives of others.

This book is composed of three parts. Part One is a physical and spiritual portrayal of my struggle to discover the truth, and my determination to survive against all odds. Part Two is a complete cancer guide covering every successful natural treatment and medical treatment to support and heal cancer. Part Three contains further valuable information for those fighting cancer, including some of my favourite healing recipes.

As a naturopath myself I am not condemning orthodox medicine. In fact, I am amazed at the skill and knowledge of surgeons in today's modern world. I do believe that orthodox medicine and natural medicine work hand in hand and one should not be completely disregarded because of the other. If doctors and natural practitioners took advantage of the amazing healing potential found within each other's medical field, there would be a lot less sick people in the world today.

I am writing this book from a firsthand perspective. As a naturopath working throughout Asia, Europe, Australia and America for many years, I treated many forms of cancer in a variety of different cultures. I worked for a number of years in a health resort in Thailand, supervising the medical department, working in coordination with doctors and nurses. I treated not only third world Thai and Asian people but many famous actors, musicians, authors, TV celebrities, artists, company directors, doctors, supermodels and journalists.

The variety of nationalities and ages was enormous, and I used every natural therapy necessary to assess and treat their various health conditions. I gave numerous lectures and wrote articles for magazines on natural health and cancer prevention, and even hosted my own 'natural health' television program.

Living in this Asian paradise was a blissful and enlightening experience. Then suddenly, without warning, my luck changed. Due to a number of factors, including exposure to a toxic chemical, my life path began to take on a completely new direction. At twenty-seven years of age I had suddenly, without warning, developed malignant cancer. After visiting six top specialists and being misdiagnosed in England, Thailand, Australia and America, one doctor finally hinted on the possibility that I may have cancer. However, he still considered this extremely unlikely.

As it turned out, I had developed a very rare form of cancer called a germ cell carcinoma, normally found in men in their teens to early twenties. No known cause of my cancer was ever offered. The tumour had grown to over twenty-two centimetres in diameter (the size of a baby) and had leaked to many other areas of my body. The task ahead of me seemed daunting to say the least. The prognosis was average and involved many months of treatment.

Being a naturopath, I wished to incorporate both therapies into my treatment and the results were amazing. After careful deliberation I chose to undertake orthodox treatment, including surgery and chemotherapy, together with natural methods of practitioner range nutritional supplements, a wholefoods diet, yoga, meditation, positive affirmations, herbs and other forms of natural healing.

A few days after major surgery, I was up stretching and doing yoga, and within ten days I had recovered and had resumed all normal movement and activity. During chemotherapy treatment I experienced few side effects besides the inevitable hair loss and felt relatively high in energy.

One of the greatest risks of the type of chemotherapy I underwent was infertility. Due to taking the right nutritional supplements and using all the supportive natural therapies available to me, my menstruation and other hormonal processes stayed perfectly on track. I stopped chemotherapy against all advice, as I knew the chemotherapy drugs were doing more damage than good. I was told I would be a 'lucky girl' if I lived past the year, yet here I am four years later, cancer-free. Faith is a wonderful thing.

I now know my experience with cancer was a lesson from God to increase my awareness and to look at my life with a deeper understanding. Recovery from cancer offers us a second chance – an opportunity to transform and change our own life, and to touch those souls that we care for. As the sun rises every day, we are given another chance to say the right things, perform good actions and open our hearts to understanding and compassion.

I believe people who develop cancer are very sensitive and caring souls who act like radars in this world of beauty and chaos, absorbing everything. To avoid this disease you can still be a radar but you must learn to be a radar who not only absorbs but also reflects negative energy. You cannot change the world, only yourself. And changing your actions for the positive will no doubt act as a ripple on the pond and change the actions of those around you.

In these pages I provide a comprehensive and informative guide that covers many of the common things you are not told in your fight against cancer. The only people who can truly understand cancer and the feelings and emotions experienced are cancer patients themselves, which is why I have written this book. This book allows you the opportunity to look through our eyes and to grasp the true empathy and understanding that springs from real life experience.

Part One

MY TRUE STORY

Chapter 1

WINDS OF CHANGE

In the following pages I will attempt to reveal the true manifestation of my illness and how, through both natural and orthodox methods, I bravely overcame this life-threatening condition. I believe my brush with cancer was caused by not only one factor, but by a culmination of different stresses which I let affect my essence and well-being. I am sure I have learnt my lesson, yet only time will tell. If I can help one person avoid this life-threatening disease or improve someone's quality of life, I have done my job.

It is difficult for me to express how having cancer affected my life. Never have I felt such emptiness, realisation, pain, hope, love, courage, hurt and depression, all at once. Having cancer or any chronic illness which touches on the possibility of death tends to evoke a myriad of mixed emotions and feelings. Anyone who has the courage to beat cancer or chronic disease has the opportunity to undergo a life-altering experience.

My intriguing story first began in the exotic South-East Asian country of Thailand. Here I lived for four years in a unique and fascinating culture, vastly different from my homeland Australia, where I was born and raised. Since I was a little girl, I had always envisioned living in far away exotic lands and immersing myself in strange and mystic cultures. It seemed my wishes were being granted and there I was, living and working with the Thai people by some strange twist of fate.

The Deputy Prime Minister of Thailand had originally summoned me to Thailand six years previously. He had visited a most esteemed monk who informed him that his destiny would involve meeting a beautiful foreign woman. This woman apparently held the key to his unusual health problems and would bring an immense amount of good luck into his life. Being a devout Buddhist with great faith in his religion, this wise man decided to follow his monk's advice. Using his own intuition to guide him in the right direction, he boarded a plane to Australia in the hope of finding the woman in his monk's vision.

I was only twenty-three years old when I first met my soft-hearted, yet extremely powerful Thai friend. One week before this chance encounter I had found a yellow piece of paper hidden on the notice board at my college, advertising a position for a 'dietician' in Thailand. Even though I was not a dietician and I was still many months away from finishing my degree, a strong impulse urged me to call the phone number listed on the piece of paper. A soft female voice answered the phone and gave me an address in Sydney where I was to meet a man who would interview me for the position. I asked myself, 'What am I doing? I know nothing about this job!' Yet my heart kept urging me to follow this path.

On entering my friend's premise, I felt a warm and comforting presence. Our eyes met and instantly we both had a strong premonition that our lives would be altered forever. Thanks to his generous offer and kind heart, I made the decision to work for him in Thailand.

As I later discovered, my powerful Thai friend's advisor and Buddhist monk had informed him that I was the foreign woman that he had seen in his visions. Upon my arrival in Thailand, he explained the unique synchronicity of events that had lead to me becoming a part of his dream to help both him and his Thai people. I treated his health with a variety of natural remedies, balanced nutritional supplements and specific yoga exercises. Within six months he was completely rejuvenated and to this day, his health has remained in good condition.

My respected Thai friend owned a prestigious and famous health resort in Hua Hin. Hua Hin is a beautiful town on the eastern coast of Thailand. I keenly undertook the position of head naturopath, nutritionist and yoga instructor. Here I treated the rich and elite, with their many diverse problems and complaints. I had never in my life seen so many people with so many problems. Most of the guests' complaints and symptoms were very deep-seated and complex.

I noticed that many guests entered my office with a facade of perfection in place, no doubt used as a coat of protection. My nature is such that others feel instantly comfortable in my presence. Within moments most people would open their hearts, revealing their true troubles, their symptoms, hurts, repressions and health problems. After all, why had these people chosen to see me in the first place? Obviously something within their souls had told them to share their pain and perhaps I had the ability to listen to them with compassion. And by opening their hearts and releasing their inner hurts, they were able to find the ability to heal and thus, start the healing process.

The clientele I was treating came from all over the world. They were the richest, most successful people in the business world. Their characters were highly developed, honed from years of experience in 'dog eat dog' corporate environments. I was amazed to find even the most athletic and so called, 'spiritual' people who had devoted their whole lives to health and fitness, seemed to have just as many hurts and deep pains in their lives and in their eyes as any normal person. These had now manifested in their bodies as real health problems and symptoms.

I worked long hours with passion, trying to help solve everyone's problems. I didn't want anyone to feel pain. It hurt me inside to see so many people hurting. I wished within my heart that I could wave a magic wand to make their pain go away.

I had learnt how to treat the cause of the problems and yes; I had a great deal of success with the minor problems and with those who were willing to help themselves. But for those people with chronic illness, long-term disease and cancer, I felt hopeless. Hopelessly lost!

I was treating up to fifteen clients every day and all with a variety of symptoms, never just one. In one hour, my clients expected me to act as a psychic, counsellor, healer and doctor all wrapped up into one package. The pressure to solve someone's lifetime of habits in one hour was immense.

I assisted in the healing of many people. My diagnosis using a combination of modern, computerised iridology and simple, age-old diagnostic techniques brought about many 'miracle-type' findings and cures. Women who had been deemed infertile were falling pregnant after six months of treatment with me. I also had great success with other illnesses deemed incurable by Western medicine. To me it was no miracle. It was simply someone listening to them and treating the cause of the problem, not trying to put a band-aid on the problem.

I gained quite a reputation internationally and people visited me from all around the world just to spend one hour with me. I was acknowledged in magazines, newspapers and television, throughout Asia and Europe. I was even offered my own television show on 'natural health', which I pursued in the small amount of time I had available. All of this attention and high expectations from hopeful souls became extremely exhausting for me.

People with more chronic and terminal illnesses began to frequent my office, hoping for some type of cure or solution to their problem. Honestly, although I'd studied all of these more serious conditions, I had never really experienced any of them myself. So when it came to these major illnesses, I felt out of my depth. I felt like a little girl giving advice to wiser souls. They had the life experience; I had the textbook learning and other therapist's advice.

Don't get me wrong, I had some fantastic advice to give, but most of this advice was from education, not from true life experience. Advice of this kind is often best given by someone who has had the true pain and suffering felt from experiencing similar illnesses. I now know that true empathy comes from life experience.

I felt something had to shift in my life. I had never realised what an earth-shattering and life-altering experience chronic disease is. How could a girl in her mid twenties who had only lightly suffered life experiences give advice to a seventy-year-old man dying of cancer? This was the type of situation in my work I was constantly being placed in. Yet, I desperately wanted to give the right advice to help. I knew it was my life path and my destiny.

One day a very kind and gentle man entered my office. He had no appointment booked, yet felt a strong desire to walk into my office to talk with me. The deep creases in his face revealed a lifetime of experience and knowledge, and yet underneath his camouflage I could detect a great sadness. After a few minutes of sitting in silence, he began to open his heart to me.

He told me about various aspects of his life, including his success in the business world and how within months, his years of dedication would end. He had been diagnosed only months before with terminal prostate cancer. The malignant cancer had spread throughout his entire body and the doctors proposed he would have only a short time left to live. His first grandchild was about to be born and he desperately wanted to start playing a more active part in his family's life.

As this man told me his story, tears began to fall from my eyes and I felt my heart aching with a strong desire to hold him like a child. Without thought, I heard words of encouragement falling from my lips. I told him that everything would be okay and not to give up. I let him know that nothing is impossible and that miracles happen every day. Yes, others had given up on him, but that didn't mean he had to give up on himself.

This courageous man ended up spending invaluable years with his family and granddaughter, much to the amazement of those who had determined his death sentence. He made me realise the miraculous power of healing and the incredible will to survive contained within the human spirit.

I continued to work six days a week, ten to fourteen hours a day, without a break for over three years. It was difficult for me to obtain a holiday, as my schedule was fully booked and I felt responsible for the welfare of my clients and department. I was surrounded by the most wonderful Thai people, and I offered free advice and help to my new family with passion and love. They in turn offered me a place in Thai society and sheltered me in a blanket of protection from any danger surrounding me in this 'eye for an eye' society. I became known as the 'good hearted Thai person with the Western face'.

Unfortunately, I began to experience difficulties in my working relationship with an employee of the resort, especially when our soft-hearted Thai owner was away on business. I felt that this person was jealous of my work and of my close relationship with the owner of the resort and with the Thai people. This person began to make my work life resemble an unpredictable roller coaster ride. Some of my contractual rights were taken away and I started to wonder if this person was searching for some way to warrant my dismissal. So here I was at my career peak, meeting the world's elite business people, actors, musicians, journalists, models and even royalty, yet nothing could balance out the unnecessary pressures I was being dealt by this person. The chance for me to enjoy the positive and fulfilling nature of my work was slowly being spoiled.

At the same time I was entertaining guests in my home and aiming to keep everyone happy, trying to find time for my demanding lover and slowly draining and exhausting myself completely. My energy was being directed away from me and into everyone else. A culmination of factors eventually forced me to make the decision to change. Enough was enough. I courageously made the decision to leave my present work and allow life to guide me in the right direction. I knew if I let go with love and complete trust, something miraculous would happen. I never realised at the time just how painful and pleasurable this miraculous event could possibly be.

Chapter 2

TROUBLE IN PARADISE

'Freedom!' I thought to myself, every day. Finally a break, after three years of working like a dog. Even though I loved every moment of my naturopathy, yoga, iridology and nutrition, working so many hours can drain your love of anything away. This is something I have now learnt from that experience.

I finally had some spare time to recover my energies and redirect my goals into future plans. This time proved short-lived as offers for work poured in from all directions. Guests continued to visit from the health resort on a private basis, as my reputation around the world had surpassed me. At this stage in my life I felt very secure, both emotionally and financially.

Visitors from my homeland continued to arrive in droves, hearing of the wonderful welcome awaiting all in my spacious home. While it was fun for a while and I enjoyed the different types of company, it also proved to be a huge drain on my energy, finances and time. Still, I continued to welcome people with open arms into my home, or should I say, 'guest house'. In my spare time I acted as tour guide and took friends and acquaintances on shopping tours, rainforest walks, motor bike treks and even gave a helping hand at healing sick visitors and counselling lost souls. These draining visits continued regularly, while I should have been recovering and reflecting on my past three years of hard work and growth.

Interestingly, so comforting and welcoming was my company that one of my good friends, Mike, made the decision to move in permanently. While at the time I didn't protest and was quite looking forward to having another natural healer living with me, later I would prove to regret this rash decision.

In the beginning Mike was quite an inspirational force, possessing a powerful personality with great knowledge. Mike and I had been wonderful friends for years and it was great to have another like-minded soul around to communicate with. Being an accomplished martial artist, body worker, natural healer and dancer, his life experiences seemed to complement my own and he brought a new optimism and friendliness to the household.

So Mike, my partner Anthony and myself, decided to embark on a totally new business venture together, unlike anything any of us had ever done before. I had been captivated for many years by the beauty and magnificence of Thai silks and it seemed both of my friends shared this interest. We decided to investigate further the possibility of combining modern Western fashions with unique and stunning Thai silks. We visited local tailors and it seemed like a feasible project, and a profitable method of obtaining a self-supporting source of income while still maintaining our creativity. However, as we realised over time, the reality proved to be far different from the concept.

After a number of weeks of searching for the right contacts both locally and in Bangkok, we all gave up hope of getting the idea and the company off the ground. Everything seemed too difficult, like pushing against a brick wall. Then, overnight, our fate changed. Within days we had a fully operational factory established in our own home and products being produced as quickly as we thought of them. It often seems when you totally give up on something and release the idea, suddenly, without expectation, it becomes manifest right before your eyes. This is what happened for us.

Life continued peacefully and steadily for a short time. We all worked hard and overcame the little glitches together without argument or complaint. Just as everything seemed okay, the ugly 'monster of dissatisfaction' reared its head and took a bite. The workers wanted more money, Mike wanted a break, Anthony was busy with his other job and I was left with a mountain of responsibility and problems to solve.

I continued to deflect the amazing work offers I was receiving from all parts of the globe in the hope that our company would succeed, and Anthony and Mike could have a wonderful career to fall back on. I started to question whether I had started this company for myself or was once again simply trying to make others happy. Nothing ever seems to succeed if your only intentions are solely to make others happy, I realised. I was learning this lesson in the most difficult way possible.

I worked continually from seven in the morning until one or two a.m. the next day. Ridiculous hours when this was exactly the lifestyle I was trying to escape. Once again I had attracted this routine back into my life. Was I a sucker for punishment? What had initially started with the intention of creating more freedom for myself was developing into a lifestyle which seemed destined to imprison me. Mike was no help; he had lost interest and seemed to be just drifting along. Anthony seemed to be absorbed in his own problems and had no time left to support and assist the company. I was left holding the 'baby', a baby I didn't even need in the first place.

On one of these long stressful days I took a moment's break and walked onto our back veranda. The day was muggy and the northerly winds had picked up dramatically. Mike was in bed, sleeping the day away. It seemed he was sleeping more than usual. I smelt a strange acetone odour in the air and looked up into the sky. There seemed to be an unusual orange-coloured mist in the sky, similar to sea spray.

I called out to Mike and asked if he could smell the strange odour and see what I was witnessing. He verified my findings and said he had also seen it the day before, and believed it had the aroma of chemicals. Immediately I had a strange feeling in my stomach and I knew something was wrong. My initial gut feeling proved to be spot-on.

The following day, the incident we had witnessed appeared in newspaper and television reports. Some deadly toxic chemicals had been uncovered, only a short distance from our home. One hundred and fifty Thai construction workers were innocently digging up the local runway to build a new airport and had uncovered the containers of toxic chemicals, obviously buried many years ago at the end of the Vietnam War. These chemicals have been linked to birth defects, serious illness, health problems and cancer.

We were all shocked. It was unbelievable. The chemical mist continued to blow over the town and the deadly chemicals remained open, whilst no clean up operation was commissioned. The construction workers were raced to hospital with various symptoms and the admission of sick people from the surrounding area into the local hospitals increased dramatically. Our entire household became ill with symptoms ranging from respiratory complaints, shortness of breath, dizziness, extreme lethargy, fever, nausea, headaches, rapid weight loss and lack of appetite.

Over the next week, Mike became a mere shadow of himself and was forced to leave the town. I suffered from a severe fever that lasted ten days and my weight dropped from fifty kilograms to a mere forty-four. I felt unwell, often becoming dizzy and suffering from regular blackout spells.

The stories in the press continued and yet no official cleanup was authorised. Instead, the stories became more and more conflicting until eventually they were covered up, to save the town from the severe loss of tourism caused by the discovery of these toxic chemicals. Local politicians and rich Thai businessmen with a vested interest in the local Hua Hin tourism began a rapid propaganda campaign to stimulate international tourism and over time, the toxic chemical discovery was completely concealed.

Local people continued to get sick and suffer from strange, unexplainable illnesses. I was forced to leave my business and home in search of a cleaner, non-polluted environment. Many other ex-pats had departed already to avoid more serious illness caused from these chemicals and I was quick on their heels. Only two weeks after the toxic chemicals were uncovered I left Hua Hin for the safer, cleaner surroundings of my home country, Australia. Due to someone else's irresponsible actions, I and many other innocent people were forced to leave our homes and suffer the dangerous consequences of chemical exposure.

At the time I was unaware how the careless actions of others could affect my life. I was to learn later, that these actions could affect the health and welfare of future generations, as well as mine.

Chapter 3

WEEDS IN MY BELLY

I heaved a sigh of relief when I reached the clean, untainted Australian soil. I took a deep breath and breathed the clean, pure air. I felt it instantly rejuvenate my soul and heal my body. My parents were shocked by my sudden weight loss. I was a stick creature compared to my former curvaceous self. I had lost a tremendous amount of weight in the previous two weeks. The toxic chemicals had exerted their damaging power and their after-effects were still being shown in the frailty of my body.

My mother took me in her arms and blessed me with her healing touch and knowledge. I ate heartily of the healthiest of organic foods and within a few weeks had returned to my former weight, and showed no apparent symptoms of illness. My partner returned to Australia and was amazed at the radiance and energy emanating from my soul. The clean air and food had dramatic healing effects on us both and in a short period of time we were dancing around, full of energy and life once again.

This period in my life was full of many joyous and happy events. My brother was to be married to a beautiful woman and both my partner and I shared in the festivities and love whole-heartedly. Feeling our hearts overflowing with love, we wished to share this amazing feeling with Anthony's family also. On a whim, we set off for their house, excited and thrilled at the possibility of sharing the adventures of our escape from Thailand and other exciting tales.

Upon arriving at my boyfriend's family home, we threw open the car doors and raced inside. It had been two years since Anthony had seen his family and he was ready to burst open with excitement. The response we received upon our arrival was distant and guarded, to say the least. Feeling surprised at their unusual reaction, we tried not to show any disappointment. Anthony's older sibling acted rudely and his parents seemed disinterested.

Both of us left after one hour to seek a more pleasant environment and I felt sick – sick in my stomach that loved ones could be so cold when we felt so loving. Out of confusion and hurt, Anthony blamed me for their reaction and I became the 'cause' of his family's problems. I felt sad, hurt and abandoned. After all of the unconditional love I had given, I was being emotionally attacked. I didn't know where to turn or what to do. My stomach felt knotted and I felt unloved by the one person in life who was meant to stand by me. I thought to myself, 'How sad life is when we blame our own unhappiness on the people we love the most.'

I cried, cried from my soul. I cried just like when I was a child, tears of hurt and pain from deep within my belly. How could he treat me like this? I had given him everything, I had supported him emotionally, spiritually and financially for years, I had even bought his plane ticket home to see his parents. He had lived the life of luxury in Thailand thanks to my kindness, or now as I clearly see it, my ignorance and stupidity. And yet he could turn around and blame me for his own family's attitude.

I remember feeling deep within myself that I just wanted to curl up and disappear. I wondered what would happen if I disappeared into thin air. Would he even care? My belly felt bloated and I noticed a sickly feeling within my stomach. Anthony told me to stop crying; he told me he understood, and if I didn't stop crying I would make myself sick. I said to Anthony in a strong way, that if this unjustified blame towards me didn't stop I could get very sick.

The battles with Anthony's family continued over the next two weeks. It was a painful time for us both, as I believed in my naivety that we had all been such good friends before. We tried several times to re-form a solid relationship with his parents, but to no avail.

One day, quite unexpectedly, an abusive argument erupted between Anthony's parents and ourselves. I found his father yelling only a few centimetres from my face and his mother wailing. It was all too much, I felt heartbroken. How could my lover allow his own parents to treat me this way? How could he stand by seeing me being hurt and not stand up and protect me? If the tables were turned, I would be to his aid like a knight to his princess. Maybe in my heart I have always lived in a fairytale world and the reality of life is not a fairytale at all.

During this stressful and rocky period in my life, my lower abdomen began to enlarge, ever so slightly at first and then larger, bit-by-bit. I continued to ignore the symptoms, yet I knew something was wrong. I felt within my heart this stress and hurt had to go somewhere. I was taking all the pain inside myself and refusing to let it go into the universe. I felt the weeds forming in my belly and yet I retained the notion that nothing could ever happen to me. I couldn't have been further from the truth. The past months filled with stress, blame, change and even toxic poison were beginning to take their toll and this last incident proved to be the straw that broke the camel's back.

Chapter 4

THE STRAW THAT BROKE THE CAMEL'S BACK

The turbulent wave of emotions had finally reached its peak and Anthony made the decision to leave Australia and head back to peaceful Thailand. I was offered an amazing naturopathy job in England and decided to follow this with passion. I felt that starting my healing work again would be good for me and give me a more solid direction in my life once more.

My stomach was still slightly enlarged and yet I continued to ignore this, putting it down to bloating from bad emotions and feeling upset. I stayed in England only a short period of time. My heart was yearning to reunite with my beautiful four-legged companions and to return to the comfort of my home in Thailand. I needed to investigate my health further and reassure myself that everything was okay. In Hua Hin (Thailand) I had access to familiar doctors and specialists, and treatment was relatively inexpensive.

On returning to Thailand I felt an instant relief. I immediately visited a gynaecologist at the local hospital as my stomach was growing larger by the day. It was beginning to appear as if I was pregnant and I had a number of pregnancy tests to rule out this possibility. The doctor performed an ultrasound examination, blood and urine tests. I felt nervous; I had never really been sick so I had little idea of what to expect.

The doctor looked nervous himself, as he had noticed a large mass in the lower left quadrant of my abdomen. He believed it to be a large ovarian cyst, eleven centimetres in diameter. He insisted he operate straight away to remove the cyst and possibly the left ovary. Shock overcame me – I felt weak and dizzy. How could I have a cyst? My menstruation had always been perfect and I had never had any signs of discomfort or pain during menstruation. I had always associated large cysts with painful periods, backaches and other noticeable symptoms.

I kept thinking to myself, 'he's wrong, he's made a mistake, they'll discover it's an ectopic pregnancy or something like that', so I ignored his suggestions and chose to seek further opinions. Two days later, with the doctor's reports in hand, I visited a top specialist in Bangkok. I showed him my reports and underwent further tests and examinations, including internal ultrasounds, internal examinations and blood tests. His results were surprising. They indicated a large ovarian cyst, fourteen centimetres in diameter, not on the left side as the previous doctor had indicated, but on the right side.

I had two different opinions; one doctor believed the cyst existed on the left side and one doctor believed the cyst existed on the right side. I felt confused and scared. This doctor thought the best treatment would be a complete hysterectomy. This was to ensure a cyst wouldn't grow on the other ovary in the future. He handed me a brochure, offering me a special price on his 'hysterectomy package', which included an operation, a private room and five star hotel meals. It was too ridiculous, the doctor trying to sell me a hysterectomy package. I burst into fits of laughter, right in front of him. Of course, I brushed off his advice and went home, dumbfounded and upset, yet slightly amused.

I quickly researched every piece of information I could find on ovarian cysts. Even though I didn't fit the classic signs and symptoms of having an ovarian cyst, I still opted to treat it naturally through detoxification, vitamins, specific herbs and foods, and aromatherapy oils. I have had success using natural therapies on my patients with ovarian cysts, so I retained a great deal of hope throughout this process. There was very little stress in my life at this stage. I removed all sources of stress and discontentment, and remained calm, positive and highly hopeful.

After three weeks of intensive treatment, the results were quite disappointing to me. My stomach seemed only slightly smaller. I needed to take this on a larger scale and I asked a close and trusted friend in America for help. He immediately flew me to California and I continued my natural treatments in greater amounts, increasing my intake of specific vitamins and herbs. In the American health food stores I felt like a kid let loose in a candy store. Every kind of vitamin, herb and homeopathic formulae available was at my disposal. I continued to treat myself naturally and after two weeks saw a greater improvement than before.

My friend arranged for me to visit a top gynaecological specialist at UCLA, California. I have always had a great fear of doctors since my mother was misdiagnosed with cancer many years ago and was given inappropriate treatment for her condition. I walked into his office nervously and was greeted by a warm hearted and pleasant soul.

Once again numerous tests were performed and he confidently proclaimed an ovarian cyst existed on the right side, twenty centimetres in diameter. I couldn't believe it had grown when all that time, my stomach felt like it had shrunk. He wanted to perform a cystectomy (removal of the cyst) and a possible ovariectomy (removal of the ovary, if absolutely necessary). My third diagnosis and I still thought something wasn't right. 'Of course he's right,' I convinced myself. 'After all, he is one of the world's top specialists.'

I walked home, holding my stomach, wishing there was some other way. I really didn't want to have an ovary removed. As they explained to me, women have their ovaries removed all the time – it's extremely common. But if it was that easy for me to get a cyst on one ovary, what was stopping it from happening to the other? And if I had my ovary removed and something happened to the other, what then? Twenty-seven years old without ovaries to produce hormones – hormones for sexuality, hormones for reproduction and hormones to keep my youth. Male doctors can sometimes forget these simple facts that are so important to women.

I went back to my suite and called my mum. I needed some wise advice, being once again so far away from home. I needed to hear her comforting voice and reassuring words. Talking to her made me feel calmer and more relaxed. So in one week,

I was destined to have this operation. I wanted to have this strange entity out of my body so I could wear normal clothes again and feel good about my body. But at the same time, I felt extremely hesitant.

While in the land of 'free information' I continued to do research about the barrels of toxic chemicals uncovered in Hua Hin, Thailand. I found a number of interesting reports on the internet from newspapers, magazines and various travel sites. Local Thai residents claimed to have been hired in 1963 to mix chemicals and spray them on forest patches in the local area. Of course, the forest had quickly been destroyed. As time passed and as parties with a vested interest in tourism and business exerted their power, the reports became fewer and more dispersed.

I consulted with several top attorneys in Los Angeles. They told me that this case was too large for them and no individual in their right mind would take on such a case. As I quietly sat pondering this problem, the phone rang and fate stepped in once again. It was the voice of a gentle, yet confident man; a talented healer from Australia. I heard his kind voice and positive words. He told me to jump on a plane and come home, as he believed he could heal me in four days.

'Four days, that's unbelievable!' I thought to myself. I was never one to ignore a challenge, so I took up his offer. Within hours I was on a plane back to Australia, feeling bright and hopeful once again. My faith was re-stimulated. At this stage I was willing to give anything a go.

As soon as I arrived in Australia, after an eighteen-hour flight, my beautiful and positive mother greeted me. She raced me around to this wise healer's home and we instantly began his unorthodox treatment. He performed an unusual technique on me called the 'raindrop technique'. This was originally derived from the North American Indians and involved a series of point holding, heat packs and stimulation. It was difficult for me to lie on my stomach, as the mass had grown so large it restricted my normal movement. He told me all forms of treatment he offered would attempt to burst the cyst and he would know within four days if the treatment would prove successful.

Before leaving his office, my mother tentatively asked him if there was any possibility her daughter might have cancer. He chuckled at the mere suggestion and reassured her that there was definitely no chance I had cancer. He had treated three to four cancer patients every day for over twenty years and in his opinion, I was simply too vibrant and healthy to even contemplate this possibility. We all breathed a sigh of relief.

In my heart I remained optimistic and full of faith. I took a number of different homeopathics, including homeopathic 'bee venom'. During this time I used a natural clay mask with four aromatherapy oils (damask rose, sweet fennel, clary sage and geranium) and let this dry on my abdomen. Hot castor oil packs were used every day to stimulate lymphatic circulation around this area of the body. In conjunction with these treatments, I repeated healing affirmations and psychological healing techniques daily, to assist with the emotional cause of my condition.

After four days, the cyst had not burst but had rather decreased in size. I noticed my abdomen getting smaller and I felt so excited that I didn't want to laugh too loud in case it wasn't real. We continued the same treatment for two weeks and over this time, my stomach got smaller and smaller. I was thrilled. I couldn't believe it and I just wanted to jump for joy.

Two more weeks passed and I came back to thank my friend and healer for his wonderful attention and help. On my last visit he asked me if I ever felt irritable around period time. I explained to him about feeling edgy one day before my period and he handed me a small bottle of homeopathics. He told me to go home and take four of these every week and the emotional cause of my illness would disappear.

I went home feeling on top of the world. My faith in natural therapies was restored; I wanted to share my knowledge and happiness with everyone. I took the tablets and planned to visit some friends living three hours from my home. I was anxious to celebrate and spread my joy. Two hours after taking the tablets I noticed my upper abdomen begin to enlarge. Very slowly it grew bigger and bigger, gradually moving down to my lower abdomen. My entire stomach area blew up into a giant ball. I now looked like I was nine months pregnant.

I couldn't believe it. I told myself that it wasn't real – that maybe it was a normal reaction to the tablets the healer had given me and it would go down later. I lay down on the couch and closed my eyes. I dreamt that upon awaking it would be gone and my stomach would be normal again. When I finally awoke the next morning, the bloating was there, larger than ever. No, No, No – it couldn't be!

I called my healer friend and explained the situation. He had no answers and offered no advice. I was on my own. I felt so disappointed; after all that hard work and effort it had come down to this. I had travelled the entire world looking for answers and the circle had led me back to the beginning. I wanted to break down and howl, but I knew it wouldn't change anything. My heart told me to push on; an answer was waiting just around the corner.

Chapter 5

IF AT FIRST YOU DON'T SUCCEED, TRY AND TRY AGAIN

I felt crushed, beaten and tired. I wanted to feel normal again and I wanted to believe that there really was an answer. I decided to see another doctor, a female doctor this time. Three days after my stomach had blown up again I walked into another specialist's office, hoping and praying for a sensible answer.

The doctor appeared shocked when she saw my stomach. She immediately requested more tests, including blood tests, an ultrasound and a CT scan. I had no energy to explain or protest and I allowed all tests to be performed without complaint. Amazingly enough, this time they believed I had hydatid disease, as a number of strange masses or cysts were showing up throughout my entire body. Hydatid disease – well, this was a new one for me. Had I been around dogs that had been exposed to parasites? Well yes, but I'd never had any other related hydatid symptoms before.

The diagnosis of my condition had gone from one ovarian cyst to a number of cysts throughout my body. What was going on, what did I have? I waited anxiously for two days, for the results of my tests. Everyone knows what a nerve-wracking experience waiting for the results of medical tests can be. I tried to keep myself busy to allow time to move quicker (although it never does) and waited for that life-changing phone call.

The following night the doctor rang and indicated that I did not have hydatid disease or cancer. I felt extremely relieved, so I assumed it must simply be an ovarian cyst. Her suggestion was for me to see another specialist in Brisbane who could accurately determine the findings of the CT scan. I agreed and was soon heading off on my fifth visit to a specialist, desperately looking for an answer.

I arrived and saw another female doctor. Another examination and my body was beginning to feel extremely violated. She explained the cyst may be a borderline tumour and was not dangerous or malignant, but needed to be removed soon. The earliest they could perform the operation was in four weeks' time. I couldn't wait four weeks. My belly button was already starting to protrude, the cyst was larger than a baby at ten months old and I had no skin left to fill the mass growing within my stomach. I needed it removed as soon as possible; otherwise I felt I could surely explode. She suggested I see another specialist who may be able to operate sooner. I agreed once again and off to my sixth specialist I went, trying to laugh at the ridiculousness of the whole situation.

The next doctor in my saga was extremely nice and accommodating. He thoroughly examined my CT scans and mentioned the possibility of a more serious form of cancer in my body. The cyst had strange projections emanating from its root, which is quite often the case with more serious forms of cancer. I was bewildered, as no one had even hinted at the probability of cancer before. He reassured me and said it was likely it wasn't but just in case, we should operate right away. Feeling a little scared and slightly doubtful, I agreed to his decision in the hope that someone could remove this abnormal mass from my belly and allow me control over my own body and emotions once again.

I had spent months detoxifying and strengthening my body through natural methods and even though I had this huge mass in my stomach, I felt I was in a safe position to undergo surgery. Being a naturopath, I knew it was important to build up my strength and reserves before the operation to ensure a rapid recovery after surgery. I took a wonderful range of energy-based natural supplements, suitable for healing and repair.

Only days later, I found myself in the hospital room waiting for the operation to commence. Here I was in the hospital, somewhere I had never been and somewhere I had vowed I would never be. I disliked the morbid colours of the walls and the disinfectant smell of the bed linen and floors. I tried to stay positive and keep smiling, and tell myself it would be all right. I had convinced myself it was nothing and I would recover quickly. After all, I was prepared for anything, I believed. Yet, was I really?

I adamantly demanded the operating doctor leave my ovaries in place and remove no necessary organs for fertility. He agreed to do the best he could. Time passed, the operation was performed and as soon as I regained the slightest hint of consciousness I asked if I still had my ovaries. I was told yes and I fell back to sleep, content and satisfied.

When I fully regained consciousness, I glanced down at my stomach and noticed tubes running from a number of different areas in my body. Strange coloured liquids were draining from inside me and into plastic collecting bags. I was beginning to feel lighter already. My brother walked into the room with a handful of flowers, wearing a courageous smile. He glanced at the tubes inserted into my skin. All hint of colour instantly drained from his face and he ran out of the room on the verge of fainting. It was quite a shock for anyone to see me like this.

During my short stay in hospital, I proved to be a huge headache to the local medical staff, as I refused to eat their devitalised foods. My family sat in the back room juicing organic fruits and vegetables, and preparing the most healing concoctions to enhance my rapid recovery. My room was overflowing with vitamins, herbs, essential oils and uplifting music. I practised yoga daily and by the third day was anxious to leave, and resume my active lifestyle.

The doctor came in to talk to me and explained what had happened. Pathology had been performed on the tissue mass which had been removed and it revealed a very rare form of cancer called a germ cell carcinoma. This type of cancer is rarely found in women and generally found in teenage to mid twenty-year-old males. It was actually one of the fastest growing and most aggressive cancers in the world.

The main cancer had burst a number of days ago and the deadly cancerous liquid had spread to other areas of my body. I now had cancer throughout my body. The tumour was so large that on its removal, more liquid had spilt and spread. Apparently they had left a sliver of my right ovary and removed a large mass off my left ovary. The doctor said my only chance of survival was to begin intensive chemotherapy straight away.

'What? Did I hear that right – did you say chemotherapy?' I asked.

I couldn't believe it; I had always been so healthy. I had never smoked, I had rarely drunk alcohol and I had eaten a very healthy diet all of my life. Now I had cancer and had the chance of dying, unless I undertook some drastic form of treatment which I had always been against. He also believed that in his experience, I would die in three to six months if I refused to undergo chemotherapy.

I didn't want to die and I didn't want to believe them. Now I felt really confused. I had to trust my own judgment, yet it was difficult when I had been misdiagnosed so many times before. How could I believe these doctors when so many errors had been made? Being a naturopath, it was going against all of my beliefs and judgments to undergo such a debilitating and barbaric form of treatment.

I had no choice, I had to dive into the pool with open arms, but this time I was taking my own lifejacket. The middle path was the way for me. After much deliberating, crying, questioning and research I reluctantly decided to undergo chemotherapy used in conjunction with all natural forms of treatment. Isn't it funny – when I had a choice between life and death what I was most concerned about was losing my beautiful, long, golden locks. I guess there's no changing the fact I have been conditioned slightly to think hair and such trivial things are so important. After facing death and the possibility of losing loved ones, I now understand the relativity of life's importance in a much clearer context.

Chapter 6

LET THE HEALING
FLOW IN

Three days after my serious operation, I began intensive chemotherapy. For the first few days I fought against it all – against the doctors, the medical system, the nurses and even myself. I told myself it was wrong, it was all a conspiracy to make money and they had mixed up the test results. Eventually I gave up fighting against the system and began fighting for my own life.

Karen, a wonderful friend of mine, visited me in the hospital on the first day of treatment. Karen is an extremely intelligent nutritionist who had worked for many years with Henry, a famous and reputable nutritionist who had developed a powerful and healing range of energy based natural medicines over many years. Together they worked out the most beneficial supplements for my needs, in the hope of protecting my body from the dangerous effects of chemotherapy and also to speed up the effects of the treatment.

The type of chemotherapy I received was the most intensive ever given. Here I was, forty-seven kilograms in total, receiving massive doses of cytotoxic drugs fit for a rugby union player. I would sit in the strange armchair having large amounts of chemotherapy drugs pumped into my veins through huge needles for up to seven hours every day, while I watched other chemotherapy patients come and go within one hour.

I felt angry. Why was I in this position when I had eaten such a healthy diet all of my life? I kept telling myself how unjust life was, how unfair and painful it could be. I kept telling myself how indiscriminate cancer could be, when someone my age and even young children were in this painful position. Yet I knew feeling like this wasn't going to help me.

As the days went on, I drew on my own inner strength to challenge this disease and beat it as quickly as possible. Beating cancer as quickly as possible became my primary goal in life. I listened to positive affirmation tapes and read inspirational books. I took large amounts of specific vitamins and herbs, and I tried to laugh and smile, and think of the beautiful things I would be doing when I was finished. I thought of the wonderful insight I would gain from this, the knowledge and empathy to help and heal others. I dreamt of running on the beach with my dogs and dancing freely with my friends. I dreamt of visiting faraway lands and rejoicing in the celebration of life with other cultures yet again.

All around me, I drew on my circle of loved ones and friends. I felt so blessed. I have the most wonderful parents who truly cherish me and two kind-hearted brothers who adore me and shower love on me every day. I looked around and in my time of need they were all there protecting and supporting me, and we were all still together. I thought to myself 'how special and how lucky I am' and in that moment I realised I had gained an insight.

My beautiful mother and father were always with me, lending their years of wisdom and unconditional love. My caring brothers also remained close by my side throughout chemotherapy treatment. They played games with me, brought me creative presents and filled my environment with joy and laughter. They would hold my hand tightly and distract me while the painful chemotherapy needles were forced into my veins. Whenever a hint of sadness washed over me, I would think of the precious love that was wrapping its arms around me every day.

Andy, a great friend of mine, regularly visited me throughout treatment. His vibrant character and unusual ways always brought a smile to my face. Bec, my lifelong friend, flew in from Tasmania and made me feel so happy as we relived all of our teenage dreams and talked about our future desires. Karen was often around, giving me the latest natural information and blessing me with her healing touch to help me to overcome this setback in my life. Even during my most painful and depressing moments, I looked around and my family and friends were always close by my side.

After six solid days of chemotherapy, my partner Anthony arrived from Japan. During this time of healing for me we had drifted apart and I was beginning to have many clear realisations about our relationship. I realised that I had stayed in a mentally abusive relationship for years with him and I had thought that somehow I could save him, and make his life better. I had forsaken everything in my life, including my health, for another person. In spite of these thoughts I was still quite excited to see him, as I really needed to feel his familiar warm touch and to hear his words of comfort. I guess I just needed something familiar to make me feel sane.

Anthony walked into the hospital at a fast pace and ran over to my side. Immediately I saw the shocked expression on his face, which he carefully tried to conceal. I suppose it was a shock for anyone to see me like this. It was quite a turn around for me. Normally I would be bouncing around, full of vibrancy and enthusiasm, a total picture of health. Now I looked like a ghost – gaunt and thin, with a number of different tubes emanating from my pallid skin. He held my hand and told me I looked beautiful. It made me laugh as I told him what a great liar he was.

He handed me some beautiful, colourful hats that he had carefully selected while in Japan. I had always loved hats and now with my inevitable hair loss, I had a real chance of wearing them much more often. We closed the curtains around us and managed to create a 'picnic' environment. We sat there and ate our favourite healthy treats, and temporarily escaped the humdrum of the hospital ward.

After the first week of chemotherapy I returned to my parents' home with Anthony. At first I felt great, so full of energy and hardly aware of any side effects or symptoms from treatment. However, as the days went by my energy levels were slowly depleted. I desperately wanted to spend more time with Anthony and do all the things we loved to do. I wanted to jump in the surf and roll in the sand, visit waterfalls and dance wildly. I guess I wanted to dive back into the past to a place that seemed easy, comfortable and familiar, at least in my memories.

Unfortunately, the surgery and chemotherapy had robbed me of my energy and drive. I was determined to feel better. I took large amounts of vitamins and herbs every day and continued to practise yoga and meditation techniques. I walked through the forest with my dogs and breathed in the clean, untainted air. In my spare time I researched and wrote about my experiences with passion, as a means of self-healing and empowerment.

Anthony and I had been apart for two months and during this period I had plenty of free time to sit and contemplate the positive and negative effects of our relationship. Even though I thought I loved him with all of my heart, his controlling and unpredictable nature had caused a great deal of stress in my life. I knew he had been unfaithful to me and yet I accepted this. I knew he would always let his family treat me without respect and yet I accepted this. I knew I would always support him financially and emotionally, yet I also accepted this.

As we had been apart for two months, Anthony desperately wanted to make love with me, even though he knew the doctors had warned me against this. My body was sore but my passion for making love was still alive and kicking. We made love, ever so gently, one night. I felt my heart reopen. It was like a promise to myself that everything would be great again.

After making love, my inner hopes were rekindled and I now had the will to defeat this enemy within my body. I also knew within my heart that this would be last time we would ever make love in this lifetime. Our paths had led in separate directions and I now had the courage to remove a negative emotional influence in my life. I realised in this moment that I had the power to close this chapter of my life with Anthony and allow a positive new door to open for me.

Anthony departed quickly and easily, and I was left with a new ray of inspiration. I wanted to live. There was no way I would let this cancer beat me. I had too many wonderful things in life to look forward to and too many beautiful people who loved me. I would not let myself down, or the people I loved.

As the weeks went by, I experienced various side effects from the chemotherapy. It was difficult having to wake up six or seven times throughout the night to go to the toilet. For the first five days after chemotherapy I always experienced a foul, rotten egg taste in my mouth. No matter how hard I brushed my teeth, I couldn't remove the taste. It made it difficult to eat, drink or even feel close to normal. Yet I continued to take natural medication and the symptoms became less and less as time went by.

My original chemotherapy treatment was set to last anywhere up to six months. I thought within my soul I could beat this sooner. I knew I could! I knew I had the will to survive, the desire to live and love and the energy to overcome this lesson. I continued to take large amounts of vitamins and to exercise and to eat organic foods, and my body felt supported. This seemed to decrease the degree of symptoms and side effects from the chemotherapy. It was a fantastic experiment and an incredible learning experience for me. I learnt more about myself, life and healing than I could ever have imagined. What I felt in pain and loss I gained tenfold in compassion and empathy.

After two weeks of intensive chemotherapy combined with my natural medicine regime, my test results showed a dramatic decrease in cancer cells, faster than ever seen before with this particular type of cancer. However, the drop in cancer cells had now plateaued and my body had begun to fight the toxic chemotherapy drugs, not the cancer cells. I visualised my body's white cells destroying the dark cancer cells every day. Whenever I found my mind wandering, I would bring it back to these positive thoughts.

Of course, I had my down days like anybody. Especially when I woke up one morning to find a pillow of blonde hair, just as I thought I'd escaped the hair loss. And when I felt so tired, I just wanted to stop breathing altogether. And when it was finally time to shave off my locks and an iridescent white head stared back at me in the mirror, then I felt sad, but the sadness never lasted for long. I kept thinking, 'Why be sad and feel sorry for yourself when you are still alive? Why be sad when you have another chance to live and do things right this time. Some people are never given a second chance, yet here you are being given exactly that.' I knew I had to make the most of every moment.

Whenever I felt sad and lost, I would adorn myself in a bright and colourful wig. At least when I looked in the mirror, sadness couldn't stare back at me. Instead I would be greeted by a bouncy, colourful image and it would make me smile. In fact, this type of character would also make others smile, especially in the chemotherapy rooms. This made me feel happy.

After about ninety hours of chemotherapy I was called into the doctor's office to discuss my results. By this stage, I had adamantly decided within my heart to stop the chemotherapy and courageously convert to natural medicine and healing to overcome my illness. I felt the chemotherapy had played its part in the initial stage of my healing. However, the cancer in my body had now become resistant to the drugs and it was now the right time to let my body take over its natural role of fighting this disease. The chemotherapy had definitely been useful in the early stages of my treatment, yet I was concerned for the welfare of the rest of my body.

I was informed that there was very little possibility that I would ever have children. The doctor also told me how the chemotherapy had killed a large number of white blood cells and I was in danger of dying if I contracted a simple cold or infection. He wished me to inject a hormone into my stomach to increase my white blood cell count. He explained that this process would prove very painful for a number of days as the bone marrow literally pushed the white blood cells into the bloodstream. My heart sank at the thought of this and tears welled up in my eyes, yet my courage rose as my decision to give up chemotherapy was confirmed.

From then on, I stayed at home and refused to go to the hospital for my chemotherapy treatment. I had decided within my heart to use my own knowledge and my body's own natural healing potential to beat this cancer. It was difficult for my loved ones to accept this, yet it was my decision and I had to trust my instincts.

The hospital and doctors called me daily. They told me I would be dead within the year if I didn't continue with chemotherapy treatment but I ignored their harsh warnings. I knew it was time to let my body's own immune system take over the process of fighting the cancer cells. All of my energy was put into making organic juices and salads, taking vitamins, herbs and natural remedies, practising yoga and meditation daily, and continuously believing I was healthy and cancer-free.

Chemotherapy was definitely a trying experience for me and I admire the courage of anyone who is going through it, or has been through it and survived. You have to have guts to agree to do something so painful and debilitating. Due to faith in natural healing and love, I managed to decrease my orthodox treatment time to less than three months, half of the time that was originally planned. My decision to fight the remaining cancer with natural therapies ultimately proved successful.

To this day I remain healthy and cancer-free. I was told I would die if I stopped chemotherapy, yet I proved everyone wrong. I was also told I would never have children yet I have also proved the doctors wrong about this – my fertility is perfect and thanks to natural medicine my reproductive system is in beautiful condition, much to the amazement of the medical institution.

Believing in yourself and believing that you truly deserve to live is the greatest tool any individual soul has in his or her fight against cancer.

Chapter 7

REFLECTIONS

Time has now passed since I had cancer and beat it. That's the wonderful thing about life – time passes and in its passing, heals everything. Why did I get such an aggressive cancer so young and why did I survive this experience? I now understand my cancer was caused from a culmination of factors. Firstly, I am a healer and I believe it is my destiny to help heal and support others. Unfortunately many healers open their arms and hearts to others without protecting themselves. I did this on a regular basis and chose to take on everyone else's pains and problems, leaving me open to sickness and disease.

In order for me to travel into the next stage of true healing, I needed a life lesson that would allow me to increase my empathy and understanding of chronic disease and cancer. I felt I had reached a crossroads in my healing and I was ready to give up. I didn't understand what people with chronic disease were feeling and hence I felt in an immature position to help them. They say you choose everything in life. Perhaps I unconsciously chose to develop cancer to allow myself to feel what others with cancer have felt, thereby opening my empathy, true compassion and understanding. You may say it's silly, that nobody chooses to be sick. Well maybe not, but it worked and I now have the ability to understand what people with cancer and chronic illness are feeling. Would I have had this empathy without this experience? I really don't think so.

I understand cancer can be caused by a number of environmental factors. It is true that I was exposed to some harmful chemicals which are known to be carcinogenic. Months after my illness, I contacted my old friend Mike. Mike had also been exposed to the toxic chemicals which had covered our town. His health had deteriorated even further and he now experienced strange and unexplainable symptoms. He deemed his condition a 'mystery' and any attempts to diagnose it failed. Before the exposure to this deadly defoliant, Mike had rarely been sick a day in his life. His illness had man-ifested shortly after exposure to the strange chemical mist.

Mike wasn't the only one affected. I know of others living near the chemical exposure site who also suffered from strange illnesses and rare forms of cancer. A sixteen-year-old boy near my home had developed breast cancer. An apparently healthy Australian woman in her early thirties was diagnosed shortly after exposure with pituitary cancer. These were just two of many cases.

Perhaps my cancer was purely a physical phenomenon. But still, I must have weakened my immunity in some way to have allowed this to have overtaken my body.

And the most significant way of weakening your body's immune system is through depressed emotions. Emotions of sadness, loss, abandonment, grief, fear, depression and hurt. Before my cancer emerged, I felt many of these emotions for sustained periods in my life. I concentrated on pleasing others, which never worked and ultimately created unhappiness and discontentment in my life. I believed my level of happiness was determined by the level of happiness of my loved ones or partner.

I couldn't have been further from the truth. It's a waste of time trying to make others happy, because ultimately they have to make themselves happy. I have learnt not to take on other people's discontented emotions and rather work on keeping myself balanced and content. I no longer react irrationally; rather, I choose to respond calmly.

Having cancer and overcoming it was definitely a growing experience. I didn't grow older from my lesson, I grew wiser. I understand more about life and I have overcome my fear of death. My arms are open to all forms of healing now and I know choosing to live is possible and choosing to die is also possible.

Through my own personal experience of working with cancer patients, I have seen that once a person chooses to die and prepares to do so, then their chosen reality has already been sealed. However, if a person reaches deep into their soul and comes into contact with their fighting spirit and truly has the desire to live, their chances of survival are completely different. Intention and manifestation are powerful tools. I understand we have all of the answers within our own soul. We have lived before, so we know all. Trusting your own intuition is so important, rather than seeking all of the answers from outside and from others.

I realise there will only be a handful of people in this world who will stand by you against all odds. I will never again waste my time seeking the approval of others. It is not important how many friends you have. It is not important to want everyone to like you. Rather, what is important is to know and understand who the special people in your life are and to concentrate on putting good energy into these relationships.

Those who have overcome cancer or chronic disease have been given a chance to begin life again or to alter their life, habits or thinking in some way. Having cancer or chronic disease should be seen as an opportunity. An opportunity to change your life, your thinking or your present situation and responses. It is important not to let the opportunities pass you by; you may not get a second chance.

I understand now my body is a temple to be cherished and loved. I used to say this before, yet I never completely lived this realisation. I believed I was invincible, because I had always been so healthy. I thought that illness happened to others and that it couldn't possibly happen to me. If your body fails you, or rather if you fail your body, then you can say goodbye to true freedom and existence.

I understand that everything happens for a reason. My life blossomed in more ways than I could have ever imagined after I beat cancer. By courageously deciding to listen to my own heart and intuition and to trust in my own healing ability, life opened its arms to me and offered me the most beautiful gifts. The gift of life, the gift of true love and the gift of friendship. I will never take these beautiful gifts for granted ever again.

This opportunity to change one's life is not restricted only to the person suffering from cancer or chronic disease. Having cancer tends to shake others, especially loved ones, out of their comfort zone and generates greater realisation about health and right living. It is an awakening experience with the ability to clear old wounds and strengthen loving bonds. In this sense, cancer can be a very life-affirming experience. How often in life are we given the opportunity to begin again?

I have now learnt to make the most of every day. To cherish the feeling of good health, to actually see and feel things, to look at a flower or animal with love and to realise we are all connected in this magical universe. Surviving cancer has given me the opportunity to share my experience with others. In this way I am now able to offer my support, love, advice and understanding to assist other people in their courageous fight against cancer. From this seed of experience, this book was born. For this I thank the universe.

Part Two

PRACTICAL STEPS TO HEAL YOUR LIFE

Chapter 8

UNDERSTANDING CANCER

Cancer Explained

To this day, cancer remains a great mystery. However, we do know this; cancer is a condition or disease that affects the body's cells. Cancer is not one single disease. There are over two hundred different types of cancer and all behave in unique ways. One thing common to all cancers is that they all begin with a change to a normal cell. Each cancer is strangely different and the cause, speed of growth and spread varies with each individual cancer.

Cells are the small building blocks of the different parts of the body. They differ in shape and function, and have the ability to reproduce by dividing – one becomes two, two become four etc. This allows tissues to grow and develop and repair after injury. In normal healthy tissues, cell division has an orderly, controlled pattern. It is regulated so that the number of cells that are actively dividing is equal to the number dying or being shed. If this orderly pattern is lost an abnormal cell may divide in an uncontrolled way, leading to a build up of tissue known as a tumour. A tumour is a swelling that can be caused by a number of conditions, including inflammation and trauma. Although they are not synonymous the terms *tumour* and *neoplasm* are often used interchangeably.

The term *neoplasm* comes from a Greek word meaning *new formation*. In contrast to normal tissue growth, a neoplasm serves no useful purpose but tends to increase in size and persist at the expense of the rest of the body. Furthermore, neoplasms do not obey the laws of normal tissue growth. For example, they do not occur in response to an appropriate stimulus and they continue to grow after the stimulus has ceased.

A tumour that invades neighbouring tissues and organs, and has spread or has the ability to spread to other parts of the body, is known as a malignant tumour. Malignant tumours are dangerous, cancerous and can spread through the blood system or lymph, forming new growths called secondaries or metastasis. The Latin word *malus* means bad; hence a malignant tumour is a bad tumour.

A tumour that remains large, yet does not spread to other areas of the body, is known as a benign tumour. A benign tumour is a good tumour. A simple example of this is a cyst.

Tumours are usually identified by the addition of the suffix *-oma* to the name of the tissue type from which the growth originates. Thus a benign tumour of glandular epithelial tissue is called an *adenoma*. The term *carcinoma* is used to designate a malignant tumour of epithelial tissue origin. In the case of a malignant *adenoma* the term *adenocarcinoma* is used.

One thing must be remembered – cancer does not just spring up in your body overnight. It takes quite a long time to develop and a culmination of factors to create a tumour, or cancerous growth. Each of us have cancer cells in our body as daily normal cells go haywire. However, our body's immune system normally steps in to clean up the damage and optimal health is maintained. If our immune system is functioning correctly, developing cancer cells are destroyed. However, if these cells grow out of control and the immune system is deficient or not working correctly or at the right speed at that time, cancer is established.

A Plausible Theory on Cancer

As humans we are made up of millions of cells, each uniquely different in shape and structure. However, one thing is common to every single cell within the body. Each cell contains amazing, life-giving structures. One of these unique structures is known as mitochondria. Mitochondria occur in the cytoplasm (fluid) of the cell and this is the primary site of cellular energy production within the body (similar to a 'power plant'). The method of energy production is known as the 'Kreb's Cycle'. This occurs in the mitochondria by means of oxidation – using oxygen, producing a substance known as ATP (Adenosine Triphosphate).

Deoxyribonucleic acid, commonly known as DNA, is our genetic information that also resides within the mitochondria. Around every cell we have a protective coating known as the cell membrane. Cell membranes regulate every substance that enters or leaves the cell, carries signals into and out of the cell and consumes seventy per cent of the cell's energy. Cancer-causing substances are able to penetrate cell membranes, breaking into the cell lining. This can reduce normal mitochondrial function and the formation of healthy DNA.

If our cell membrane is strong and stable, certain carcinogens are unable to enter and are usually destroyed by the immune system, if it is functioning correctly. However, if cell membranes are weak and the immune system is deficient, a cancer-causing substance is able to enter and cause damage to the cell. This damage also affects cellular energy production and damages the mitochondria and DNA sequence. When the cell replicates itself to heal and repair tissue the replicated cell will be damaged, possibly leading to the initial formation of cancerous cells. If the immune system still hasn't stepped in due to deficiencies, the cancerous cells may continue to reproduce, eventually causing a tumour to form.

Therefore, to prevent and also to beat cancer, the cells throughout the body need to be normalised. This includes strengthening cell membranes, regulating ATP production in the mitochondria (the cell's 'power plant') and enhancing immune system function. Certain substances enhance the function of the mitochondria, such as carnitine, alpha-linolenic acid (LNA), co-enzyme Q10, gingko biloba and vitamin C.

Likewise, avoiding cancer-causing substances, eating a healthy, nutrient-rich diet, positive emotions, regular intake of antioxidants and immune system support are essential ingredients in preventing and beating cancer.

What Are Your Chances of Beating Cancer Today?

Your chances of fighting and overcoming cancer in today's world are extremely good, particularly if detected early. New improved techniques of detecting cancer have led to a decrease in mortality. In most cases, cancer is <u>not</u> a death sentence, as it was in the past. If detected early, survival and quality of life after treatment with both (and/or) orthodox medicine and natural methods is greatly improved.

It is difficult to beat cancer if it has been detected in the very late stages and has spread throughout the lymph and blood system. However, it is not impossible. Miracles occur every day; I know of many people including myself, who have overcome cancer even after it has spread to a number of different body areas. Remember, God and the universe often gives you a second – and sometimes a third and fourth – chance to right the wrongs done to your body and mind. Think of cancer as a message from God to repair the delicate pattern of your soul and internal bodily health through love, nurturing, understanding and acceptance, and as a way to bring those aspects of your life that are out of balance back into balance.

Causes of Cancer

There are many causes of cancer (for a more detailed list of causes, refer to Chapter 9, Alarm Bells). Some common carcinogens and pre-cursors of cancer are environmental toxins, chemicals, pollution, cigarette smoke, alcohol abuse, artificial additives in foods, radiation, viruses, man-made electromagnetic fields of high frequency, hereditary factors, bad dietary habits such as a high fat intake, an insufficient fibre intake, excess sugar, inadequate antioxidant and immune system nutrients, excessive sun exposure, stress and psychological and emotional factors.

In adults, it is believed that at least sixty per cent of cancers are due to environmental causes. However, this is unlikely to be true for childhood cancers. More than half of the cancers today are preventable. For instance, more than thirty per cent of lung cancer deaths can be avoided by not smoking! That's an amazing statistic, yet one we prefer to ignore, particularly if we are smokers. Cancer is becoming more common every day and environmental toxins and pollutants are ever-increasing in our society.

Many people live by the saying 'ignorance is bliss'. This may be true for those who ignore their own health and manage to stay healthy, but for those who develop cancer, life certainly takes on a less than blissful existence. The pain and suffering that you experience with cancer and cancer treatment makes you want to know answers and to take affirmative action to change your world.

A normal healthy body has the ability to detoxify chemicals and toxins. If our bodies are unable to do this, due to any number of reasons, disease and in some cases cancer will result.

Methods of Detecting Cancer

Methods of diagnosing cancer have improved dramatically in the past few years. With the rapid progress of technology we now have new, more advanced methods of detecting cancer in the early stages. The methods used in the diagnosis and detection of cancer are determined largely by the location and type of cancer suspected. Common methods of diagnosing cancer are described below.

Biopsy

A biopsy involves surgically removing a small section of suspected cancerous tissue. A pathologist then examines it under a microscope for abnormal cells. The extent of the operation depends on individual circumstances and varies with the type of cancer and area of the body affected. X-Ray guided needle biopsies are simple and effective and can be done under a local anaesthetic. For a liver biopsy, a small needle is inserted into the liver through a numbed area of the skin.

Blood Test

Blood tumour marker tests are only used for certain types of cancer. The most common being colon or rectal cancer (tumour marker CEA – carcinoembryonic antigen), prostate (PSA – prostate specific antigen), ovarian cancer (CA 125 and CASA), multiple myeloma (paraprotein), testicular cancer (HCG and/or AFP hormones), germ cell carcinoma (alpha-beta proteins) and choriocarcinoma (HCG and/or AFP). None of these blood tests are specific, as many of these substances are normally present in the blood in small amounts anyway. For instance, a woman menstruating will show higher than normal levels of CA125, as will conditions such as endometriosis and inflammation.

Endoscopy

Endoscopy involves using an internal telescope instrument to view internal organs. A specialist can insert a tube through the mouth into the gullet (oesophagoscopy) and/or stomach (gastroscopy) or through the back passage or anus into the lower bowel (colonoscopy). You are able to watch this on the screen with the doctor and it is also possible to take a biopsy with this equipment.

Magnetic Resonance Imaging (MRI)

This is one of the newest methods. It works by making use of the fact that different molecules produce different patterns of magnetism, which can be recorded on sensitive equipment. MRI scanning is relatively harmless and revolutionary.

Nuclear Scanning and PET Scans

The doctor injects a radioactive 'tracer' substance and after a waiting period, special equipment scans the organ to pick up radioactive emissions. This must be analysed carefully, as other conditions can give a similar appearance.

PET scan technology has been available for many years. However, since the year 2000 it has become more available. It helps to evaluate in the staging and response to medical treatments in lung cancer, solitary pulmonary nodules, colon cancer, oesophageal cancer, malignant melanoma, head and neck cancer and lymphomas. It involves using a combination of bone scanning and CT Scanning at the same time. You are given a radioactive material that is absorbed and then metabolised at the specific tumour sites. A camera then takes images of the entire body to detect the size and location of the tumour.

Pap smear
A pap smear involves the doctor inserting a small instrument into the vagina and taking a small scraping of cells from the wall of the cervix. A pathologist then examines the cells under a microscope for abnormal cells. This is used to detect cancer of the cervix and other abnormalities.

Self-awareness
It is very important to be aware of common warning signs and symptoms of cancer.

Self-examination
This is useful for many types of cancer, especially breast cancer, skin melanomas, testicular and prostate cancer. Self-examination can be performed by you at home. Early detection and screening can ensure you catch cancer in the early stages and prevent further illness.

X-rays and Other Imaging Techniques
This incorporates a wide range of techniques which produce an image of the body's internal structure. CT Scanning, also known as computerised tomography, involves taking repeated X-Rays, each one at a greater depth than the next one. The person being tested lies flat on a table and is passed under a doughnut shaped machine while the machinery spins around them. For the clearest images, an injection of dye is given or barium is drunk. Clear views can be obtained of soft tissues as well as dense bone matter. Some people find this procedure quite uncomfortable and claustrophobic.

***

Common methods of detecting individual types of cancer through modern diagnostic methods include:

Bladder Cancer
Urine tests, CT scans, x-rays and ultrasound

Bowel Cancer
Rectal examination, Sigmoidoscopy (the inside of the bowel is examined using a tube with a light attached), barium enema (x-ray of the bowel which can show abnormalities), colonoscopy (special flexible tube examines the whole bowel), CT Scan.

Brain Tumours
MRI or CT scan of the brain and blood tests.

Breast Cancer

Breast self-examination, blood tests, mammograms, x-rays, CT scans, bone scans and thermography. A PET scan can help to determine the staging of this condition.

Cervical Cancer

Pap smears, blood tests, pelvic examinations and/or biopsy. X-rays, CT scans and sigmoidoscopy will help to determine the direction of treatment.

Endometrial Cancer

Biopsy or pap smear of the endometrium, physical examination including a pelvic examination, dilation and curettage, transvaginal ultrasound, CT scan and ultrasound.

Germ Cell Carcinoma

X-rays, blood tests, CT scans and ultrasound.

Hodgkin's Disease or Lymphoma

Biopsy of enlarged lymph node, blood tests, evaluation of bone marrow with a microscope.

Kidney Cancer

Chest x-rays, CT scan of the abdomen, urine sample, fine needle aspiration of the tumour, ultrasound.

Leukaemia – There are a number of different types of leukaemia. Tests for each type include:

Acute Myeloid Leukaemia (AML) – blood test, bone marrow test, chest x-ray
Acute Lymphoid Leukaemia (ALL) – blood test, bone marrow test, chest x-ray
Chronic Myeloid Leukaemia (CML) – blood test looking for raised white blood cell count, bone marrow test, analysis of blood and bone marrow under a microscope
Chronic Lymphoid Leukaemia (CLL) – blood test looking for raised white blood cell count, bone marrow test, analysis of blood and bone marrow under a microscope

Liver Cancer

Blood tests (AFP- alpha feto protein), ultrasound or CT scan, MRI, biopsy and angiography. Fine needle aspiration or a trochar biopsy of the liver.

Lung Cancer

Chest x-ray, sputum sample study, bronchoscopy, microscopic examination of cells, and blood tests. If lung cancer is established, CT chest scans and bone scans are performed. PET scans can be used to stage the tumour.

Non-Hodgkin's Lymphoma

Biopsy of enlarged lymph node, evaluation of blood or bone marrow under a microscope, CT scan of the chest, abdomen and pelvis.

Oesophageal Cancer

Endoscopic examination, biopsy, barium swallow or upper GI x-rays, endoscopic ultrasound and CT Scan or MRI.

Oral Cancer

Oral examination and microscopic examination of cells.

Ovarian Cancer

A detailed pelvic examination, ultrasound or CT scan of the pelvis, blood tests (CA 125 and CASA – a tumour marker). If ovarian cancer is suspected, a tissue diagnosis is taken by using FNA or trochar biopsy of the tumour, examination of the fluid in the abdomen or surgery with removal of the tumour.

Pancreatic Cancer

CT scan or ultrasound, guided needle biopsy of the pancreas, endoscopy and biopsy, and blood tests.

Prostate Cancer

Self-examination, x-rays, CT scans, biopsy, blood test (PSA – Prostate Specific Antigen) and digital rectal examination. Staging of prostate cancer is determined through CT Scans or MRI of the pelvis and abdomen, and bone scans.

Skin Cancer or Melanoma

Skin examination by doctor, noticeable changes in mole or freckle, biopsy of the mole or affected site, blood tests.

Stomach Cancer

Upper endoscopy, biopsy, MRI, barium upper GI radiographs and endoscopic ultrasound.

Uterine or Endometrial Cancer

Pelvic examination, biopsy, pap smear and curette.

Be Aware of These Signs in Detecting Cancer

The most important method of diagnosing and preventing cancer is to be your own best doctor. This means listening to your body, becoming aware of any changes in normal bodily functions and to not live with feeling slightly unwell or off balance. The body is a finely tuned instrument which gives you regular signs as to its discord – listen to your body and take affirmative action by consulting with a doctor or natural therapist the moment you notice any of these changes. Prevention of disease is a much easier path than trying to cure disease, once it is established.

Cancer will not go away if you ignore the symptoms. It is more likely to spread further, especially if your lifestyle and dietary patterns remain unchanged. Pain is not an early warning sign of cancer – cancer is often well advanced before any pain becomes noticeable. If you notice any changes in your normal body functions, seek further advice from a health professional. Common risk factors, warning signs and symptoms for various types of cancer are listed in Table 9.1 in Chapter 9, 'Alarm Bells'.

What Options Do You Have for Orthodox Treatment?

Orthodox medical treatment for cancer will vary with each person depending on the severity and type of cancer you have. The goals of orthodox treatment methods fall into three categories:

1. Curative
2. Palliative
3. Adjunctive

The most common types of conventional or orthodox treatment used to treat cancer are surgery, chemotherapy, radiation treatment, biological treatments, hormone treatment, blood cell and bone marrow transplantation and cancer drugs. In recent years, immunotherapy has been added to the list of treatment modalities. A combination of a number of these different orthodox treatments may be used, according to your particular cancer.

In some cases only one type of treatment is used. This again depends on the type of cancer. If any of these forms of medical treatment sound overwhelming, you're absolutely right. If you plan to undertake any of these forms of cancer treatment, be prepared and informed as to the side effects and complications. These can be many and varied.

New, more advanced cancer treatments are being studied and implemented every day. Always seek a number of opinions about your treatment and choose a doctor who specialises in your specific type of cancer. If you do not wish to undertake any of the orthodox cancer therapies offered to you, seek more advice. Knowledge is important. Find out about your type of cancer and other methods people have used to treat this. I believe it is wise to use alternative medicine in addition to orthodox treatment, to give your body the full support it requires. Try to choose a doctor who is open and accepting of both options.

Are There any Side Effects Associated With Orthodox Treatment?

Orthodox medical treatment of cancer is not without any long-term or short-term side effects. Many books about cancer forget to mention these relevant side effects and doctors often do not mention them, either. Doctors may feel telling patients every-thing could dissuade them from having valuable treatment against cancer, due to the many side effects associated with its use.

It is your right as a human being to know EVERYTHING about the treatment you will undertake and any side effects associated with its application. It's no wonder many people, especially elderly people, decide not to follow through with normal medical cancer treatments, as the side effects can often make them feel much worse than when they actually have the cancer itself. Refer to individual chapters on chemotherapy, surgery and radiation therapy for a full list of side effects and natural remedies to counteract these. Natural medicine works fantastically in the prevention and alleviation of many of the side effects experienced with conventional cancer treatment.

What Options Do You Have for Natural Alternative Treatments?

It must always be remembered that you are not without choices. As a human being, you always have options and a right to choose which treatment best suits your needs. No one can force you into doing anything you do not wish to do. Ask questions, seek other opinions and know there can be many solutions to one problem. There are some amazing natural healers in this world, including YOURSELF.

Many natural healers specialise in cancer treatment and alternative methods of beating cancer. It is important to find a natural health practitioner who has many years of practical experience with a condition such as cancer. Natural remedies are excellent in building up the body's immune system, fighting cancer, helping to find the original manifestation of your problem, balancing the body's emotions and easing or eliminating many of the side effects associated with orthodox medical treatment. Some natural therapies being used to fight cancer include juice therapy, cancer orientated diets, sound/music therapy, colour therapy, mind/body therapy, herbal treatment, vitamin and mineral therapy, nutritional support, meditation, yoga, relaxation techniques, emotional cleansing, positive visualisation, metabolic treatment and many more!

Incorporating Both Orthodox and Alternative Remedies into Your Treatment Regime

There is nothing more beneficial when fighting cancer, than incorporating both natural and orthodox medicine into your treatment regime. A natural wholesome diet rich in cancer fighting nutrients and foods is a great way to begin. This assists the body both in cancer prevention and during orthodox treatment. During chemotherapy and radiation therapy many of the side effects experienced are due to malnutrition. If an appropriate diet can be undertaken during cancer treatment, including lots of high-density nutrients, malnutrition can be avoided and elimination of the cancerous mass can be quicker than usual.

Other ways to combine the two include undertaking meditation, relaxation techniques or yoga during treatment. This relaxes the mind and helps to maintain a positive attitude to decrease the tumour size further. Vitamin and mineral therapy is extremely beneficial, providing the body with necessary anti-oxidants and energy-giving nutrients to combat harmful cancer cells and to provide higher levels of energy. Side effects experienced during chemotherapy, surgery or radiation therapy can be reduced or completely avoided with the use of certain vitamins, minerals and herbs.

It is important to never limit yourself to only one type of therapy. By using a combination of orthodox and natural remedies, a great attitude, positivity, laughter and a wholesome diet, your good results in fighting cancer will be realised faster than expected.

Even though I am a naturopath with total belief in alternative therapies I decided not to close my mind to orthodox medicine, realising that each has its place in this world and in my own particular healing needs. I used surgery and chemotherapy along with every natural therapy I felt was most beneficial and suitable to my needs.

Originally my treatment was planned for six months, as the cancer was larger than a newborn baby and had spread to many sites. After three months of treatment with both orthodox and natural medicine, I was completely cancer-free, stunning doctors, family and friends. It is amazing what a totally open mind with the desire to heal can accomplish. Never doubt the power of your mind!

Being Actively Involved in Your Own Treatment

It is your body and your disease. Never give away your power to anyone – especially not the power to heal your body. You can ask doctors, specialists, natural therapists and healers for advice and treatment options but ultimately, you are the one with the power to make the decisions to heal your body. Keeping your empowerment will enable you to also keep your self-confidence and motivation.

How can you take a more active part in your healing process? Firstly, ask your doctor or specialist plenty of questions; it is your right to know everything. The more you know the more control you have over your own destiny and outcome. Never go into your healing or treatment in the dark. Find out everything you can about your type of cancer and the most effective forms of treatment to heal your cancer. Ask for articles, research papers and information from your health practitioner concerning treatment of your cancer. Ask questions and obtain more knowledge about your disease. It is your right to know the results of all tests – it is your right to be one hundred per cent informed about every procedure and its possible side effects.

If you have made the conscious decision to undertake orthodox cancer treatment, please don't forget the benefits of incorporating natural therapies into your program. Set yourself a schedule for taking your vitamins, performing your creative visualisations, meditation and yoga and allow plenty of free time for yourself. Never overcommit yourself – this is your time to rediscover what you truly love and enjoy in life.

Every day is truly precious; don't let another moment pass you by without feeling the beauty in every breath of life giving energy. It is a wonderful feeling to take charge of your own destiny and to have an active part in your own healing process.

Some Common Myths about Cancer

Cancer only happens to the elderly

Cancer can affect anyone at any age, even newborn infants. It is more common in the elderly, as cells become weaker as we age. This may be avoided if you keep your body in good condition with harmonious living techniques. However, we can all be affected by cancer, as there are many different causes and precursors that are not predetermined by age. We must be aware at any age.

Cancer is always a death sentence

In the past many cancers were deadly, as successful treatment was unknown. Today, cancer is becoming easier to detect and thus early treatment can be commenced. Advanced methods of treatment and a greater understanding of the causes of cancer also improves our chances to beat it. Even though cancer is becoming more common every year, more people are recovering every year. There is a vast array of options and useful information out there to assist in beating this modern-day illness. Natural methods of healing are also proving extremely successful in reversing cancerous growths.

Cancer only happens to negative, depressed people

Some of the happiest, most relaxed people in the world develop cancer. Our environment is becoming more toxic every year, radiation levels are increasing and additives in foods pop up everywhere. We are continually exposed to a deadly concoction of toxins, including car fumes, fluoride in drinking water and cigarette smoke, to name just a few. However, negative emotions can weaken the immune system, which will increase the possibility of developing cancer. Many people are simply negative or pessimistic by nature and venture through their entire lives without developing cancer. However, a positive attitude definitely plays a strong role in cancer prevention.

Cancer Prevention

Prevention is the most important tool we have in our fight against cancer. Some cancers are preventable, this is a proven fact. However, it can be difficult to prevent something if we do not know what actually causes it. Cancer is a condition in which cells grow abnormally. We do know that certain conditions lead to the onset and development of cancer. So how do we keep our cells in a healthy state and prevent toxins/carcinogens from affecting our cells and causing cancer?

Following a healthy lifestyle, incorporating a wholesome diet rich in antioxidants and regular exercise, with a positive attitude and stress-free living is a great way to start. Avoiding known carcinogens or cancer causing agents is very important (refer to Chapter 9, 'Alarm Bells' for a list of cancer causes).

It is difficult to completely avoid stress as we live in such a fast-paced society that a degree of stress is required, in order to live adequately. However, we can learn techniques to enable us to deal with and release stress much more effectively. One of the most important preventative tools is to avoid excess in your life. An excess of anything can lead to stress on your body's cells, which will eventually lead to the onset of disease and possibly cancer.

Chapter 9

ALARM BELLS

No one knows exactly why cancer cells behave the way they do. We do know however, that a number of causative factors are responsible for the growth of certain types of cancer. The causes of cancer are abundant and diverse.

As mentioned in the previous chapter, every day we are exposed to thousands of different environmental, dietary, man-made and plant-made toxins. Our body's immune system is designed to detoxify these chemicals and maintain a balance in health, preventing illness. Due to any number of factors, our body's immune functions may become weakened or find it difficult to detoxify as normal. When our body is unable to perform these regulatory functions, disease results.

In the United States alone, one person dies from cancer every minute. Another three million people have cancer and one out of three will eventually die of some form of disease. 1 334 100 new cancer cases are expected to be diagnosed in the year 2003 in that country. Cancer is now the second most common cause of deaths in the United States, running dangerously close to cardiovascular disease. There are more than one hundred different varieties of cancer today. Over 170 000 cancer illnesses in the United States alone are preventable.

In Australia in 1999, 82 135 new cancer cases were reported and there were 34 695 deaths due to cancer, not including non-melanoma skin cancer. Globally, cancer rates are expected to rise by at least fifty per cent to fifteen million new cases in the year 2020, according to the 'world cancer report'.

The most common types of cancers worldwide in men are lung cancer (which is mainly due to tobacco smoking), prostate cancer and colorectal cancer. The most common cancer worldwide for women is breast cancer followed by lung cancer, colorectal cancer and uterine cancer. These statistics do not include skin cancer, which is on the rise and is extremely prevalent in countries such as Australia.

These are scary statistics, ringing strong alarm bells for all of us. Different types of cancer are more prominent in different cultures and countries. This alerts us to the fact that many factors in our environment do contribute to the development of cancer, more than genetic factors. It is necessary to become aware of these risk factors and limit our exposure to them as much as possible. Repeated exposure to carcinogens over a lengthy period increases the risk of cancer developing. It is important to be aware of contributing factors to cancer development, to prevent both ourselves and our loved ones from developing this life threatening condition.

Common Causes of Cancer

As stated earlier, if you maintain a healthy and strong immune system by eating a healthy diet rich in antioxidants and immune stimulating nutrients, and avoid known carcinogens as much as possible, your chances of avoiding cancer are very high. A positive, stress free attitude go hand in hand with dietary factors in avoiding disease and cancer. However, it is necessary to be aware of known carcinogens which may lead to the onset of cancer.

Carcinogens are substances or agents that produce or incite cancer. Continued exposure to carcinogens will eventually weaken the body's immunity and open the pathway for disease. Recent evidence suggests that at least one third of the cancer deaths predicted to occur in 2003 will be related in some way to nutrition, obesity, carcinogens and lifestyle factors that could be prevented. Likewise, most skin cancers can be prevented by limiting our exposure to the sun's rays. The majority of cancers today arise from damage to genes or DNA (genetic information within a cell) due to internal factors such as hormones or carcinogens in foods or external factors such as repeated exposure to carcinogens. Following is a list of the substances or carcinogens that may provoke or exacerbate the development of cancer:

Alcohol Abuse

Alcohol abuse accounts for at least three per cent of all cancer cases today. It is believed alcohol acts as a promoter of carcinogens. Women who drink heavily have a higher chance of developing breast, liver, larynx and oesophageal cancer and men who drink heavily have a higher incidence of developing cancer of the liver, larynx, oropharynx and oesophagus. A combination of heavy alcohol drinking and smoking is dangerous. Alcohol is thought to strip the oily lining of the cells in the mouth and throat, allowing the cancer-causing agents in tobacco smoke to get inside and accentuate the development of cancer of the throat, larynx, tongue, mouth and oesophagus. Alcohol abuse alone is believed to contribute to cancer of the oropharynx, oesophagus, liver, larynx and even breast cancer.

Emotional Factors

Psychological, emotional and behavioural factors such as long, unresolved bitterness may contribute to the development of cancer. Chronic, poorly managed stress and tension contributes to a suppressed immune system by altering adrenal, hormonal balance, leading to disease and possibly cancer. Other emotions that may lead to the manifestation of disease include resentment, deep seated anger, the loss of a loved one, sadness, depression and unresolved hurts in a person's life.

Environmental Causes

Environmental causes are believed to contribute to a vast majority of different cancers. Below are some suspected environmental cancer-causing agents.

- Aromatic hydrocarbons such as benzene, benzo (a) pyrene, dibenzo (a) anthracene and 1-nitropyrene are produced by incomplete combustion of fossil fuels. Benzene is used to make other chemicals which are then used to make resins, rubbers, lubricants, dyes, detergents, drugs, pesticides, nylon and synthetic fibres. It is also a natural part of crude oil, gasoline and cigarette smoke. Benzene is a cancer causing agent that may lead to leukaemia and cancers of other blood forming organs. These hydrocarbons are known to be breast carcinogens.

- Cadmium, mercury, lead and other heavy metals, from environmental exposure.
- Chloroform (chlorine vapours produced in hot showers) is another risk factor. In studies, animals that ate or drank water containing chloroform developed cancer of the liver and kidneys, indicating that this chemical may be a possible cancer risk.
- Chronic exposure to electromagnetic frequencies omitted by power lines, unshielded video, computer terminals, television, radio waves and electric blankets all increase the risk of developing cancer.
- Asbestos is the name given to six fibrous minerals that occur naturally in nature. However, asbestos is tough and fibrous and is commonly used in building materials, friction products such as brake pads, heat resistant fabrics, packaging and even in some talc products. Asbestos has been classed as a 'carcinogen' that may cause cancer in some people. In fact, a combination of cigarette smoking and asbestos dramatically increases one's chances of developing lung cancer.
- Excessive exposure to gamma rays can cause various forms of cancer.
- Excessive ultraviolet exposure from the sun and sun lamps.
- Formaldehyde is a proven carcinogen.
- Iatrogenic causes from x-rays and chemotherapeutic drugs (unless used in conjunction with the amino acid – glutamine).
- Industrial and agricultural chemicals and pesticides (including chlordane and heptachlor). Chlordane is a man-made pesticide that was used on crops such as corn and citrus. It was banned in the US in 1988, however it can stay in soils for over twenty years. It causes serious health problems and small amounts of chlordane given to mice leads to liver cancer.
- Many types of cough medicine may be carcinogenic (high chloroform content).
- Pink fluorescent light increases the risk of some forms of cancer. White fluorescent light is thought to be safer.
- Polyvinyl chloride (PVC) is strongly suspected of causing some forms of cancer (particularly brain tumours).

Food Processing Methods

Barbecuing, frying and overheating of dietary oils causes the production of carcinogenic benzopyrene and toxic polyhydrocarbons (PAH), which are strongly linked to cancer when ingested or inhaled in excessive amounts. Food irradiation also increases the risk of cancer, as does the smoking of foods.

Hereditary Factors

It is thought that approximately five per cent of cancers are inherited. An inherited faulty gene puts an individual at a higher risk of developing cancer. A few rare types of cancer can be inherited, such as cancer of the eye (retinoblastoma), found in children. Children inherit this cancer-causing gene from one of their parents. With kidney cancer, there is often a history of the disease in the family. Breast cancer and cancer of the bowel exhibit strong hereditary factors.

Oestrogens

Excessive manufacture of oestrogens (2-Hydroxy Oestrone), except during pregnancy, or a long-term intake of oestrogen drugs, may create cancerous conditions in the body. This risk can be increased with excess fat consumption and by leading a sedentary lifestyle. You can decrease this potential risk by increasing your intake of cruciferous vegetables and soy products, decreasing fat intake, decreasing body weight, increasing exercise and increasing flaxseed oil, fish oil and vitamin C.

Overexposure to Sunlight

Overexposure to sunlight is a major cause of malignant melanomas on the skin. Queensland has the highest rate of skin cancer in Australia, due to its close proximity to the equator. The risk is greater in fair-skinned people who have had periods of sunburn throughout their life.

Poor Dietary Habits

Poor dietary habits account for thirty-five per cent of cancer cases. Food carcinogens may include:

- A high intake of bacon, corned beef, maize oil, cottonseed oil, sassafras oil, champignon mushrooms and excessive pepper can cause or exacerbate cancer.
- Burnt or browned foods such as burnt toast and fried pork.
- Eating meats containing antibiotics and other growth enhancing agents may provoke cancer.
- Excess quantities of capsaicin (found in chillies) may lead to cancer. (Although moderate consumption has many health benefits and may prevent cancer).
- Excessive fat intake, mainly rancid, oxidized fat and altered vegetable oils.
- Excessive intake of caffeine.
- Excessive intake of simple sugars tends to feed cancer.
- Food additives or contaminants, including artificial additives, artificial colours, flavourings, artificial sweeteners (saccharin), propyl gallate, sulphites, BHT, BVO, BHA, MSG, sulphur dioxide, food colouring Amaranth (Red Dye No. 2), Benzopyrene, cyclamates, Hydrazines and piperine may be harmful. (For a further list of dangerous artificial additives, refer to Part Three of this book.)
- The herb chaparral in excessive amounts can contribute to the development of some forms of cancer. (However, chaparral can also be used to help heal cancer if given in correct dosages.)
- High triglyceride levels and trans-fatty acids contribute towards cancer onset.
- Inadequate antioxidant and immune system nutrients.
- Low fibre intake. If the bowel's transit time is slow and bile is permitted to remain in the colon, detrimental bacteria convert cholic acid into the powerful carcinogen, apcholic acid. Likewise, the fermentation of food in the colon due to habitual overeating or long-term constipation causes toxins to retain within the bowel area possibly increasing one's risk of developing colorectal cancer and other illnesses.
- Excess intake of mould carcinogens found in mould-contaminated foods such as corn, some grains, some nuts, peanut butter, bread, cheese and peanuts. Aflatoxin is a highly carcinogenic mould found on peanuts.

- Nitrites are extremely potent carcinogens that convert into nitrosamines and have the ability to cause cancer in any part of the body, particularly the stomach and bowel. Foods cured, pickled, smoked and packaged all contain nitrites. Meats which contain nitrites include bacon, sausage, hams, salami and luncheon meats.
- Toxic metals such as arsenic found in shellfish and grapes treated with arsenic pesticides in large amounts may prove dangerous.

Recreational and Prescribed Drugs

Recreational drugs and prescribed drugs, such as marijuana, LSD and valium, in large amounts may also contribute towards the growth of cancer cells. Long term use of marijuana is believed to suppress the body's immune system. Marijuana use has been linked to cancer of the testes and cervix.

Tobacco Use

Tobacco use contributes to twenty to thirty per cent of cancer cases. A person who smokes two or more packets of cigarettes a day is 20 to 25 times more likely to develop cancer. Cigarette smoking represents the single most avoidable cancer-causing agent in the world. Tobacco smoking is carcinogenic because it contains many harmful chemicals, including polynuclear aromatic hydrocarbons. Around ninety per cent of lung cancer cases are contributed to tobacco smoking. In the past 30 years, the rate of males smoking cigarettes was much higher than females. This was the primary reason why lung cancer was more prevalent in males. However, in recent years, the amount of women smoking has increased dramatically. This has caused a scary increase in the number of women being diagnosed with lung cancer. Smokers also have an increased risk of cancer of the mouth, stomach, anus, pancreas, penis, nasal passages, throat, oesophagus, kidney ovaries, cervix, testes and bladder.

Viruses

Viruses are rare but possible causes of cancer. Liver cancer may be linked to the incidence of hepatitis B and C. Cancer of the cervix may be due to a virus known as human papilloma virus. Human immunodeficiency virus (HIV) and helicobacter may be other viruses that could increase one's risk of developing cancer.

The above list of known and suspected carcinogens shows the more common types of cancer causing agents. For a full list of suspected carcinogens, please refer to the following websites:

1. http://ntp-server.niehs.nih.gov/ – This website is an initiative of the National Toxicology Program that provides an 'annual report on carcinogens'. It is a unit of the US Department of Health and Human Services that provides a comprehensive list of potentially toxic chemicals to research agencies and to the public.
2. http://atsdr.cdc.gov/ – This website is presented by the Agency for Toxic Substances and Disease Registry. It provides an amazing list of potential cancer-causing agents, what products they are found in and what health conditions and types of cancer they may cause.

The Most Common Risk Factors and Warning Signs of Cancer

Following is a table indicating risk factors and warning signs of various types of cancer. Most forms of cancer can be prevented, so take affirmative action today and be aware of ways to prevent cancers and their associated warning signs. Consult with a medical professional if any of these warning signs occur. Ask your doctor for regular early detection cancer-screening tests recommended for your age and sex.

There are also many fantastic natural diagnostic methods available today to warn you against pre-existing cancerous conditions. Iris diagnosis done by a professional Iridologist/Naturopath with advanced computerised equipment is a wonderful method of pre-detecting weaknesses in the body to prevent illness and disease from occurring in the future.

Table 9.1

Type of Cancer	Risk Factors	Warning Signs
All Cancers	Carcinogens, emotional factors, toxins etc.	Unusual bleeding or discharge, sores that fail to heal, lumps that grow on or under the skin, obvious change in a wart or mole, chronic fever, unusual bruising, unusual changes in bowel habits, weight loss, persistent difficulty in swallowing, recurring indigestion, nagging cough or hoarseness
Bladder and Kidney	Exposure to certain chemicals such as benzidines, aniline dyes (in rubber), naphthalene (in unfiltered cigarettes), smoking, excessive consumption of caffeine and/or artificial sweeteners, a history of schistosomiasis, obesity, frequent urinary tract infections, kidney dialysis	Blood in the urine, pain and burning with urination, increased frequency of urination, persistent unexplained fever, anaemia, fatigue, weakness, weight loss
Brain tumour	Chronic exposure to man-made electromagnetic fields from certain machinery devices, radiation, certain chemicals – solvents, pesticides, nitrosamines (found in processed or cured meats)	Severe and persistent headaches, dizziness, lethargy, unexplained weakness of one part of the body, visual disturbances – blurred vision, nausea, vomiting, seizures, altered mental status, altered speech, paralysis

Table 9.1 continued

Type of Cancer	Risk Factors	Warning Signs
Breast	First childbirth after age 35, having no children, family history of breast cancer in first degree relative, radiation exposure before the age of 30, pesticide exposure, smoking, lack of exercise, high pesticide exposure, early or late onset of menstruation, late onset of menopause, high alcohol and/or caffeine intake, high fat diet, diabetes, high sugar intake, long period of oral contraceptive pill use or hormone replacement therapy use, excessive oestrogen, either made by the body or taken as a drug, obesity	Lump(s), thickening and any other physical changes in the breast such as dimpling or retraction (turning inward) of breast tissue, thickness of swelling of a nipple, itching, redness and/or soreness of the nipples not associated with breastfeeding, unusual discharge
Cervical	More than five complete pregnancies, early age intercourse, a history of gonorrhoea or genital warts, multiple sex partners, infertility, prolonged use of oestrogens, long term use of oral contraceptives, high tobacco intake or marijuana use (cervical cancer). Cervical Herpes Simplex II and Human Papilloma virus, long-term deficiency of folic acid, Vitamin A and C, High dietary fats and obesity (uterine)	In early stages, no signs. Bleeding between menstrual periods, unusual discharge, painful menstruation, heavy periods, painful intercourse, bleeding after intercourse, atypical cells found via pap smear, fatigue, abdominal pain or bloating.
Colon (bowel) and rectum	Lack of dietary fibre and calcium, polyps, family history of colon cancer, continued constipation and/or diarrhoea, a build-up of toxins in the colon, high fat diet, high red meat intake, excess food intake, excess alcohol intake, lack or overproduction of bile, obesity, chronic inflammatory bowel disease such as ulcerative colitis, physical inactivity, holding onto anger and negative emotions, inherited illnesses, common over 50 years old	Rectal bleeding, dark blood in the stool, blood mixed with mucous, either combined or separate from the stool, changes in bowel habits, persistent diarrhoea and/or constipation. A sense of urgency or feeling of incomplete emptying of bowel, persistent cramping or abdominal pain, appetite loss, fatigue, weight loss, nausea, vomiting, abdominal swelling, pain or discomfort.

Table 9.1 *continued*

Type of Cancer	Risk Factors	Warning Signs
Endometrial and Uterine	Never having been pregnant, post menopausal, family history of this type of cancer, diabetes, obesity, history of high blood pressure, early menstruation, irregular menstruation, high animal fat intake, infertility or no children, tamoxifen, long-term use of oestrogen replacement therapy, long term exposure to abnormal hormone levels	Early signs – abnormal painless vaginal bleeding between menstrual periods, unusual discharge, painful menstrual periods, heavy periods, pelvic pain, weight loss, unexplained loss of appetite, fatigue. Late signs – cramping, post coital bleeding, lower abdominal pressure, enlarged lymph nodes
Laryngeal	Heavy smoking, alcohol consumption	Persistent cough, hoarse throat, a throat condition that won't heal
Leukaemia	Hereditary factors, radiation exposure, high frequency power lines, pesticides, chronic viral infections, benzene, the antibiotic chloramphenicol	Paleness, fatigue, weight loss, repeated infections, easy bruising, bone and joint pain, nosebleeds, other haemorrhages, fever, anaemia, enlargement of spleen or liver or lymph glands, night sweats, paleness, night sweats, low platelet count
Liver (hepatoma)	Intake of aflatoxins (fungus found in peanuts, peanut butter, corn, rice), high alcohol intake, intake of pyrrolizidine alkaloids, polyvinyl chloride, tamoxifen, hepatitis B and C, cirrhosis, thorium dioxide, birth control pills, anabolic steroids, arsenic, tobacco use, iron overload, throrotrast (used many years ago in radiation studies)	Signs and symptoms often occur in the later stages. Pain or enlargement in liver area right sided under ribcage, jaundice, generally feeling unwell and exhausted, unexplained weight loss, anorexia, aching abdominal pain, flatulence, nausea, early satiety (fullness), jaundice, anemia
Lung / bronchogenic	Smoking, exposure to asbestos, nickel, cadmium, chromates or radioactive materials, such as radon, chronic bronchitis, history of tuberculosis, exposure to certain chemicals such as pesticides, herbicides and PVC, more than 5 cups coffee/day, high caffeine intake, high alcohol intake, chemotherapy drugs such as bleomycin and cyclophosphamide, high cholesterol, excess margarine and fats	Persistent cough, sputum with blood, chest pain, fatigue, exhaustion, shortness of breath, wheezing, dull intermittent poorly localised retrosternal pain, change of voice, hoarseness, weakness, weight loss

Table 9.1 *continued*

Type of Cancer	Risk Factors	Warning Signs
Lymphoma – Hodgkin's disease	Hereditary factors, immune system dysfunction, high mercury or polyvinyl chloride intake, some cases may be linked to a viral cause, such as EBV or HIV	Painless, enlarged rubbery lymph nodes, itching, night sweats, unexplained fever and/or weight loss, pruritus, anaemia, spleen and liver enlargements, frequent infections, low platelet count, itching, fatigue
Mouth and throat	Irritants inside the mouth, broken tooth, ill-fitting or broken dentures, excessive alcohol intake, smoking, chewing tobacco	Chronic ulcer of the mouth, tongue or throat that does not heal, hoarseness
Myeloma (Cancer of the Bone Marrow)	90% of cases occur in people over 40, more common in men, exposure to chemicals (dioxins, solvents, cleaners), radiation, risk may increase with infections such as HIV, hepatitis, herpes virus infections, Epstein Barre virus, cytomegalovirus	Bone pain concentrated in the back is one of the first symptoms. Weight loss, feeling of weakness, recurrent infections, anaemia
Non-Hodgkin's Lymphoma	Hereditary factors, immune system dysfunction, high mercury or polyvinyl chloride intake, some cases may be linked to a viral cause	Signs and symptoms similar to Hodgkin's except for early involvement of oropharyngeal tissue, skin, gastro-intestinal tract and bone marrow
Oesophageal	Ageing – common between the age of 45 to 70, tobacco, long-term heavy drinking, diet deficient in fruits and vegetables as well as Vitamin C, A and B2, lye ingestion	Difficulty swallowing, a feeling of food stuck in the mouth or throat, slight pain or discomfort in the chest, weight loss
Ovarian	Not having had children, high fat diet especially animal fats, most develop after menopause, fertility drugs, clomiphene citrate, menstruation early age, first child after 30, talcum powder, family history, exposure to pesticides (organo-chlorines, creosote, sulfallate chlordane, lindane triazine herbicides), infertility, asbestos exposure, smoking	Often no obvious symptoms until in the later stages. May experience pelvic discomfort, ovarian swelling, leg pain, bleeding in between cycles, prolonged swelling of the abdomen, digestive problems such as gas, constipation, bloating, long term stomach pain

Table 9.1 *continued*

Type of Cancer	Risk Factors	Warning Signs
Pancreatic	High alcohol intake, tobacco use, diabetes mellitus, coffee has been linked – over 2 cups of coffee per day, history of liver cirrhosis, chronic pancreatitis, exposure to chemicals such as gasoline and insecticides	Pain at the back of the abdomen, unexplained jaundice, loss of weight, blood clots in the legs, anemia, fatigue, nausea, vomiting
Prostate	Recurring prostate infection, history of venereal disease, diet high in animal fat, high intake of milk, meat and/or coffee, genetic predisposition, frequency of sexual activity, use of male hormone testosterone in treatment of impotence, vasectomy, being over the age of 50, cadmium, rubber, long term nutritional deficiencies – especially of lycopene, vitamins E and D, and selenium, high cholesterol for many years	Weak or interrupted urine flow, burning while passing urine, difficulty in starting urine stream, blood in urine, bone pain, swelling of legs, continuous pain in the lower back, pelvis and/or upper thighs, need to urinate frequently at night
Skin	Exposure to the sun, sun lamps and tanning booths, especially for those with fair skin, history of moles (malignant or otherwise), moles on the feet or in areas irritated by clothing, scars from severe burns, family history of skin cancer, fluorescent lighting, microwaves, UV radiation, high alcohol intake, long term use of oral contraceptive pill (more than 5 years), vitiligo, weak immunity	Tumour or lump under the skin, resembling a wart or an ulceration that never heals, moles that change in colour or size, flat sores, lesions that look like moles, scars and sores that won't heal, large moles with irregular shapes or borders, dark black moles, bleeding moles.
Stomach	Pernicious anaemia, lack of hydrochloric acid and dietary fibre, high-fat diet, chronic gastritis, stomach polyps, high intake of pickled foods, white champignon mushrooms, nitrosamines and nitrites found in cured meats, high intake of smoked foods, salted fish, tobacco and alcohol abuse, helicobacter pylori infection, genetic predisposition, atrophic gastritis	Indigestion and pain after eating, anorexia, weight loss, lack of appetite, vague discomfort in the abdomen, abdominal pain, fullness in the upper abdomen, heartburn, indigestion, nausea, vomiting, swelling of the stomach. Often asymptomatic until late stages.

Table 9.1 *continued*

Type of Cancer	Risk Factors	Warning Signs
Testicular	Undescended testicle, excess caffeine, long term marijuana use, chronic irritation by infection or other inflammatory process, vasectomy, family history of testicular cancer may increase the risk, exposure to certain chemicals. Commonly found in miners, oil, gas and utility workers. Common age is 15 to 40 years old.	Lumps, enlargement of a testicle, thickening of the scrotum, sudden collection of fluid in the scrotum, pain or discomfort in the testicle or in the scrotum, mild ache in the lower abdomen or groin, enlargement or tenderness of the breasts, changes in urinary function, tiredness/lethargy
Vaginal	Diethylstilbestrol, vaginal adenosis, human papilloma virus, cervical cancer, smoking	Abnormal vaginal bleeding, abnormal discharge, pain during intercourse, continuous pain in the pelvis

Errors in Diagnosis

No form of diagnosis is 100 per cent effective in detecting cancer. Mistakes are often made in diagnosis, as screening methods are still largely based on the medical practitioners' experience and personal knowledge. I am a perfect example of misdiagnosis, as are many friends of mine. In my search to discover what exactly was out of balance in my body, I attended a number of highly respected medical institutions throughout Europe, America, Asia and Australia and was misdiagnosed six times by specialists in their respective fields.

A good friend of mine was misdiagnosed by doctors for over one year and hence given the wrong medication, further exacerbating her condition. These are but two cases out of millions throughout the world. Diagnosing cancer in many cases is similar to a guessing game; chances are they will find it, but how long it will take is the real question. And at what cost to your health?

No diagnostic tool is completely accurate. Many blood tests that are deemed specialised in detecting cancer in the body find it difficult to discriminate between cancer and inflammation, and other similar conditions. It is impossible in many cases for doctors to determine what the actual problem is until they actually open you up to operate. This can be dangerous, as cancer is a fear-based condition and cancer cells tend to spread through the body rapidly and easily, if given the right environment to do so. By opening you up to explore they run the risk of spreading the cancer further to other areas of the body, which is obviously why chemotherapy, radiation therapy and cancer drugs are so often employed in follow up treatment of cancer.

It is important to never let a doctor turn you away. We all have strong intuitions and most people know their own bodies very well. If you feel something is out of balance or not quite right, don't be afraid to see a medical practitioner and ask for tests. If they refuse to listen to you or laugh at you, never give up. Seek a practitioner who is understanding and empathetic to your needs. Chances are if you think something isn't quite right in your body, you're absolutely right.

A close friend of mine had no symptoms at all, yet felt something wasn't quite right in his body. He went to see a doctor and asked him to run some blood tests. Of course, the doctor thought he was crazy, but reluctantly acknowledged his wishes and ran the appropriate blood tests. He later discovered he had the early stages of prostate cancer, which had only begun a few months earlier. Listening to his intuition and trusting his gut feeling saved his life, and the future happiness of his family.

As most medical practitioners only spend 10 to 15 minutes with every patient, it is difficult for them to fully take the time to listen to your problems. Never leave until you are completely satisfied with the outcome and their diagnosis. Many cancer deaths today are due to misdiagnosis, which allows the cancer to spread further and in many cases, makes it difficult to cure. Become aware of the symptoms for each type of cancer and if you are experiencing any of these, consult with an open-minded practitioner. Don't let any medical practitioner make you feel like you are being a hypochondriac. It is your health and listening to your intuition could mean the difference between life and death.

Chapter 10

WHAT THE DOCTOR MAY NOT TELL YOU ABOUT CANCER AND MORE

C ancer is an extremely common condition in today's society. The treatment for cancer, especially in less affluent countries is already pre-determined by the doctor. This is also the case in many Western countries like Europe, New Zealand and Australia. It is almost guaranteed if you have any type of cancer you will most likely need an operation to remove the cancerous growth or tumour, followed by chemotherapy, radiation therapy or cancer drugs to prevent further cancer from occurring in the future or to remove the remainder of the cancerous cells in the body.

In countries more advanced in technology such as America, an alternative treatment may be offered. The doctor may remove a portion of the tumour and send this off for testing to see which type of chemotherapy drug or other cancer treatment will have the greatest effect on the cancer. New anti-cancer drugs are being developed all over the world (US and Australian scientists being in the forefront) and are proving successful in treating many forms of cancer. However, at the present moment, these forms of treatment are ridiculously expensive and only affordable by extremely wealthy people.

In less affluent countries we have limited options, although we have a large range of highly skilled alternative therapists and talented doctors to assist in treatment. Treatment is based largely on past experience, research and success with treating particular types of cancer.

A great amount of secrecy surrounds the diagnosis, treatment and recovery of cancer. Many doctors are afraid to tell patients the entire truth concerning their cancer and treatment, and patients are not well informed enough to ask the right questions concerning their disease. One of the most important tools and aids any person can attain in their fight against cancer is KNOWLEDGE. Knowledge is power and self–empowerment is necessary in fighting and overcoming your disease.

I myself had a very aggressive form of cancer, with very little information available due to its rarity in women. This made me feel helpless and at the mercy of doctors and their treatment prescribed. Before the operation I was given a consent form to sign which would allow the doctors to basically do as they wished while I was under anaesthetic. At twenty-seven and with a desire to have a family, this was a very scary thought. I was signing a form giving the doctors permission to remove my reproductive organs.

Fortunately, I have been involved in the medical field for many years as a qualified naturopath and I knew where to access the most useful information. Thank God for the internet and caring practitioners. On my consent form, I only allowed my very skilled doctor to remove the tumour and I instructed him to leave all of my reproductive organs in place. This was mostly acknowledged, hopefully allowing me the opportunity to have children in the future and the doctors the opportunity to use their skills to their full advantage and to realise there are usually surgical alternatives available.

Never sign a consent form until you research the facts concerning your type of cancer or until you ask your doctor the right questions and are happy, confident and satisfied with the treatment being offered. Remember, you are a person and you have rights!

My heart goes out to the many women and also men from previous generations who were at the mercy of barbaric medical doctors. It was common practice many years ago for doctors to immediately give women hysterectomies, even if their other reproductive organs were perfectly okay. Today, these women are suffering the consequences from the ignorance of the 'old school doctors' from that generation. Many of today's doctors tend to be much more open to alternatives and if asked, may provide the patient with alternative treatments currently available.

What You May Not Be Told About Surgery

Cancer almost inevitably involves some type of surgery – although not always. For example, cancer of the cervix is normally removed with laser treatment, depending on the severity of the cancer.

Before surgery, very little information is given to the patient as to the side effects, symptoms, emotions experienced and lack of movement felt after surgery. It is important to find out how you can be best prepared for surgery to ensure a rapid and successful recovery. Yet again, remember to ask as many questions as possible concerning your treatment.

Some common questions and answers concerning surgery are below. Refer to Chapter 11, Understanding Surgery, for a further in-depth look at surgery and more helpful information on what to expect.

Q. Will my bowels function normally after surgery?

A.   NO, not immediately. The doctors give you a surfactant before the surgery to clean out the bowels and basically shut them down. You may find it difficult to go to the toilet for a number of days after the surgery. This can be very painful, as gas accumulates in the bowel due to lack of movement. Many believe this is more painful than having a child and very little orthodox treatment is given to ease this pain. Solid food should be avoided until the first gas release, as it simply makes the gas worse. Peppermint herbal tea, ginger tea, aloe vera juice or chamomile tea is very good for flatulence and gas.

Q. Will my body movement be normal after surgery?

A. NO, not immediately. It can often take three months to fully recover from cancer surgery, depending on a person's age and health before surgery. As the skin and muscle tissue are being cut open and internal/external stitches inserted, body movement is often very painful and limited following surgery. Pain relief is given in the form of drugs. However, this can limit your movement further. It is advisable to work with a physiotherapist on gentle exercises to rebuild muscle strength and to avoid damaging the wound. Yoga and Tai Chi postures are also very useful. Remember, the healthier you are before surgery, the healthier and quicker you will recover after surgery.

Q. Will my energy levels return to normal after surgery?

A. YES, in time. Anaesthetics and other drugs, coupled with the stress of a major operation, tend to exhaust the body's energy levels. You must give your body time to regain its energy levels by sleeping as much as the body requires, and by supporting the body with good nutrition and natural supplements.

If you have taken time to enhance your body's immune system, strength and energy levels before surgery, you will find your energy levels will improve rapidly following surgery. For many people it can take up to three months to fully regain energy levels after surgery. If you provide the body with the right nutrients, including a high protein intake, plenty of fresh fruits and vegetables, nuts and seeds, the appropriate natural supplements and adequate rest, your energy levels will improve much faster.

Q. Are there any other medical procedures I should be aware of?

A. YES. You are rarely informed that a catheter may be inserted into your body to drain fluid. This is a long metal or plastic tube inserted into the body (anywhere from three centimetres to 10 centimetres long) and used to drain unnecessary fluid out of the body. When this is removed, you are given little warning. In my case the nurse held me down and quickly pulled the metal tube out. It became stuck due to the skin healing around it and she merely pulled harder a second time. I was offered no pain relief or warning. No doubt I screamed 'blue murder', as the pain was quite intense.

A tube connected to a bag may also be inserted into your vagina/penis to eliminate urine. A drip is put into your wrist, to feed your body with the right nutrients, saline and pain medication, usually morphine, although pethidine is also used. Therefore, be aware – you may wake up with many tubes running from your body into bags and this can be shocking for you and also your family and friends. To be forewarned is less of a shock for all involved.

Q. Can I choose which way the wound is cut?

A. YES. As a patient, you have rights! If you wish the doctor to cut horizontally or vertically, or to perform less invasive keyhole surgery, you must ask him if this is possible. For many women who like to wear bikinis or mid-riffs, having a vertical scar down the middle of the body can cause psychological and confidence problems in the future. Ask your doctor if it is possible for him to cut horizontally and as low as possible for aesthetic reasons. If you are worried about scarring, there is plastic surgery available later and also many natural treatments available to lesson the effects of scars. Remember also that you will lose sensation around the area where the skin has been cut for a period of time.

Q. Should I do anything prior to the operation to aid in a faster recovery?

A. YES. This is very important. Try to build up your strength, health and nutritional levels prior to the operation. If you are a smoker it would be advisable for you to give up smoking before surgery, as nicotine robs the body of valuable oxygen and nutrients required for healing, not to mention the stress it places on the heart under anaesthetic. It is important to eat lots of good protein, as protein assists in tissue healing. Do deep breathing exercises to improve haemoglobin levels, aerobic and strengthening exercises, stretching, yoga and positive visualisations and affirmations. Never go into an operation tired or negative. It is important to be as energised as possible and to always visualise the most positive outcome.

Q. Will I feel more emotional than usual?

A. YES. On finding out you have cancer right through to the treatment and the acceptance of your condition, your body's emotions may feel like they're being put through a washing machine. Medication and anaesthetics tend to congest the body's organs, which creates emotional imbalance. You may feel sadness, anger, blame, confusion, denial or fear – a whole multitude of emotions. Use this time to grow stronger, accept your condition and find ways to overcome the causative factors in your life that led to the onset of your cancer. Never give up! There is a lesson in every experience in life and having cancer will enable you to grow stronger and become more aware in every facet of your existence.

Q. How will I feel if any of my organs are removed?

A. If part or any of your organs are removed during surgery, it feels like part of who you are is being taken away. No one understands this unless it happens to him or her. If you are unaware of this and you wake up to find your ovaries are gone or your prostate is gone, it is an extremely traumatic and debilitating experience. You may not feel like a full woman or man anymore, in more ways than one.

This is why it is so important to be 100 per cent aware of what the doctor plans to do and to be completely in agreement before the operation. Seek other opinions and also never forget to seek alternative methods and therapies – there may be another way. Counselling, support from loved ones, compassion and understanding all go hand in hand to overcoming these overwhelming life experiences.

What You May Not Be Told About Chemotherapy

Chemotherapy is often given after cancer surgery and as with surgery, very little information may be provided with regard to what to expect. Below are some common questions and answers about chemotherapy. Refer to Chapter 12, Understanding Chemotherapy, for an in-depth look at this treatment and further helpful information on what to expect.

Q. What exactly does chemotherapy involve?

A.   Chemotherapy is administered to people of all ages. It is the most common medical treatment used to fight cancer. The most common method of giving these toxic drugs is by a drip inserted into either the wrist or the back of the hand, although they can be given by other methods.

Firstly a saline solution is passed through the drip into your body, followed by anti-nausea drugs and a mild steroid. Then the cytotoxic chemicals used to kill the cancer cells are administered and lastly the drip is flushed with saline. A large amount of fluid and cytotoxic agents pass through the body via the drip. The length of treatment and the amount and type of drugs used depends on the type of cancer being treated, the severity of the cancer and the age and inherent strength of the patient.

Q. Is chemotherapy painless?

A.   NO. The needles used are larger than normal blood testing needles. They are usually inserted directly into the veins on the back of the hand or wrist. The pain you experience during this process depends largely on the skill of the nurse involved. Always ask for a very experienced and empathetic nurse, at least for your first few times. If any of the chemotherapy drugs leak out because the needle isn't inserted properly then you will experience burning and pain. More than pain, you may experience discomfort due to the many side effects.

Drugs are given to counteract these side effects, but these also cause more side effects. Look for natural alternatives to ease the side effects involved with chemotherapy and natural methods to enhance the actions of the chemotherapy treatment. Glutamine, a powerful amino acid, is very effective in reducing the side effects and pain associated with chemotherapy.

Q. Are there many side effects involved with chemotherapy?

A.   YES. Side effects commonly experienced include nausea, vomiting, lack of appetite, weight gain or weight loss, fluid retention, sore joints, a furry taste in the mouth, bruising, lowered immunity, hair loss, irritability, emotional distress, mouth ulcers and acne. Long-term side effects may include infertility, secondary cancers, kidney damage and lung damage (Although these are rare, as symptoms are monitored and chemotherapy treatment is not as severe today as it was in the past). Most chemotherapy drugs suppress bone marrow function and the formation of blood cells, which can lead to anaemia (low iron levels) and leukopenia (low white blood cell count).

Q. Will I definitely lose my hair?

A.   NO. Patients do not always lose their hair. It depends on the chemotherapy drugs the doctors choose to use, the type of drugs being used, the length of the treatment. Chemotherapy affects each person differently. There are no set rules as to who will suffer which particular side effects. Often if you are young, the doctors choose a more intense chemotherapy program and if this is the case, you will most likely lose your hair. Etoposide or Vp16, a common chemotherapy drug, does cause temporary hair loss. One saving grace is that hair loss is temporary and the hair tends to grow back when treatment is stopped.

Q. If I lose my hair, will it grow back the same?

A.   No. Not exactly the same. Often the hair will grow back much thicker, shinier, and healthier, and often a different texture. Many times it grows back curlier, as chemotherapy affects and deforms the hair follicle, making it grow curly and sometimes a different colour altogether. In the beginning, it grows back just like baby's hair. In a way, after chemotherapy is completed, the overall appearance of your hair and skin is similar to being 'reborn as a baby'.

Q. Can I still have children after chemotherapy?

A.   In most cases yes, although this cannot be guaranteed. In the past, the chemotherapy drugs used were extremely toxic and this often led to infertility. Today treatment is less intense and with time, everything should return to normal. Try to support and protect your reproductive organs during chemotherapy with the right nutritional supplements. Most likely you will not be fertile for one to two years after chemotherapy. It can affect the transport of the eggs to the fallopian tubes and often doctors suggest IVF treatment for a successful pregnancy. For men and women, it is suggested to remove healthy sperm and eggs before chemotherapy to be safe. Before, during and after chemotherapy, it is advisable to use nutritional supplements and a healthy diet to support your reproductive system.

Q. Should I drink lots of water during chemotherapy?

A.   YES. Try to drink two to three litres of water during treatment. This is very important, as one of the most common side effects of chemotherapy is damage to the kidneys. By flushing the kidneys with adequate water you will prevent kidney damage. Chemotherapy tends to fill you with large amounts of fluid, yet dehydrates you at the same time.

Q. Is there anything else I should be cautious of during chemotherapy?

A.   YES. It is important to maintain your immunity levels during treatment. Chemotherapy kills white blood cells as well as cancerous cells, making your body's immune system prone to infections, fevers and other illnesses. Keep your immune system strong by avoiding substances which weaken your immunity, i.e. stress, alcohol, smoking, recreational drugs, fats and sugar. Maintain a good and varied diet, rich in nutrients and supplements.

Q. Are there any other procedures I should be aware of during chemotherapy?

A.   YES. The nurse will perform a blood test every day to check on nutrient levels, red blood cell count, white blood cell levels and kidney function. You may feel like a pincushion. It is all part of the process in avoiding long-term side effects. They say you become used to needles. I highly doubt this; you may become more tolerant, but that doesn't mean you'll ever grow to like them – would anybody?

What You May Not Be Told About Radiation Therapy

Radiation therapy is also often given after cancer surgery. Just as for surgery and chemotherapy, very little information may be provided with regard to what to expect. Below are some common questions and answers about radiation treatment. Refer to Chapter 13, Understanding Radiation Therapy, for an in-depth look at this treatment and further helpful information on what to expect.

Q.   What is Radiation Therapy?

A.   Radiation therapy involves using large amounts of ionizing radiation (such as x-rays, radium or radioactive cobalt) for short periods of time on the cancerous area of the body. This process involves bombarding the malignant cells with radiation at the specific site to destroy the harmful cancer cells. It is performed in a number of different ways according to the type and severity of the cancer being treated. For instance, in endometrial cancer, some doctors insert a tooth-pick-like device into the vagina and pass radium through for 48 hours.

　　In other forms of cancer, tattoos are placed on the body, the radiologists exit the room to avoid exposure and the patient is given radiation therapy for 30 seconds over a number of continuous days.

Q.   How does radiation therapy make you feel?

A.   Radiation therapy can be quite a degrading experience for the person involved. Many people who have undergone radiation therapy feel like rag dolls being played with. The nurses place permanent tattoos on the body, which may take years to disappear in some cases. The body is dosed with large amounts of radiation which in most cases lead to long-term side effects. Psychologically it is one of the hardest forms of therapy to deal with and overcome, as the physical and mental side effects are often long term and in some cases, permanent.

Q.   Will I have permanent scarring from Radiation Therapy?

A.   YES. In most cases. Because radiation affects all rapidly proliferating cells it usually causes some adverse effects. Tissues that are most frequently affected are the skin, the mucosal lining of the gastro-intestinal tract and bone marrow. Radiation tends to kill the affected and surrounding tissues. The tissue may experience permanent blackening or have a burnt appearance.

I know of one case of a man who had radiation therapy for twenty-one days in a row and came through with no permanent or noticeable burning. He was taking large doses of the nutrient lycopene, which is believed to prevent burning. Radiation can induce bone marrow depression, leading to a decrease in white blood cells and platelet production. This can increase the risk of infections and bleeding.

Q. Are there any other side effects caused by this treatment?

A. YES. As in chemotherapy, there are similar side effects of nausea, vomiting, loss of appetite, weight loss, lassitude (lack of energy), temporary hair loss and sore throat or mouth, depending on the area being zapped with radiation. Drugs are given to counteract these side effects, which generally lead to more side effects.

There are many natural alternatives available to assist with preventing these symptoms. Loss of tissue sensation in the area is common and in some cases it may take years to return to normal. Taking the right nutritional supplements, eating a nutrient-packed diet, exercise and a positive attitude will rectify this condition faster than expected.

***

Conventional cancer treatment is not without risks or harmful side effects. It is advisable to seek many opinions, know your options, seek alternative approaches and therapies and be well informed about every aspect of your condition. It is your body, your mind and your life, so you ultimately have the right to choose what works best for you. A specialist can give advice as to which treatment they feel will be most successful for your condition but once again, doctors are only human and are not always free from error. You are putting your life into someone else's hands, and I'm sure they will not accept responsibility if something does go wrong.

Knowledge and understanding is the key. It is your responsibility to understand your condition as much as possible. Find a good, open-minded medical or experienced natural health practitioner to guide you in the right direction and to support your decisions.

Chapter 11

UNDERSTANDING SURGERY

Preparing For and Recovering From Surgery

For many people the prospect of undergoing surgery seems terrifying, to say the least. As much as we may detest this thought, sometimes surgery is the best available answer to improving our quality of life. Often there are other options so if you are planning to undertake surgery, try to seek second and third opinions first. Find out about effective alternative approaches to treating the problem. If you have decided that surgery is the most viable option for you, it is important to prepare your body for it to ensure a faster recovery, optimal healing and reduced side effects.

By taking nutritional supplements you will increase your body's healing process and ensure less post-surgery discomfort and pain. Your general health following surgery depends largely on your general health before surgery. That is, the healthier and stronger you are before your surgery, the quicker and more successful your recovery will be after surgery. It is also important to go into surgery feeling as relaxed as possible, visualising the most positive and beneficial outcome. The mind is one of the body's most powerful tools in healing. Practise creative imagery before surgery and try to imagine a wonderful and successful result from surgery.

Surgical Techniques

Surgery can be a traumatic experience on the body and mind. New techniques can minimise the trauma caused from surgery. Laparoscopic surgery, or keyhole surgery, is less traumatic and ensures you a faster release from the hospital. You are also left with only a very small scar or wound. Likewise, instead of the common vertical cut that doctors regularly use in all types of operations, ask your doctor if it would be possible for him to cut horizontally, below your bikini line. In many cases this is entirely possible and leaves you with less psychological trauma later.

Herbal Remedies

Herbal remedies and herbal teas are highly recommended before and after surgery. Herbs enhance healing and stimulate the body's natural defences, particularly immune system function. Try some of the following herbal teas to encourage more rapid healing:

- Echinacea tea boosts the body's immune system and increases production of white blood cells to fight disease.
- Ginseng improves recovery time after surgery. It also boosts energy levels and alleviates depression. Ginseng is used throughout China to decrease pain.
- Goldenseal is a natural antibiotic and helps to prevent infections. It also helps to stimulate a healthy appetite and can ease a nasty case of gastritis. Do not take for more than one week at a time as it may disturb normal intestinal flora.
- Milk thistle protects the liver from a toxic build-up of drugs, chemicals and anaesthetics used in surgery. Often following surgery it can take some time before the bowels function normally again. Milk thistle helps to relieve constipation caused from liver and gallbladder congestion.
- Pau d'arco is a natural antibacterial, detoxifying and immune-stimulating herb. It speeds up the healing process, cleanses the blood and aids in the prevention of candida and thrush.
- Rosehip tea is a wonderful spring tonic that aids general debility and exhaustion. It is a good source of natural vitamin C and enhances healing.
- Chamomile is a natural carminative and relaxes the body's nervous system, easing the stress of surgery.
- Dandelion herbal tea aids good liver and kidney function, helps to eliminate excess fluids and cleanses the blood system.

Nutritional Advice

Nutritional Supplements are very important as they tend to enhance healing and recovery. Eat a healthy diet rich in vitamins and minerals before surgery and make sure you eat plenty of protein-rich foods. Protein is needed to repair cut tissues and muscles, and to rebuild the body's energy levels. Good sources of protein include nuts, seeds and fish, particularly salmon, tuna, mackerel, cod, sardines, organic chicken breast, organic turkey, grain-fed lamb and red meats in moderation. It is best if you can obtain organic meats, free from antibiotics, fertilizers and pesticides.

Dietary Advice
✓ Ensure that you drink at least two to three litres of water per day to ensure that your body does not become dehydrated.
✓ Check for any signs of anaemia pre-surgery. To check for anaemia, place your hand down flat on a table and push your nails down. If the pink colour returns quickly, generally your iron levels are quite good. If your nails are a whitish colour this may indicate low iron levels. If anaemic, take an iron, vitamin B12 and folic acid supplement before surgery (do not take following surgery).
✓ Support the immune system with the appropriate nutrients or herbs as suggested in table 11.1.
✓ Increase intake of onions and garlic for their natural antibiotic properties.

✓ Avoid aspirin or NSAIDs (non-steroidal anti-inflammatory drugs) prior to surgery, as they can cause excessive bleeding.
✓ To improve detoxification of anaesthetics, supplement with liver herbs or nutrients and a good antioxidant containing vitamin C, E and beta-carotene.
✓ Take a protein powder or eat plenty of protein foods before and after surgery to enhance healing.
✓ Ensure that you maintain good digestion by supplementing with a good digestive enzyme, hydrochloric acid supplement or by taking apple cider vinegar – one to three tablespoons per day in water.

Table 11.1 shows nutritional supplements that are useful for healing.

Homeopathics

Arnica is a great homeopathic which aids in wound healing and prevents bruising. Arnica can be taken (up to 6 c) the night before surgery. Take every two hours following surgery. Alternate doses of arnica and hypericum (up to 6c) during waking hours. These remedies diminish pain and reduce the need for medication.

Essential Oils

Aromatherapy oils are oils obtained from flowers, roots or leaves of plants in their purest form. They are very useful for relaxation, healing, cleansing and uplifting the moods and emotions. In hospital it is beneficial to use oils to aid relaxation and uplift the emotions, as depression can often occur after surgery. Essential oils can be added with water to an oil burner and burnt throughout the day and night. Useful oils are listed below.

- Lavender – Relaxes the nervous system, brings a sense of peace and calmness, good for headaches, nausea, insomnia, shock and uplifts moods. Externally, great for burns.
- Bergamot – Great for uplifting the moods, aids depression, anxiety and nervous tension, and enhances creativity.
- Clary Sage – Specifically for depression, aids positivity, helps to eliminate fear, paranoia and delusions.
- Patchouli – Uplifts the moods, enhances creativity and increases acceptance.
- Jasmine – Sedates the central nervous system, aiding relaxation.
- Basil oil – Relaxes the entire nervous system and enhances appetite, clears the head and can be used for weakness, indecision and hysteria. It is good for people who need protecting due to a debilitating illness or for low resistance conditions.
- Lemongrass – Relaxes the nervous system slightly, and brings a sense of happiness and positivity.
- Tea Tree oil – Great for cuts and external wounds, and acts as an antiseptic.
- Eucalyptus – Great for colds, flu's and lowered immunity. Also improves breathing and clears airway passages.

Table 11.1

Supplement	Dosage	Comments
A multi-vitamin supplement to include zinc, calcium, magnesium, silica, vitamin D, vitamin A, beta-carotene	Calcium – 1500 mg/day, zinc – 50 mg/day, vitamin A – 10000 – 50000 IU/day Take 1 tablet daily with food	Important for tissue repair. Vitamin A is needed for protein utilisation in tissue repair and as a free radical scavenger
Amino Acid complex or protein powder	Free form amino acid powder or protein powder. As directed on label. Refer to recipes in Part 3 of this book – protein/energy shake.	Accelerates tissue repair and recovery, maintains a healthy nitrogen balance, speeds up the healing of wounds
Bromelain	350 – 700 mg/day in divided doses	Bromelain has anti-inflammatory properties, which can help reduce swelling and pain associated with swelling
Coenzyme Q10	90 mg day or up to 270 mg/day if on chemotherapy/radiation treatment	Destroys harmful free radicals, improves tissue oxygenation, antioxidant, speeds up the healing process
D-L Phenylanine (amino acid)	3 tablets daily on an empty stomach with fruit juice. Take one hour before meals or take as directed in powder form	Decreases post surgical pain, only take if you are experiencing a great deal of pain
Essential fatty acids (evening primrose oil, fish oils, DHA/EPA)	As directed or 3 teaspoons/day Fish oils – 1000 – 3000 mg per day	Important for healing of tissues and proper cell growth, prevents and decreases inflammation – also found in flaxseed oil, mackerel, salmon, sardines, tuna, cod, halibut
Garlic	500 mg 3 times/day	A natural antibiotic that boosts immunity, helps to prevent infections
Glutathione	100 mg per day	Powerful self-generating antioxidant that helps recycle vitamins C and E, and helps to detoxify anaesthetics

Table 11.1 *continued*

Supplement	Dosage	Comments
L-Arginine	1000 mg/day in divided doses	Promotes wound healing, involved in collagen synthesis – also found in almonds, cashews, garlic, ginseng, peas, and pecans
L-Glutamine	500 mg 3 times /day	Speeds the healing of wounds, detoxification – also found in cottage cheese, most protein sources, ricotta cheese, rolled oats
Lipoic acid	100 mg per day	Essential for cellular and muscular energy production, which aids in faster healing
Lysine	500 – 3000 mg/day	Increases immunity, aids formation of collagen and elastin, promotes healing – also found in chicken, fish, lamb, milk, mung bean sprouts, oat flakes
Selenium	50 mcg/day or higher. This is usually available in a tablet or as a liquid. Obtain Sodium Selenite on prescription from your doctor.	When combined with vitamin E, selenium has a synergistic effect in the treatment of tissue damage due to restricted blood flow
Vitamin C and bioflavonoids	3000 – 10000 mg/day in divided doses. Take large doses after surgery. If you take too much Vitamin C before surgery, it may wake you up from anaesthetic.	Aids in tissue repair and accelerates healing of wounds, boosts the body's immune system, antioxidant, detoxifies toxins and anaesthetics. Do not take the day before surgery, take immediately after.
Vitamin E	Only take small amounts before surgery, as it may thin the blood – 200 IU/day. The day after surgery you can increase to 750 IU – 1500 IU/day.	Improves circulation, repairs tissues and reduces scar formation; neutralises free radicals generated during surgery and protects from toxic effects of chemicals used in anaesthesia

Table 11.1 *continued*

Supplement	Dosage	Comments
Vitamin E oil	Apply topically to the wound after stitches have been removed, as often as you feel comfortable	Promotes healing and prevents scar formation – cut open a capsule to release the oil
Vitamin K	As directed	Aids in effective blood clotting
Zinc	50 mg – 100 mg/day	Necessary for good wound healing and tissue repair, great for stress, involved in over 80 enzyme reactions in the body – also found in almonds, ginger, sunflower & pumpkin seeds, oysters, liver and fish

Australian Bush Flower Remedies and Bach Remedies

Emotions have a powerful impact on a person's ability to recover from illness. Negative emotions are known to weaken our body's immune system through a number of internal metabolic reactions, as outlined in Chapter 19 – Mind Medicine. Therefore, to increase your ability to heal following surgery, you must ensure that you maintain a positive attitude before surgery by eliminating any niggling fears, anxieties or emotional blocks in your life.

Two useful combination remedies for pre and post surgery are the Australian Bush Flower Remedy – 'Emergency Essence' and the Bach Flower Remedy – 'Rescue Remedy'. Both these combination remedies are used to alleviate panic, distress and fear. They ease these feelings, provide comfort until your surgery and ease stress following surgery.

Creative Imagery Exercise to Ensure a Successful Surgery and a Healthy Self

If you truly wish to be healthy and cancer-free then why not use the power of your mind to create this. Visualise yourself regaining perfect health, vitality and happiness. If you can see the surgery in your mind, the tumour, the treatment proposed and the white blood cells, then visualise a positive outcome from treatment, visualise yourself in a state of 'ideal health'. Imagine yourself performing fun activities that you would love to do if you were perfectly healthy. Try to actually feel the 'wellness' of your body and mind. Picture yourself at the healthiest and happiest time in your life. Bring these images into the present feeling exactly that way and watch the magic of your visualisations unfold. Another positive step is to bring your favourite photo of yourself looking healthy and vibrant into the hospital and keep this beside your bed. If a beautiful, healthy and vibrant image greets you everyday, then this image will enter your subconscious mind creating a mirror image of yourself in real life. Never underestimate the incredible power of your mind...

Other Recommendations

- If you smoke, stop smoking. Smoking interferes with recovery from surgery and decreases overall healing time. Smoking increases the body's needs of various vitamins and minerals, which are already needed in extra amounts at this time.
- Many operations require that the patient be shaved. If this is your case, ask to be shaved the day of surgery as this decreases chances of infections.
- Before surgery you are given a detergent type mixture, to cleanse the bowel of any wastes. The bowels are also shut down. You can ask to clean the bowels yourself, which can be done naturally with fibres, enemas or colonic irrigation. It is important to add adequate fibre to your diet to ensure better intestinal tract function.
- Try to de-stress as much as possible before the operation. Surgery is very stressful, both mentally and physically. It would be advisable to have a good therapeutic massage with relaxing aromatherapy oils before surgery (if this is suitable for your condition – refer to chapter 28 – Bliss and Harmony).
- The use of affirmations, imagery and self-hypnosis can aid recovery and accelerate healing. Listen to relaxing and positive music before and after surgery.
- Transform your hospital room into a healing environment (refer to Chapter 14 – Transform Your Hospital Environment). Bring your favourite music; surround yourself with bright colours, beautiful smells, loving family and friends and your most treasured items, to enhance your healing environment.
- Surgery performed on women with breast cancer should be done during the luteal phase (day twenty-one to thirty-six) of the menstrual cycle. Generally this is associated with a much better healing outcome, particularly in oestrogen receptive negative tumours.

Chapter 12

UNDERSTANDING CHEMOTHERAPY

Chemotherapy Explained

Chemotherapy is a form of cancer therapy which uses drugs to treat cancer. These specially designed drugs are commonly called cytotoxic ('cyto' meaning cell and 'toxic' meaning to 'injure' or 'kill'). Many of these drugs are obtained from natural sources, such as plants. Other cytotoxic drugs are man-made. There are over sixty different drugs used in chemotherapy and many of these are used in different strengths and combinations.

Combination chemotherapy has been found to be more effective than treatment with a single drug. Doctors combine drugs with different mechanisms of action, different metabolic pathways, different times of onset of action and recovery, different side effects and onset of side effects. The cytotoxic drugs are inserted into the body by a number of different methods, and work at destroying cancer cells, as well as normal healthy cells.

How Chemotherapy Works

Chemotherapy drugs enter the bloodstream and travel throughout the body to most tissues. The drugs kill certain cells but mostly cells that are rapidly dividing i.e. cancer cells. This means that the drugs affect both cancer cells and normal cells (this is the reason hair loss often occurs).

Generally the effect on normal body tissues is temporary and they recover quickly from the drugs because of the body's normal process of repair and healing. Cancer cells recover slowly and with more difficulty than normal cells. By the time the person is ready for the next chemotherapy treatment, the body's normal cells have mostly recovered, yet the cancer cells have not. They are then killed with further treatment. If the chemotherapy treatment can kill all of the cancer cells, the cancer is curable. However, this is not always the case.

Important Note

Chemotherapy as a form of cancer therapy does not work on all types of cancer. At first, the use of chemotherapy drugs may cause an initial disappearance of weaker cancer cells killed directly by the cytotoxic poisons and by the body's own immune system. Hence, the tumour may seem as if it is regressing. When this happens, you may feel a little better for the next few weeks.

If the chemotherapy is continued during this period, the immune system becomes weakened even further. There may be a fall in white blood cells. In many cases, the tumour may become resistant to the chemotherapy drugs and it may begin to grow again. If this occurs, the oncologist generally changes the type of cytotoxic agent being used. However, the second course of drugs is usually less effective than the first.

Finally, the body's immune system is so weakened, that it becomes susceptible to infections or even secondary tumours. Energy levels fall, symptoms increase and the doctor often recommends a small break from treatment to allow the body's white blood cells to regrow. However, this can be dangerous as it can cause the stronger cancer cells to increase.

Alternatively, they may recommend injections of a hormone to push white blood cells out of the bone marrow. Either way, the body is in a dangerous position. The body's immune system is extremely weak and may be unable to fight off the onslaught of cancerous cells.

Therefore, chemotherapy as a traditional and conventional form of cancer treatment is only effective on particular types of cancer.

How Chemotherapy is Given

Chemotherapy is usually given in a series of cycles rather than as a continuous treatment. The length and cycle of treatment is dependent on the severity and type of cancer being treated. Chemotherapy drugs are given in either tablet or capsule form orally, as injections into muscles (intramuscular) or under the skin (subcutaneous), into the spinal fluid (intrathecal) or much more commonly into veins (intravenous), as discussed earlier, in Chapter 9.

Sometimes the intravenous injection can be given over a few minutes or it may be given in a larger volume of fluid over some hours in a drip or infusion. Sometimes more than one drug is used at the same time. It is often given on outpatient terms, meaning that it is not usually necessary to stay in hospital during treatment.

Why Chemotherapy is Given

Chemotherapy is given to either cure or improve the future for those with cancer. It may be given to cure the cancer or as an added treatment to increase the effectiveness of surgery and radiotherapy (radiation treatment) by killing possible remaining cancer cells. It may be used as a treatment to reduce the symptoms of cancer and to improve the quality of life. Chemotherapy is still given today as a treatment for cancer, as doctors are following long-term protocol in conventional cancer treatment. This is what they understand and are taught in their training, so many doctors fear diverting from the normal cancer therapy treatments used over the last fifty years.

Chemotherapy and other orthodox medical cancer therapies such as radiation therapy and cancer drugs are a high income provider for the medical institution. Many of the answers to healing cancer are already found within 'nature' in the form of herbs, holistic medicine and nature cure. Some doctors dissuade clients from undertaking natural treatment to beat their cancer as it would take a huge money-generating source away from them that is provided by medical cancer treatments.

Toxicity of Chemotherapy Drugs

Chemotherapy drugs are extremely toxic. They are actually carcinogens (cancer-causing substances) in their own right. They attempt to kill cancer cells, yet at the same time they kill normal healthy cells. Chemotherapy drugs tend to remain in the body for long periods of time after treatment. Having a toxic carcinogen like this in the body can often lead to the onset of secondary cancers such as non-Hodgkin's lymphomas, kidney and bladder cancer. Therefore, if you do decide to undergo chemotherapy, it is extremely important for you to detoxify these harmful carcinogens from your body following completion of treatment, to ensure that they will not create secondary cancers. An intense detoxification regime after chemotherapy is essential in the prevention of secondary tumours.

With cancer, the body's liver is already in the process of detoxifying harmful substances and cancer cells from the body. By putting another harmful carcinogen such as chemotherapy drugs into your system, you are simply giving the liver another volatile toxin to deal with. If the liver is overloaded, aberrant cancer cells may escape into the bloodstream and lodge in other areas of the body, causing another tumour to form elsewhere in the future. As mentioned above, if you do decide to undertake chemotherapy or radiation therapy at any stage in your life, it is essential that you detoxify these harmful cancer-causing substances from your body to ensure that you remain cancer-free.

Chemotherapy and Pain

Chemotherapy can be painful, depending on the empathy of the nurse who is treating you. In my experience, I found the actual chemotherapy to be painful about 75 per cent of the time. Nurses will often give excuses as to the patient having 'tough veins' or 'flattened veins' or some other excuse but really, how effectively the drip needle is inserted depends on the degree of experience, empathy and care the nurse exhibits.

Chemotherapy drugs are very cold. Keep warm when having chemotherapy and ask for a hot pack to be placed on your arm to aid with the extreme cold. And always make sure you warm up the area with a hot towel or hot pack first to soften the veins. Use a vitamin E cream or lotion to soften up your skin and veins – this can make the needle insert easier. A test dose of more allergic cytotoxic drugs is given with a needle directly into the upper arm. This is very painful, similar to your inner veins being stung by a bee. People say you get used to the needles. This is not true, you never get used to having large needles inserted into your arms and copious amounts of toxic drugs inserted into your veins.

If the nurse hasn't positioned the drip correctly, you will experience some aching in the arm and often bruising around the insertion point. Always ask for experienced nurses to perform the insertion of your drip.

The most painful experience with chemotherapy is the debilitating side effects associated with its application, which normally don't become apparent until shortly after chemotherapy is given. The side effects from placing cytotoxic drugs into your body are many and varied, according to each individual, and may affect you both mentally and physically.

Continuing Your Normal Life During Chemotherapy

Many people continue their normal schedules and work their chemotherapy treatments around their work and social life. This depends on the amount of chemotherapy you are having. If you are having large amounts of chemotherapy, you will find your energy levels will decrease more and more over time. The side effects and energy decrease are cumulative, often getting worse as the weeks go by. As you have more and more chemotherapy treatments you will find your energy levels will decrease, even though it doesn't seem that way in the beginning. However, if you keep up a healthy, nutritious diet and supplement with the correct nutrients you should be able to avoid most side effects and maintain relatively good energy levels.

I would recommend ceasing the majority of work during chemotherapy and concentrating this time on healing. In many cases, a hectic schedule and tense work commitments may have been a contributing factor towards your cancer development. Everyone is affected by chemotherapy very differently. It is best to judge for yourself and see how you feel as time goes by. Don't feel obligated to anyone during this period – try to make as much free time for yourself as possible and healing will occur much quicker.

Will Chemotherapy Work for You?

Cancer cells, once exposed to a chemical agent such as chemotherapy, have the unique intelligence to create methods to improve their ability to cope and survive. This can result in a resistance to chemotherapy, which acts as an obstacle to treatment success. Cancer cells not only develop a resistance to the particular chemotherapy drugs being used, but also to other toxic drugs and chemicals that they have not yet encountered. Therefore, chemotherapy may initially seem to decrease cancer cells, however, as the cancerous cells develop their own methods of protecting against these drugs, the chemotherapy treatment will, in many cases, hit a plateau.

The effectiveness of chemotherapy depends largely on the condition of the cancer cell. If the tumour is hypoxic (lacking oxygen) or the mitochondrial function within the cell is compromised, chemotherapy is often of little value. Initially you may see a rapid decrease in the size of the tumour, however this is only a reflection of destruction of the weakest cancer cells, leaving the more resistant super-survivors to re-establish themselves and grow their own 'city network' again.

To be successful, chemotherapy needs to kill all cancer cells, otherwise it is just a technique for allowing the strongest cancer cells to survive and replicate themselves. Apart from this, chemotherapy leaves harmful toxins within the body that act as carcinogens and if not detoxified may cause the onset of secondary and more aggressive cancers.

Determining Whether Chemotherapy is Working

Certain medical tests and natural diagnostic tests can indicate how successful the chemotherapy treatment is. Blood testing, physical examinations, scans and x-rays are all orthodox diagnostic methods used to indicate how well treatment is working. There are also a number of alternative therapy tests that can offer insight into your present health condition, for example, Live Blood Analysis, Magnagraph testing and Computerised Iridology.

Never hesitate to ask the doctor about your results and what they indicate about your progress. Lack of side effects from the chemotherapy is not an indication that the treatment is not working. Side effects vary from person to person and treatment to treatment depending on many factors and what you are actively doing to assist your treatment.

Use the modern diagnostic techniques to monitor your condition and always ask your health practitioner how effective your treatment is and how your condition is improving. The doctor may tell you in the beginning, 'we need to get your tumour markers down to 0 to ensure you are in remission'. Later you may find out this isn't the case, as some doctors, perhaps even out of a misguided concern for your wellbeing, tend to keep you in the dark about your condition, assuming you don't have the knowledge to comprehend or understand your own illness. Never let any doctor keep you in the dark, ask for details about everything, write down questions to ask at your next appointment and never be swayed from knowing everything about your condition.

Raising Self-esteem During Treatment

Chemotherapy can be a humiliating and debilitating experience at any age. As human beings, we love and cherish our hair. It is believed the most traumatic experience in life for any man is to lose his hair. Imagine how terrifying this thought is for a woman, when we put so much energy into looking and feeling great for both our own self-confidence and for others. Many chemotherapy drugs often result in hair loss or hair thinning.

To maintain good levels of self-esteem and self-respect during treatment, prepare yourself for this outcome by cutting your hair into a short style. If you still wish to keep your locks, have your own hair made into a wig. There are some excellent wig specialists, who will style and colour a wig exactly to your needs and to suit your face shape. It's actually fun to have the opportunity to try so many wigs on and experiment with different styles, lengths and colours. My favourite wig was a cute little pink bob style – I had always wanted to be daring and have pink hair. Opportunity knocked.

Hats, scarves, bandanas and colourful turbans are all available to decorate your head and uplift your spirits. I found using coloured henna paints, glitter pencils and body art painted in beautiful swirls and designs on my head, to be uplifting and creative. For younger people, there are some great tattoos, Indian bindis and other forms of body art available to give you a boost.

Ask a friend to draw some wonderful inspirational artwork on your head. If you experience a drop in self-confidence from other side effects like weight gain, weight loss, exhaustion or pimples, take action and use natural remedies to avoid and rectify these problems. Alternative remedies can be highly effective in eliminating many side effects and in decreasing the duration of treatment. Great activities to improve confidence and positivity include affirmations, meditation, breathing exercises, maintaining a good posture, yoga, tai chi and guided imagery.

Be around people who are positive, understanding and accepting of your condition. Keep your sense of humour; see funny movies, be around positive people, laugh and have lots of fun. One thing is certain in life, nothing remains the same. The world and life's effects are ever-changing. Time passes and in its passing you will find yourself in a completely different environment and in a completely different stage in your life, filled with happiness and good health.

Types of Chemotherapy Drugs/Side effects/ How Given

Table 12.1 outlines the types of drugs used in chemotherapy, how they are given, the types of cancer they are used for and a brief list of side effects associated with each drug. Further useful information on side effects and how to combat them follows.

There are hundreds of different types of chemotherapy and anti-cancer drugs being used in orthodox cancer treatment today. To find a more comprehensive list of short-term and long-term side effects and complications involved with their application, refer to a current MIMS manual. MIMS manual is a drug guide used by health professionals in Australia and information from them can be obtained from your doctor, upon your request.

The Side effects of Chemotherapy

As you can see, there are a diverse range of side effects involved with the application of chemotherapy medications. Side effects vary according to the dosage being used, the type of chemotherapy drug employed and the length of treatment. Here is a more comprehensive description of the most common side effects experienced today:

Constipation/Diarrhoea

These are not common side effects, yet they do occur. Anti-nausea drugs and steroids used during chemotherapy can cause constipation. It may take a few days after completing treatment before your bowels return to normal. Diarrhoea may also occur as the microflora in the bowel is destroyed and the microvilli (hair-like projections along the bowel wall which are essential for proper absorption) are damaged. In fact, the microvilli and absorption of nutrients can be compromised for up to two years following chemotherapy, unless a natural, rejuvenation program is followed.

Table 12.1

Type of Drug	Name	Method	Type of Cancer	Short-term Side Effects	Long-term Side Effects
Alkylating agent	Busulphan (Myleran)	By mouth; oral pill – IV is used in some cases	Chronic Leukaemia (bone marrow transplanta-tion)	Low blood cell counts, low platelet counts, anaemia, hair loss, sore mouth, diarrhoea	Dark skin, lung stiffness and damage, bone marrow depression, alopecia, hemorrhagic cystitis
	Chlorambucil (Leukeran)	By mouth	Ovarian, breast cancer, leukaemia	Low blood cell counts, loss of menstrual periods, possible nausea, vomiting	Small risk of leukaemia, lung damage
	Cyclophospha-mide (Endoxan or Cytoxan)	IV, or by mouth in pill form	Breast, bone, ovarian, cervix, lung cancer, Lymphoma, bladder, leukaemia, soft tissue sarcoma, multiple myeloma	Vomiting, nausea hair loss, skin pigmenta-tion, mouth ulcers, bladder irritation, sore mouth, diarrhoea, anaemia, low white blood cell counts, red urine	Bladder cancer, small risk of acute leukaemia, lung damage, irritation and bleeding of the bladder
	Melphalan (l-pam, Alkeran)	Orally, in pill form	Multiple myeloma, breast, ovarian	Low platelet counts, anaemia, diarrhoea, appetite loss	None known – long term side effects are highly dependent on the amount of administration

Table 12.1 *continued*

Type of Drug	Name	Method	Type of Cancer	Short-term Side Effects	Long-term Side Effects
	Nitrogen mustard (Mustine)	IV	Lymphoma Hodgkin's disease	Nausea and vomiting, low blood counts, anaemia, hair loss, infertility	Small risk of leukaemia, vein damage, severe tissue damage if drug leaks from the injection site
	Cytarabine (Cytosine, Ara-C, Arabinoside)	IV, SC, spinal fluid injection	Acute and chronic myeloid leukaemia, lymphoma	Low blood cell counts, low platelet counts, anaemia, hair loss, sore mouth	Damage to the brain if used in high doses
	5 Fluorouracil (5-FU)	IV and cream for skin cancer	Breast, colon, stomach, pancreas	Low blood cell counts, diarrhoea, sore mouth, stomach pain, anaemia, skin that is sensitive to the sun	Excessive tear formation from the eyes (this may only be temporary)
Anti-metabolic agent	Methotextrate	By mouth, IV	Breast, bladder, head, lung, cervix, bone, lymphomas leukaemia, neck, arthritis	Mouth ulcers, low blood cell counts, malaise, nausea, vomiting, anaemia, hair loss, sore mouth, diarrhoea	Kidney damage, lung inflammation, lung damage, nerve damage, liver damage
	Bleomycin	IV, IM	Lymphomas, breast cancer, germ cell carcinoma	Fever, allergic reactions, skin rashes	Lung damage, skin blisters

	Drug	Route	Cancer treated	Side effects	Side effects
Plant alkaloid	Dactinomycin	IV	Wilm's tumour of the kidney	Nausea, vomiting, diarrhoea	Hair loss, sore mouth
	Etoposide (Vp-16)	IV	Cancer of testis, lung, ovaries, lymphomas	Low blood cell counts, nausea, dizziness, hair loss	Low blood counts – temporary
	Vinblastine (Velban)	IV	Lymphoma, testes, breast, Hodgkin's Disease, gestational trophoblastic disease	Low blood cell counts, anaemia, hair loss, sore mouth, diarrhoea	Nerve damage, damage to veins, paralysis of bowels, severe damage to tissues if leaks from injection site.
	Vincristine (Oncovin)	IV	Leukaemia, lymphoma, Hodgkin's disease, breast, myeloma, soft tissue sarcoma, neuroblastoma	Constipation, low platelet count, hair loss, anaemia, bowl paralysis, diarrhoea	Numbness and weakness of limbs, nerve damage, damage to veins
	Taxol (Paclitaxel)	IV only	Breast, ovarian, lung, testicular, melanoma, head and neck	Low white blood cell and platelet counts, hair loss, sore mouth, fluid retention, anaemia, allergic reactions	Numbness of limbs, liver damage

Table 12.1 *continued*

Type of Drug	Name	Method	Type of Cancer	Short-term Side Effects	Long-term Side Effects
Other	Asparaginase	IV	Acute lymphobla-stic leukaemia	Severe allergic reactions	None reported
	Dacarbazine (DTIC)	IV	Malignant melanoma, soft tissue sarcoma, Hodgkin's disease, neuroblastoma	Low blood cell counts, vomiting, anaemia, hair loss, sore mouth, diarrhoea	Transient liver damage
	Cis Platinum (Cis-platin or CDDp, or Platinol)	IV	Testes, ovaries, lungs, head and neck, endometrial, breast, stomach, lymphoma	Vomiting, hair loss nausea, ringing in the ears, low blood counts, diarrhoea, anaemia	Deafness and other hearing damage, kidney damage, permanent pins and needles in hands or feet
	Procarbazine	By mouth	Hodgkin's disease	Low blood counts, high blood pressure	None reported
	Adriamycin (Doxorubicin)	IV only	Stomach, breast, sarcoma, lymphoma, multiple myeloma, bone tumour	Sore mouth, difficulty in swallowing, diarrhoea, low white blood cell and platelet counts, anaemia, red urine	Heart problems, damage to veins, tissue damage
	BiCNU (Carmustine)	IV only	Multiple myeloma, brain, melanoma, lymphoma, bone marrow transplant	Low white blood cell and platelet counts, anaemia, hair loss, sore mouth, diarrhoea	Kidney and lung damage if used in high doses

	Drug	Administration	Cancers treated	Side effects	Other
	Hydroxyurea (Hydrea)	By mouth in capsule	hronic myelocytic leukemia, polycythemia, head and neck, sickle cell disease	Low white blood cell and platelet counts, anaemia, hair loss with long-term use	None known
Steroid hormone	Tamoxifen (Nolvadex, Genox)	By mouth	Breast cancer	Hot flushes, menstrual changes, weight gain, emotional changes	Increased clotting tendency of the blood, knife-like chest pains
Newer Drugs	Carboplatinum (Paraplatin)	IV only	Ovarian, lung, testes, head and neck, leukaemia	Low white blood cell and platelet counts, anaemia, hair loss, nausea, diarrhoea	Nerve damage
	Ifosfamide	IV only	Testis, bone lymphoma, soft tissue sarcoma	Low white blood cell and platelet counts, anaemia, hair loss	Bleeding from bladder – Mesna is used to counteract; possible bladder damage
	Mitoxantrone	IV	Leukaemia, lymphoma, breast, ovarian	Low white blood cell and platelet counts, anaemia, hair loss, sore mouth, diarrhoea, blue urine	None known
	Herceptin (trastuzumab)	Orally – by mouth	Metastatic breast cancer	Anaemia, fever, chills, nausea, vomiting, fatigue, skin rash, low blood pressure, headache, low blood counts, fluid retention, hair loss, diarrhoea	Cardiac dysfunction

Table 12.1 *continued*

Type of Drug	Name	Method	Type of Cancer	Short-term Side Effects	Long-term Side Effects
	Irinotecan (Camptosar, CPT-11)	IV	Recurrent colon cancer	Severe diarrhoea, low white cell counts	Lung damage
	Navelbine (Vinorelbine)	IV, oral form	Non small cell lung cancer	Nausea, vomiting	Liver damage, nerve damage
	Rituxan (Rituximab)	IV	Low grade lymphoma	Fever, chills, nausea, vomiting, fatigue, rash, low blood pressure, asthma, shortness of breath, fluid retention, low cell counts	None reported
	STI-571 (Gleevec)		Chronic myeloid leukaemia	Fluid retention, low cell counts, anaemia, stomach irritation	Liver damage
	Taxotere (Docetaxel)	IV	Breast and non small cell lung cancer	Low blood cell counts, fluid retention, weight gain	None reported
	Topotecan (Hycamtin)	IV	Ovarian, lung, leukaemia, non Hodgkin's lymphoma	Low blood cell counts, fatigue, anaemia, hair loss, nausea, vomiting, sore mouth, diarrhoea	None reported

IV – means intravenous – the drug is given by injection directly into a vein, usually by a drip. SC – means subcutaneous – the drug is given by injection under the skin IM – means intramuscular – the drug is given by injection into the muscle.

Effects on the Cells

Most chemotherapeutic drugs suppress bone marrow function and the formation of blood cells. A decrease in red blood cells can make you anaemic and you may feel tired, lethargic, dizzy and breathless. If this occurs, your doctor will suggest a blood transfusion to build up your stores of red blood cells.

A decrease in white blood cells can lead to infections. If you have any signs of infection such as fever over 38 degrees, chills, coughs or a burning feeling when passing urine, call your doctor immediately. The doctor usually prescribes a hormone injection to increase white blood cells. This involves injecting a hormone into your stomach or abdomen over a 10 day period, to push white blood cells out of the body's bone marrow. Intense bone pain and aching joints are associated with this. Other options may include a delay in your next treatment or a reduced dose of chemotherapy in the next course.

If your platelet count is low, bleeding may occur. Platelets are needed to clot the blood. If you are bruising easily, bleeding from gums, nose or bowel, or notice blood in your urine, consult your doctor immediately. A platelet transfusion is given to counteract this.

Effects on the Mouth

Chemotherapy drugs affect the cells lining the mouth and throat, often causing soreness, dry mouth, mouth ulcers, difficulty in swallowing, furry/slimy/coated tongue, pimples on the tongue and a metallic taste in the mouth. Difficulty in swallowing or chewing can lead to a loss of weight and malnutrition and will slow down the recovery.

Fluid Retention

Fluid retention is a common side effect caused by use of anti-nausea drugs and steroids. It is also inevitable, with so much fluid being put into the body with treatment. Look for natural diuretics in foods, herbs and supplements to remove unwanted fluid. Drink plenty of water.

Hair Loss

Not all chemotherapy drugs cause hair loss. This side effect is only temporary and following cessation of treatment your hair will tend to grow back healthier, shinier, thicker and often curly. Hair loss can occur at any time during treatment, but is most likely to happen within the first three to four weeks. It occurs as the drugs impair the proliferation of the hair follicle. Many people will experience hair thinning, not complete hair loss.

Kidney Damage

This is a side effect, which is closely monitored by regular blood testing of creatinine levels before onset of treatment. Some of the chemotherapy drugs, particularly

Cisplatin, can cause permanent kidney damage if not monitored correctly. It is important to drink adequate amounts of water and to eat kidney-supporting foods.

Lethargy/Tiredness

Chemotherapy treatment tends to deplete energy levels. This is cumulative as the drugs build up in your system. Often the doctor tells you if you have plenty of energy after the first session of treatments this will determine your energy later. This is generally not true. Energy levels get worse with more and more treatments.

Loss of Appetite

This is a secondary side effect of nausea, vomiting, worry or stress. A yellow coating can become obvious on the tongue, which is slimy and has a foul taste. This often leads to a decrease in appetite.

Lung Damage/Shortness of Breath

Lung damage and shortness of breath is another side effect which is closely monitored. The effects of lung damage (primarily scarring of the lungs) are long term and may last for many years. If you experience any shortness of breath, tell your doctor immediately.

Nausea/Vomiting

This is the most common side effect related to chemotherapy. The nausea is due to the stimulation of an area in the brain known as the trigger zone (vomiting centre). Today doctors are using and testing much more potent anti-nausea drugs to combat the ghastly nausea and vomiting of chemotherapy which often leads to weight loss and malnutrition. Today's most common anti-nausea drugs are Zofran and dexamethasone (a steroid). According to doctors, Zofran has revolutionised chemotherapy. It may make you feel better while the drugs are being put into you but hours after treatment, the nausea generally returns with a vengeance.

There are also a number of side effects related to the use of these drugs and steroids including constipation, pimples, thrush, exhaustion, weight gain/loss, fluid retention, emotional instability and sleeplessness. Doctors will often prescribe milder anti-nausea drugs after treatment like Maxalon. There are a number of different brands of anti-nausea medications, all giving a Band-Aid effect and carrying their own side effects. Maxalon can make you feel like a zombie.

Reproductive System

The rapidly proliferating structures of the reproductive system are particularly sensitive to the actions of cancer drugs. Many women who are still experiencing menstrual periods will experience irregular menstruation during treatment. In some women, menstruation stops completely. If this happens, hot flushes may also occur. Men may have decreased sperm numbers and motility. Some drugs used ¦ cause temporary and sometimes permanent infertility.

Feeling tired or unwell during treatment may also decrease ability. I found my menstruation was perfect, both during an(believe this was due to a healthy, supportive diet rich in the appropriate supplements, herbs and natural therapies. Some combinations of chemotherapy drugs offer only a 30 per cent chance of fertility after treatment.

Weight Loss/Gain

Chemotherapy affects each person very differently. Some people may experience weight loss due to difficulty in swallowing or nausea, while others may experience weight gain due to the use of steroids in treatment.

Natural Treatments Used to Counteract the Side Effects of Chemotherapy

Broken Capillaries

Diet
- Eat foods rich in bioflavonoids including berries, cherries, buckwheat, citrus fruits, lemons, plums, grapefruit, blackberries, blackcurrants, green peppers, broccoli, tomatoes and apricots.

Vitamins and Nutrients
- Bioflavonoids increase the strength of capillaries, especially the bioflavonoid, rutin. They prevent rupture of the blood vessels and maintain collagen structure. Take vitamin C powder with bioflavonoids daily @ 1000 to 5000 mg of Vitamin C powder containing bioflavanoids including 500 mg of rutin.
- Bromelain accelerates the healing process of the skin. Take 250 to 750 mg per day.

Herbal Teas
- Rosehip herbal tea is rich in bioflavonoids.
- An excellent astringent for capillaries and veins is witch hazel – apply externally (distilled witch hazel can be purchased from a chemist).
- Horse chestnut increases the strength and tone of veins and capillaries and is an excellent circulatory tonic.

Constipation

Diet
- Drink 6 to 8 glasses of water per day.
- Eat a diet rich in fibre foods including whole grains, fruits and vegetables, nuts and seeds, and brown rice. Good foods include prunes, dates, figs, pears, sweet potatoes, brussel sprouts, cabbage, kale, apples, endive, dandelion greens, beets and okra.

Avoid spicy foods, full fat dairy products, fried foods, white flour products, processed foods, coffee, sugar and fats.

- A good formula to make up for breakfast is prunes, soaked overnight in water with 1 teaspoon of blackstrap molasses/1 teaspoon of oat bran/1 teaspoon agar-agar and ½ cup of natural acidophilus yogurt.
- A healthy breakfast cereal made from ½ part slippery elm, 1 part oatbran, 1 part lecithin granules, 1 part psyllium husks, 1 part LSA mix and ½ part crushed pumpkin seeds mixed together is a fantastic way to begin the day.

Vitamins and Nutrients

- Take a good fibre supplement containing psyllium husks, guar gum, apple pectin or modified citrus pectin, ricebran, soya bran or oatbran. Lactobacillus Acidophilus or fructo-oligosaccharides helps to put friendly bacteria into the bowel.
- Essential fatty acids or flaxseed oil is needed for good digestion and stool formation. (This is essential if stools are hard and dry.)
- Vitamin C (3 grams/day) and glutamine repairs intestines damaged by chemotherapy.

Herbs

- Aloe vera juice has a healing and cleansing effect on the digestive tract and aids in forming soft stools. Drink ½ cup in the morning and night. OR
- Mix – 1 teaspoon of senna leaves/cascara bark/fennel seeds/chamomile – infuse 1 cup or 1 tablespoon of flax seeds ground – swallow with a glass of hot water. OR
- Dandelion herbal tea is useful not only in alleviating constipation but also in enhancing kidney and liver function. OR
- Infuse 1 teaspoon of psyllium seeds in a cup of boiling water and drink twice daily. OR
- Use 1 dessertspoon of whole linseeds and boil in 600 ml of water for 25 minutes. Strain and mix with equal amounts of water and orange juice or lemon juice. OR
- Alfalfa tablets (3 to 5/day) may also prove useful.

Hydrotherapy

- Epsom salts (magnesium sulphate) baths help to stimulate bowel movements.

Cramps

Nutrients

- Muscle cramps are often caused from a magnesium deficiency. Take a good magnesium powder (600 – 2000 mg/day) in combination with calcium to alleviate cramping.
- Cramping can also be a result of sodium, chlorine or zinc deficiency. Vitamin B3 alleviates muscle cramps caused from poor blood circulation.
- Many forms of cramps respond well to vitamin E use. Take at least 450 IU per day.

Herbs

- Chamomile, ginger, lavender tincture and baths, or valerian may alleviate muscle cramps.

Hydrotherapy

- Epsom salts (magnesium sulphate) baths help to relieve cramps.

Depression

Diet

- A balanced, healthy diet is very important in preventing and alleviating depression. Avoid white flour products, caffeine, alcohol, tobacco, sugar and refined foods.

Vitamins and Nutrients

- Take 50 mg of zinc with vitamin B6 (50 mg) and magnesium (500 – 1000 mg/day).
- Take 800 – 1000 mg/day of glutamine.
- Other important nutrients include NAD (activated B3) or alpha keto gluterate for low energy levels.
- The amino acid tyrosine is excellent for depression related to stress.
- Phenylalanine is good for pain related depression.
- Take histidine for depression linked with anxiety.

Herbs

- Useful herbs include oats, lemon balm, passionflower, vervain, skullcap, basil and St John's wort. St John's wort at 1000 – 2000 mg/day is excellent for depression.
- In Wales, borage is known as the 'herb of gladness' – make this into a tea and drink twice daily, or chop plenty of borage into your salads.
- The herb damiana eases depression (steep 1 teaspoon of leaves in 1 cup of boiled water for 10 minutes. Strain and drink upon arising).

Lifestyle

- Exercise stimulates the production of powerful mood elevators such as endorphins and norepinephrine. In addition, stretching, yoga, tai chi, positive affirmations, meditation, swimming and playing games help to break the cycle of negative thinking that contributes to depression.

Diarrhoea

Diet

- Make sure you drink plenty of water, fruit and vegetable juices, and herbal teas to replace lost fluids and avoid dehydration. Drink the cleansing vegetable broth regularly (refer to recipes in Part Three of this book).
- Choose plain, bland foods and eat small frequent meals.
- Eat banana, pineapple or papaya juice, oatbran, ricebran, raw foods and yogurt.

- Avoid dairy products and coffee.
- Watermelon juice should be drunk regularly.

Vitamins and Nutrients
- Essential fatty acids aid in forming healthy stools. Eg DHA/EPA, flaxseed oil.
- Take acidophilus powder or capsules to replace friendly bacteria.
- Psyllium husk or a fibre formula may be beneficial.
- Glutamine repairs intestines damaged by chemotherapy. Take 1 to 4 gm per day.

Herbs
- Use cinnamon in tea (1 teaspoon per cup) or on food. OR
- Goldenseal, citrus seed extract, oregon grape, barberry root bark, pau d arco or raspberry leaves are useful. OR
- Slippery elm bark is soothing to the digestive tract. OR
- Charcoal tablets (4 tablets/hour with water until diarrhoea subsides).

Herbal Teas
- Try either chamomile, dandelion tea, peppermint, pau d'arco, papaya or raspberry leaf tea to ease diarrhoea.

Effects on the Mouth

Once again, diet is an important factor. Mouth ulcers, metallic taste in the mouth, a furry or coated tongue, sore throat and dry mouth are common symptoms experienced. Mouth ulcers are often caused from a zinc deficiency.

Diet
- Eat plenty of clear vegetable soups with brown rice. Use a food blender to blend foods. Avoid extremes of temperature and highly spiced foods.
- Avoid alcohol and cigarettes.
- Figs contain demulcents, which soothe the mouth, oesophagus and digestive tract.
- Suck on natural ice blocks or ice cubes made from fresh juice. Natural fruit sorbet helps to keep your mouth moist and feeling fresh.

Vitamins and Nutrients
- Glutamine helps to protect the body's mucosa and prevents mouth ulcers. Glutamine soothes and relieves the pain of and quickly heals sores in the mouth.
- Vitamin E reduces the occurrence of oral mucositis @ 250 iu to 500 iu/day.
- Zinc and L-lysine are useful in healing mouth ulcers. Take 4 ml of zinc liquid per day or an 80 mg zinc tablet or suck on zinc and L-lysine lozenges.
- B complex vitamins are essential in preventing mouth ulcers.

Herbs
- Add 5 to 10 drops of myrrh oil or myrrh tincture and add to a glass of water. Use as a mouthwash – good for healing mouth ulcers.

- Another powerful and useful herb for healing/preventing ulcers is red sage.
- Aloe vera juice is also very soothing and healing on mucous membranes. Drink ¼ cup morning and night.

Other Advice
- Brush teeth with a soft toothbrush. Use a small amount of bicarbonate soda/water after eating (¼ teaspoon in ½ glass of water).
- Use a natural lip balm or beeswax to keep lips moist.

Gastritis/Indigestion
Diet
- Eat a balanced, healthy diet rich in alkaline forming foods and low in acidic foods (refer to chapter 37, Acid/Alkaline Foods).
- Include in the diet fresh pineapple (which contains bromelain) and fresh paw paw (which contains papain). These are great sources of digestive enzymes.
- Add acidophilus yogurt to the diet.
- Try using brown rice or barley broth (Use 5 parts water to 1 part grain and boil mixture, uncovered for 10 minutes) Strain, cool the liquid and drink throughout the day.
- Avoid caffeine, carbonated beverages, fried foods, potato chips, snack foods, sugar and salty or spiced foods. Never eat if you are upset or over-tired.

Vitamins and Nutrients
- Glutamine helps to repair intestines damaged by chemotherapy.
- Bromelain acts as a proteolytic digestive enzyme, which helps with the absorption of nutrients from foods. It also has anti-inflammatory properties to help reduce inflammation.
- Acidophilus is necessary for normal digestion (½ hour before meals or as directed).
- Vitamin B complex plus extra vitamin B1 and B12 are essential for normal digestion.

Herbs
- Slippery Elm – take up to 5 grams of powdered bark in capsules, or mix with water, before meals.
- Anise seeds help to relieve a sour stomach – chew the whole seeds or grind and sprinkle on food.
- Other useful herbs include calamus, lemon balm and fennel.

Herbal Teas
- Meadowsweet, Marshmallow, Ginger, Parsley, Chamomile and Peppermint tea all ease indigestion or gastritis.

Hair Loss
Diet
- Eating a healthy, wholesome diet rich in fresh fruits and vegetables, fish, nuts and seeds, vegetable and fruit juices will help to maintain healthy circulation to the

head area. Eat foods rich in silica, folic acid and biotin, including brewers yeast, sunflower seeds, walnuts, oats, lentils, soybeans and brown rice.

Vitamins and Nutrients
- Folic acid (800 mcg/day) is very important.
- Co-enzyme Q10 up to 270 mg/day enhances oxygenation throughout the body.
- Lipoic acid is also beneficial.
- A good B complex vitamin supplement rich in vitamin B3, vitamin B5, vitamin B6, biotin and inositol is important for hair growth and health.
- Vitamin C (3000 to 5000 mg/day) aids in improving circulation to the scalp.
- Vitamin E and zinc are also very useful.
- L-cysteine and L-methionine may prevent hair from falling out.

Massage
- Regular head massage will aid in good blood circulation to the head.

Yoga
- Certain yoga poses will help to maintain good circulation to the head, particularly the shoulder stand and the headstand postures. A slant board does a similar job.

Note
- With certain types of chemotherapy drugs, it is impossible to prevent hair loss. The cytotoxic drugs are designed to kill rapidly dividing cells in the body. The hair has some of the fastest dividing cells. However, after chemotherapy, hair often grows back thicker, healthier and shinier.

Insomnia
Diet
- Avoid a high intake of tea, caffeine, alcohol, nicotine, sugar and white flour products.
- Foods that help to encourage a more restful sleep include lettuce, warm milk, thyme, honey, bananas and turkey.

Vitamins and Nutrients
- Take a good Calcium/Magnesium supplement before bed.
- If you have difficulty falling asleep tryptophan can be useful (this should be prescribed by a practitioner). Try taking a combination supplement that contains 75 to 150 mg of 5 HTP (5 Hydroxy tryptophan) on an empty stomach, one hour before bedtime.
- If you wake during the night and have difficulty going back to sleep a histidine formula is more suitable.
- If restless legs are keeping you awake, a folic acid or vitamin E deficiency may be the cause.

- If you have a burning sensation in the legs try a supplement with choline and vitamin B1 to help relieve the symptoms.
- A mineral deficiency of copper, iron or zinc can also cause insomnia.

Herbal Teas
- Some great herbal teas to promote a peaceful and relaxed sleep includes valerian, hops, passionflower, jamaican dogwood, catnip, kava kava, skullcap, wild lettuce and chamomile.
- Ground anise seed mixed with honey in warm milk is an age-old cure for insomnia in Germany and Russia.

Lifestyle
- Progressive muscle relaxation can help. Isolate each of your muscle groups, tense for a count of 5 and then relax for 15 to 20 seconds before moving on. You should slowly fall into a blissful dreamland with this relaxing exercise.

Kidney Damage
Diet
- To prevent kidney damage it is important to drink at least 8 to 10 glasses of pure water every day.
- Eat more foods that are beneficial to the kidneys such as watermelon, lemons, celery, cucumber, parsley, green leafy vegetables, cranberries, papaya, asparagus, watercress, garlic and soybeans.
- Reduce intake of chocolate, meat, table salt, tea, coffee, animal protein and dairy products.

Vitamins and Nutrients
- Vitamin B6 helps to reduce fluid retention at 50 mg/twice daily.
- Calcium, vitamin A, vitamin C and bioflavonoids (2000 – 6000 mg/day) are also useful.
- L-Arginine helps to reduce pressure in the kidneys and also helps to stimulate the body's immune system.
- L-methionine (as directed) improves kidney circulation.

Herbs
- Buchu tea, celery and parsley tea, dandelion root, uva ursi, marshmallow tea, red clover, watermelon seed tea (Place fresh watermelon seeds in a pot of water, bring to the boil and simmer for 10 minutes. Strain and drink.) and nettle tea all help good kidney function. Dandelion root protects the kidneys and the liver.

Lethargy/Tiredness
Diet
- Eat a wholesome diet rich in fresh fruits and vegetables, whole grains, nuts and seeds, and fresh fruit and vegetable juices diluted with water.

- Make sure you eat adequate protein, including deep water fish, nuts and seeds, legumes, cottage cheese/flaxseed oil mix, soybeans, organic chicken breast/thigh and grain-fed red meat. (no more than 3 times/week.)
- Add a protein supplement to your juice or smoothie or alternatively, try making a protein/energy shake.
- Avoid energy robbing foods like sugar, alcohol, fats, caffeine, white flour products and highly processed foods.
- Try to eat one fresh salad daily with a variety of different coloured vegetables. For extra energy, make up a salad dressing from organic flaxseed oil and pure apple cider vinegar.
- Try not to skip any meals and eat a wholesome breakfast that includes a protein source such as egg (no more than 3 to 4 a week), cottage cheese or fish. Porridge eaten in the morning provides a long-term source of energy.
- Energy boosting foods include bananas, grapes, cabbage, kelp, carrots, dates, figs, oatmeal, onions, peas, prunes, raisins, soybeans, cayenne pepper, spinach, borage and strawberries.

Vitamins and Nutrients
- It is recommended to ask your doctor for regular injections of vitamins, particularly B group vitamins such as B complex, vitamin B12 and vitamin C. This guarantees that your body is receiving adequate nutrients to produce energy. Alternatively, take a good B complex supplement rich in vitamin B1, B3, B5, B6 and choline.
- Check for vitamin B12, iron and folic acid deficiency.
- Check for any signs of Candida – if present, supplement with lactobacillus acidophilus and avoid yeast foods.
- It can be difficult to absorb nutrients as orthodox therapy tends to destroy the microvilli, digestive enzymes and hydrochloric acid. To improve absorption in the gut, take digestive enzymes and hydrochloric acid supplements with meals (if deficient). This increases absorption of nutrients, giving the body the correct nutrients to make energy.
- Bee pollen, a few granules daily for 3 days, often has a marked effect on energy levels.
- Free form amino acid complexes are great for improving energy levels.
- Spirulina, barley grass, wheatgrass or chlorella are great whole foods sources providing abundant energy-giving nutrients.
- Vitamin C and the amino acid tyrosine will aid energy levels by boosting adrenal gland function.
- Acetyl L Carnitine, alpha keto gluterate, lipoic acid and coenzyme Q10 (180 – 360 mg per day) are key nutrients in energy production in the mitochondria of the cell.
- Vitamin B3 in its active form, NAD (nicotinamide adenine dinucleotide) is extremely useful in boosting energy production.

Herbs
- Ginseng root, licorice root (do not take if you have high blood pressure), gingko biloba, damiana, yerba mate, star anise, cayenne pepper, oatseed and gotu kola leaf.

- A tea brewed from burdock root, dandelion and red clover promotes healing by cleansing the blood and enhancing immune system function (2 to 4 cups/day).

Note
- One of the most common causes of fatigue during chemotherapy is diminished absorption of nutrients in the gastro-intestinal tract. If your digestive system is only absorbing fifty per cent of nutrients, the body switches to survival process and puts its energy in maintaining vital body system functions rather than producing optimal energy.

  During cancer and cancer treatment, it is highly recommended to supplement with digestive enzymes (to increase absorption), apple cider vinegar (to maintain good hydrochloric acid levels in the stomach to absorb proteins that help to create energy) and try taking a supplement containing (aloe vera, fructo-oligosaccharides, glutamine, glucosamine, slippery elm and a soft, soluble fibre) to maintain the health of your microvilli in the bowel area. This guarantees optimal absorption of valuable vitamins and minerals from your diet allowing for improved energy production.
- Try to get regular exercise and go to bed early. Remember, the hours slept before midnight are twice as valuable as the hours slept after midnight.
- Detoxification of the liver is important. If the liver is congested with toxins and drugs, the body is unable to produce energy efficiently.

Loss of Appetite
Vitamins and Nutrients
- Free form amino acid supplements (3½ grams/day).
- Vitamin B complex increases the appetite and maintains energy levels.
- Check zinc levels – low zinc levels can cause a lack of taste and appetite. Zinc (80 mg/day) is recommended.
- Check for hydrochloric acid or digestive enzyme deficiency (commonly depleted during orthodox treatment). If levels are low, supplement with hydrochloric acid supplements or apple cider vinegar or digestive enzymes.
- Swedish bitters is also useful for stimulating the appetite.

Herbs
- To stimulate a poor appetite use fennel seed, centaury, ginger root, ginseng, papaya leaves or peppermint leaves.
- Calamus (also known as Sweet Flag), is an excellent tonic for the gastro-intestinal tract and a great appetite stimulant. Pour 1 cup of boiling water onto 1 to 2 teaspoons of the dried herbs/seeds and let infuse for 10 to 15 minutes. Drink 30 minutes before meals.
- Gentian root is an excellent bitter that stimulates the appetite and digestion via the gentle stimulation of digestive juices. Gentian combines well with ginger and cardamom. Put ½ teaspoon full of the shredded root in a cup of water and boil for 5 minutes. This should be drunk warm 15 to 30 minutes before meals.

Other Advice
- Gentle exercise can stimulate appetite.

Lung Damage
Diet
- Eat plenty of yellow, white and orange vegetables such as pumpkin, sweet potato, carrots, apricots, squash, garlic, radish, onions, ginger, cauliflower, bamboo shoots, lotus root, green leafy vegetables and onions.

Vitamins and Nutrients
- Coenzyme Q10 improves oxygenation (90 – 270 mg/day).
- Beta-carotene and vitamin A (50 000 IU/day), vitamin C and vitamin E. Silica is also useful.

Herbs
- Astragalus, Echinacea, pau d'arco, horsetail, mullein and myrrh are all very useful herbs for strengthening and protecting the lungs.

Lifestyle
- Practise deep breathing exercises daily to oxygenate and heal the lungs. Other useful exercises include yoga, tai chi, martial arts, chi gung, aerobic exercise and swimming.

Maintain Weight
Diet
- Try to eat nutrient-dense, protein-rich foods. Good sources of protein include fish (salmon, mackerel, sardines, tuna, halibut, cod), organic chicken breast/thigh or turkey, legumes, soy products, brown rice, organic/grain fed meats (red meat no more than 3 times/week) and nuts and seeds. Drink energy/protein drinks, fruit shakes and smoothies.
- Making vegetable soups with legumes, vegetables and a protein source is a great way to maintain weight and energy levels.
- To stimulate the appetite eat plenty of alfalfa sprouts – these miracle sprouts have long been proclaimed as an excellent appetite stimulant.

Vitamins and Nutrients
- Free form amino acid supplements (3½ grams/day) or protein powder.
- Vitamin B complex supplement is also very helpful.
- Malabsorption in the gastro-intestinal tract can cause rapid weight loss as nutrients are not being absorbed to maintain body mass. If lowered absorption is present, supplement with either digestive enzymes, bitters or hydrochloric acid supplements.

Nausea/Vomiting

Diet

- Try to eat small amounts of food often. Eat six small meals a day instead of three large ones. Take at least one bite of food each hour to keep food in your stomach. An empty or full stomach can cause discomfort.
- Avoid greasy, fatty or fried foods. Plain foods are better tolerated than spicy foods.
- Do not eat large amounts of food prior to treatment.
- Regular sips of cool, clear drinks are useful, especially if you don't feel like eating solid food. Drink plenty of liquids, especially energy-dense vegetable juices, fruit juices, ice cubes and soups.
- Fresh salads are easy to digest.
- Barley water is also useful.
- Try blending your meals into liquid form, warming and eating like soups.
- Treat yourself to your favourite healthy foods. Small meals eaten frequently will prevent nausea and maintain energy levels.

Beneficial Foods

- Ginger is great for nausea. You can chew on ginger or use it in your soups or cooking.
- Mustard seeds in cooking have also been used to decrease nausea.
- Olives helps to dry the mouth and minimise excess liquid that adds to stomach queasiness.
- Crackers or dry toast in the morning is helpful if you can't face a large meal.
- Eat fresh fruits such as papaya, pineapple, apples, grapefruit and watermelon if you feel queasy in the stomach.
- Try drinking water mixed with baking soda to ease nausea. This reportedly works by neutralising stomach acids. Alternatively, try a glass of water with a teaspoon of apple cider vinegar.

Vitamins and Nutrients

- Try supplements containing slippery elm, glutamine, glucosamine, fructo-oligosaccharides, acidophilus, citrus pectin, aloe vera and pysllium husk – take 1 teaspoon in water 3 to 4 times/day. These nutrients in combination provide quick relief from the dreaded nausea; they also help to protect and repair the gut lining and prevent diarrhoea and constipation.
- Take 120 mg of zinc and 50 mg of vitamin B6 per day

Herbs

- Ginger root (1 to 3 grams of the dried root per day) will decrease nausea.
- Cinnamon sticks and cardamom seeds (approximately 8 seeds) may alleviate nausea. Use a nut or coffee grinder, place mixture in a jar and use one teaspoon in boiling water.
- Goldenseal root (1 or 2 capsules 3 to 4 times/day – do not take for more than one week) is believed to ease nausea.

- Swedish Bitters formula (contains gentian, calamus, angelica, turmeric and many more) – 1 teaspoon in 60 ml of water, sipped over 20 minutes.
- Cloves taken as an infusion or take 1 to 2 drops of essential oil on food or clove powder sprinkled onto food.

Herbal Teas

- Ginger tea made with fresh grated ginger (1 teaspoon in boiling water) is very helpful in easing nausea.
- Other useful herbs include peppermint tea, meadowsweet tea, grapefruit (the tea is made from fresh grapefruit peel), peach tea, chamomile tea, raspberry leaf tea (600 ml of boiled water poured over 2 rounded teaspoons of dried raspberry leaves or chamomile leaves. Steep, strain and drink throughout the day.)

Homeopathics

- Ipecac is effective (prescribed by a homeopath).

Reproductive System Effects (to prevent infertility/sterility)

Diet

- Eat a healthy, natural diet rich in fresh fruits, vegetables, nuts and seeds, whole grains, adequate protein and fresh fruit and vegetable juices.
- Avoid alcohol, tea, cigarettes, fried foods, sugar, full fat dairy products, processed foods and caffeine.
- For males, increase intake of oysters and mussels (these contain high amounts of zinc) to protect the prostate and sperm. Onion juice and honey mixed together encourages the production of sperm in men.

Vitamins and Nutrients

- Selenium is very important (400 – 800 mcg/daily). Deficiency of selenium leads to reduced sperm count, linked to sterility in men and infertility in women. The best type of selenium can be obtained from your doctor in a liquid form, called Sodium Selenite.
- Vitamin C (2000 – 6000 mg/daily) is important in sperm production.
- Vitamin E (400 IU – 1000 IU/day) is required for balanced hormone production and to carry oxygen to the sex organs.
- Zinc (80 mg/day) is needed for healthy functioning of reproductive organs.
- A mineral supplement containing iodine, manganese, copper and zinc would be helpful.

Herbs

- For men – Siberian ginseng (100 mg three times/day before 4 p.m.). Astragalus protects the immune system and aids with sperm motility.
- For women – False unicorn root and vitex agnus castus in tincture (1 teaspoon 3 times/day) or royal jelly (1000 to 2000 mg/day). Other useful herbs for

hormonal balancing include licorice root, wild yam, dong quai, yarrow or sarsaparilla.

Thrush/Fungal Infections

Diet
- Eat natural, low fat acidophilus yogurt (good brands include Jalna or Hakea).
- Avoid sugar, refined carbohydrates, bread, yeast products, cola, processed foods and fried foods as fungi thrives on these, particularly sugar.

Vitamins and Nutrients
- Take a natural acidophilus or bio-bifidus powder 30 minutes before meals.
- Vitamin C with bioflavonoids (5000 mg/day), zinc (50 to 80 mg/day) and vitamin E (400 to 800 IU/day) all enhance immune system function.
- Vitamin B complex, plus extra vitamin B5 is needed for correctly balanced 'friendly bacteria' in the body.

Herbs
- Tea tree diluted with water, used as an enema. Add 5 drops of tea tree oil to a hot bath.
- Take 2 capsules of garlic, 3 times daily.
- Drink 3 cups of pau d'arco tea daily.
- Grapefruit seed extract is extremely useful.

Urinary Tract Infections (Cystitis)

Diet
- Drink at least 2 litres of pure, filtered water. Drink 1 glass of water every hour.
- Avoid white flour products, alcohol, carbonated drinks, chocolate, processed foods, caffeine, nicotine and sugar.
- Eat more watermelon juice, celery, cucumber, lemons and green leafy vegetables.

Vitamins and Nutrients
- It is important to support immune function as urinary tract infections occur more readily when the immune system is lowered. Vitamin C plus bioflavonoids (4000 to 5000 mg/day), acidophilus (as directed on label), calcium (1500 mg/day – reduces bladder irritability) and magnesium (750 – 1000 mg/day – aids in the stress response).
- Other useful nutrients include vitamin E (500 – 750 IU/day), zinc (50 mg/day), natural beta-carotene (15000 IU/day) and potassium.

Herbs
- Cranberry is the best herbal remedy for cystitis. Quality cranberry juice produces hippuric acid in the urine, which acidifies the urine and inhibits bacterial growth. Other components found in cranberry juice prevent bacteria from adhering to the

lining of the bladder. Drink 1 to 2 cups of cranberry juice daily. If pure cranberry juice is not available, cranberry capsules can be used.
- Other beneficial herbs include birch leaves, goldenseal (do not take for more than one week), cornsilk, marshmallow root, celery, buchu and couchgrass.

Lifestyle
- Slip into a hot bath and pour ¼ cup of pure apple cider vinegar into the bath. Alternatively, use garlic cloves in the bath.

For a further list of natural treatments for side effects, refer to Chapter 13 'Understanding Radiation Therapy'.

Table of Natural Remedies to Speed Up the Actions of and Reduce the Toxicity of Chemotherapy

Table 12.2

Nutrient, Herb or Food	Actions
Adenosine (200 to 300 mg/day)	Improves white blood cell production and recovery
Astragalus (3000 to 6000 mg/day)	Protects against the toxic effects of chemotherapy, protects the bone marrow, boosts immunity, strengthens and protects the lungs, boosts energy, helps the body to produce interferon
B complex vitamins	Enhance effects of chemotherapy, reduce the side effects of chemotherapy drugs, protects digestive system
Bromelain (300 mg x 4 capsules per day in divided doses)	Improves the effectiveness of chemotherapy drugs
Cabbage, cauliflower, brussel sprouts and broccoli	Contain potent cancer fighting nutrients
Calcium and vitamin D	Improves response to drugs that treat Hodgkin's disease, bone cancer and lung diseases
Cat's claw (Uncaria tomentosa)	Reduces the severity and side-effects of chemotherapy and radiation treatment
Co Enzyme Q10 (270 mg/day plus)	Maintains the health of cells, preserves white blood cells, improves oxygenation to cells and tissues. Oxygen saturated cancer cells find it difficult to survive.
Cysteine and N-acetyl cysteine	Amino acid which protects against the toxic side-effects of chemotherapy, protects against kidney and bladder damage, reduces nausea

Table 12.2 *continued*

Nutrient, Herb or Food	Actions
Echinacea	Increases white blood cell production
Fibre foods or supplements	Assist with elimination of toxins
Fish oils, omega-3 fatty acids, DHA/EPA	Improves the killing of cancer cells, reduces the side effects of many drugs, anti-inflammatory actions
Genistein	Improves the killing of tumour cells
Glutathione	Protects kidneys and liver against toxic effects of chemotherapy, decreases the side-effects associated with chemotherapy, particularly cisplatin
Glutamine (this is very important – take 1 to 4 grams per day)	Powerful amino acid that supports and enhances the effects of chemotherapy for the treatment of cancer, helps to reduces side effects associated with chemotherapy – in addition, the size of tumours may decrease by 45% compared to 25% without sufficient glutamine, protects mucous membranes and the gut lining to maintain healthy digestion
Lipoic acid (600 to 1200 mg per day)	Reduces drug resistance and the side effects of vincristine sulphate, cisplatin and boosts immunity
Maintain fluid intake	3 to 4 litres per day – chemotherapy causes dehydration and water helps to eliminate toxins
Niacin and nicotinamide	Enhances chemotherapy, triples the time that (activated B3) chemotherapy stays in the blood, increases anti-tumour activity of chemotherapy drugs, decreases toxicity of drugs
Pancreatic enzymes (take up to 18 tablets per day, in between meals in divided doses) For digestion, take 2 tablets with each meal	Remove blocking antigens from cancer cells, improve survival, decreases inflammation, improves gut absorption, preventing malnutrition, may increase survival time
Quercitin (500 mg – 1500 mg/day)	Anti-inflammatory, enhances chemotherapy treatment
SOD – Superoxidedismutase	Reduces side-effects and toxicity of chemotherapy
Selenium (400 mcg – 800 mcg/day. Ask your doctor for prescription sodium selenite. Take 2 to 4 drops/day or as prescribed).	Reduces tissue damage in ovarian cancer and metastic endometrial cancer, reduces the side effects of chemotherapy, protects reproductive organs

Table 12.2 *continued*

Nutrient, Herb or Food	Actions
Vitamin A and carotenes	Enhance the body's immune system, reduce the toxicity of chemotherapy, protect the lung and mucous membrane linings, enhances the effectiveness of chemotherapy drugs
Vitamin C (5 grams/day)	Increases survival time in melanoma patients, enhances effectiveness of drug treatment – people who are given vitamin C in adequate doses often only need half the normal amount of therapy, reduces side effects of chemotherapy, boosts white blood cell function and general immunity, helps to detoxify harmful substances from the body
Vitamin E (800 to 1600 IU/day) – begin this at least 2 weeks prior to treatment	Enhances inhibition of oestrogen dependent tumour growths, may prevent baldness associated with certain, chemotherapy drugs, reduces the side effects of chemotherapy, improves the effectiveness of chemotherapy drugs to prostate cancer and melanoma, reduces the occurrence of mouth ulcers
Vitamin K	Improves in killing tumour cells and enhances 4 out of 15 chemotherapy drugs

A Final Note

If you are concerned that vitamins might interfere with your conventional treatment, take your supplements eight to twelve hours after chemotherapy or six hours before chemotherapy. The above table includes a large number of different nutrients and herbs capable of reducing the toxicity of chemotherapy and also to increase the actions of chemotherapy. Many of these nutrients can be found in high quality combination supplements from your natural health practitioner or health food store.

Chapter 13

UNDERSTANDING RADIATION THERAPY

Radiation Therapy Explained

Radiation therapy, also known as radiotherapy, is a widely used method of orthodox cancer treatment. It is commonly employed as a modern treatment for persons afflicted with cancer, in an attempt to kill the malignant tissue that is involved with cancer. It can be used singularly, as the primary method of treatment, or it can be used prior or post surgery, or in conjunction with chemotherapy.

External beam therapy uses a complicated machine called a 'linear accelerator' to generate radioactive beams or rays, to damage and kill dividing cells.

Alternatively, a radioactive variant (isotope) of a common element, such as radium or iodine, can be implanted into or close to the cancerous tissue, or injected in. This type of internal treatment is called brachytherapy. It deals mainly with the problem site and therefore with one part of the body, usually where the tumour was first discovered.

Unlike surgery, radiation therapy does not involve an operation and removal of the part affected. It resembles chemotherapy in that it can damage tumour cells. Unfortunately damage to surrounding healthy tissue usually occurs, in particular to bone marrow and the mucosal lining of the gastrointestinal tract. Radiation acts at the cellular level, causing cell death. Radiation exerts its greatest effect on rapidly proliferating cells.

How Radiation Therapy Works

Radiation Therapy consists of an orderly arrangement of steps:

1. Planning
2. Treatment
3. Care and supervision during the course
4. Care and support of reactions and side-effects
5. Periodic review to check on progress

Radiotherapy uses a source of ionizing radiation, such as x-rays, gamma rays, radium or radioactive cobalt (Cobalt-60 or Iodine-131) delivered to the cancerous tissue to kill malignancies. The idea is to bombard the diseased tissue with radiation in the precise area that will destroy the tumour, and hopefully only cause minimal damage to surrounding tissues.

How Radiation Therapy is Given

Planning – In planning for radiation therapy, surface marks are drawn on the skin in red or purple so that the beam of radiation can be aimed at the tumour. These marks are miniature tattoos that are left on throughout the course of the treatment and may take a long time to disappear after treatment. Measurements are taken and doses calculated through diagnostic x-ray exposures with metallic markers. A prescription is then written for the radiographer to follow with treatment.

Treatment – The application of radiotherapy is painless and rapid (often only 30 seconds in length). The linear accelerator (most commonly used x-ray generator) is activated as all operators leave the room. The patient must lie perfectly still to ensure the radiation hits the correct area. Treatment is required several times and usually given daily for a period of three weeks or more. Alternatively, a radioactive variant can be inserted into the body, or injected. An example of this is the insertion of a radioactive element into the vagina for forty-eight hours to kill any cancerous cells.

Care and Supervision – It is recommended that the person receiving radiation therapy should see the doctor and radiographer every week, to check on side effects and results of treatment. Blood tests are taken regularly to monitor blood cell counts, as with chemotherapy.

Why Radiation Therapy is Given

Radiation therapy is commonly used before scheduled surgery to shrink tumours to more operable sizes. It is also used after surgery, to ensure removal of any remaining cancerous tissue and to prevent the onset of further cancerous growths in the future. It is also employed as a method of removing and shrinking small tumours present in the body. Some particular types of cancer respond better to radiation therapy rather than chemotherapy or other cancer drugs.

Radiation Therapy and Pain

The actual session of radiation therapy is not painful. It is the side effects and reactions from radiation therapy that can cause associated discomfort, illness and pain. The most noticeable side effects are nausea, vomiting and damage/scarring/burning to tissues. The side effects depend largely on which area of the body is being zapped.

It is important to maintain a good diet, rich in supporting and selective nutrients to ensure that only limited reactions and side effects occur. Radiotherapy can also be very invasive to your body and therefore may cause many emotional reactions.

Continuing Your Normal Life During Radiation Therapy

Continuing your normal life during radiation therapy is totally dependent on your lifestyle and work requirements. It is advisable to take time out for yourself and relax totally during this period. Lassitude or lack of energy is a major side effect of radiotherapy, so you will definitely feel more tired than usual. The energy drop is very cumulative, tending to get worse over time. Your body requires as much support as possible to ensure rapid healing, so try not to do too much. Concentrate this time in your life for healing your body. The more rest you receive, the quicker your body will heal.

Side Effects of Radiation Therapy

Reaction to radiation therapy varies from patient to patient. Symptoms can range from lassitude (lack of energy), to decreased appetite, nausea, neuropathy (numbness or tingling), vomiting and temporary hair loss (if radiation is given to the head). Later reactions include inflammation due to cellular damage and symptoms vary according to the site being treated. For example, you may experience a sore throat or mouth if this area is being treated, or diarrhoea if the abdomen is being treated.

The major side effect of radiation therapy is scarring. This is a severe reaction and is unforeseeable, as doctors still do not fully understand differences in individual's tolerance levels. Sterility is possible if the testicles or ovaries are being treated. Cancer induction is also possible, as radiation is another type of carcinogenic substance being exposed to the body. Deformity may be another risk.

Radiotherapy can cause internal bleeding and often destroys the microvilli (minute projections from the intestinal wall that are the primary site of absorption) for up to two years. It often produces toxicity and free radicals, weakens the body's immune system, reduces white blood cell count and disrupts the body's sodium/potassium ratio, leading to fluid retention.

Natural Treatments to Counteract the Side Effects of Radiation Therapy

Burning and Scarring

Diet
- Eat foods rich in vitamin E, B complex, beta-carotene, essential fatty acids, zinc and germanium.
- Eat plenty of fish (salmon, sardines, tuna, cod and mackerel), tomatoes, sun-dried tomatoes, salt-free tomato paste and powder, berries, whole grains, green leafy vegetables, grains, wholesome soups and nuts and seeds.

Vitamins and Nutrients
- Superoxide dismutase, or SOD, administered by injection improves the condition of tissues that have been hardened by radiation therapy.

- Lycopene in large doses helps to protect against scarring and burning. Take double of the recommended dosage, at least 3 to 4 weeks before radiotherapy treatment.
- Vitamin A (50000 IU/day) is needed for tissue repair and mucous membrane protection, or 30 to 60 mg/day of beta-carotene or a carotenoid complex containing alpha-carotene and beta-carotene aids.
- Vitamin E at 600 to 1600 IU/day is needed for healing and to prevent scarring.

Herbs
- Calendula (marigold) successfully treats the damage caused to skin by radiation therapy or exposure. (Calendula ointment applied topically heals wounds smoothly, quickly and perfectly.)
- Aloe vera juice protects against skin injury, helps to prevent burning/scarring and soothes burns.
- Use vitamin E oil externally and internally (break open a Vitamin E capsule and apply directly to the affected area).

Damage to Cells
Diet
- Alkylglycerols (found in shark liver oil) counteract the decrease in white blood cells that occur as a result of radiation treatment.
- Asian mushrooms such as reishi, shitake, maitake and ganoderma all protect and enhance the production of healthy cells.

Vitamins and Nutrients
- Lipoic acid increases white blood cell production.

Herbs
- European mistletoe facilitates the regrowth of red blood cells after radiotherapy.
- Echinacea helps to improve function and production of white blood cells.
- Garlic causes decreased loss of white blood cells.
- Ginseng stimulates resistance and boosts the immune system, improving the function of white blood cells.

Decreased Appetite

Decreased appetite can be due to the killing of the microvilli in the bowel, nutrient deficiencies, stress, anxiety, nausea or vomiting. It is important to address these symptoms first to help improve your desire to eat. Try to keep eating to maintain constant energy levels and to support your body's healing process.

Vitamins and Nutrients
- To increase appetite use free form amino acid supplements (3½ grams/day).
- Vitamin B complex increases the appetite and maintains energy levels.
- Check zinc levels – low zinc levels can cause lack of taste and appetite. If zinc levels are low take zinc at 80 mg a day plus.

Herbs

- To stimulate a poor appetite use fennel seed, ginger root, ginseng, alfalfa, papaya leaves or peppermint leaves. These can all be made into herbal teas. Alfalfa sprouts assist in stimulating the appetite.

Fluid Retention

Diet

- Eat potassium-rich foods. Avoid salt, processed foods, fried foods and salted foods, as these cause the body to retain fluid. Use sea salt or Herbamere as an alternative to table salt.
- Good foods to remove fluid build up include watermelon, celery, cucumber, lemon juice, lettuce and green vegetables.
- Drink plenty of pure fresh water, at least 8 glasses of pure water daily.

Vitamins and Nutrients

- A potassium supplement aids fluid retention.
- Vitamin B6 at 100 mg/day can help to eliminate excess fluids from the body.
- The celloid SS (sodium sulphate) also helps in fluid removal. Eat a diet rich in potassium foods. Avoid salt, fried foods and processed foods, as these cause the body to retain fluids.

Herbs

- Good herbs include bucchu, juniper, dandelion and cornsilk. These herbs may be taken as herbal teas. I found dandelion tea one of the best teas for removing excess fluid from the body.

Impotence

In 80 per cent of cases, impotence is caused by reduced blood supply to the penis due to narrowing of blood vessels in the penis area.

Vitamins and Nutrients

- The amino acid, glutamine may alleviate impotence.
- Vitamin E is very useful.
- Phosphorous deficiency can be an underlying cause of male impotence.

Herbs and Foods

- Celery seeds (added to water and applied as a wash before intercourse) can stimulate a full erection.
- Tribulus, an Ayurvedic herb, is renowned for alleviating impotence.
- Damiana, sarsparilla and ginseng are believed to assist with impotence.
- Yohimbe alleviates impotence (scientific research – yohimbe alleviated male impotence in 62% of males whose impotence was due to physical malfunctions and in 42% of males whose impotence was due to psychological reasons. Use 6 mg/day over 10 weeks). (Hyperhealth, 1995)

Internal Bleeding

Vitamins and Nutrients

- Rutin, a bioflavonoid found in buckwheat, prevents excessive bleeding.
- Vitamin K assists with blood clotting.
- Glutamine can prevent damage to the microvilli and intestines.

Lethargy

This is largely caused from the killing of the microvilli in the intestines. Microvilli are needed to absorb nutrients from food. If these are destroyed, no nutrition is being gained from food and the body is unable to create natural cellular energy as normal.

Diet

- Eat a wholesome diet rich in fruits and vegetables, whole grains, nuts and seeds, and fresh vegetable and fruit juices.
- Make sure you eat adequate protein, including deep water fish, nuts, legumes, cottage cheese, soybeans, seeds, chicken breast and red meat (no more than 3 times per week).
- Add a protein supplement to your juice or smoothie, or try making a protein/energy shake.
- Energy boosting foods include borage, grapes, nuts, cayenne pepper, figs, honey and kelp, bananas, cabbage, carrots, dates, oatmeal, onion, peas, prunes, raisins, soybeans, spinach, borage and strawberries.
- Try to eat one fresh salad daily with a variety of different coloured vegetables. For extra energy make up a salad dressing from organic flaxseed oil and pure apple cider vinegar.
- Try not to skip meals. If you are feeling nauseous, try pureeing your foods in a blender.
- Eat a wholesome breakfast that includes a protein source such as an egg (no more than 3–4 a week), cottage cheese or fish. Porridge is a long-term source of energy.
- Avoid energy-robbing foods like sugar, alcohol, fats, caffeine, white flour products and highly processed foods.

Vitamins and Nutrients

- It is recommended to ask your doctor for regular injections of vitamins, particularly B group vitamins such as B complex, vitamin B12 and vitamin C. This guarantees your body is receiving adequate nutrients to produce energy. Alternatively, take a good B complex vitamin supplement, rich in B1, B3, B5, B6 and choline.
- Check for vitamin B12, iron and folic acid deficiency.
- Check for any signs of Candida – if present, supplement with lactobacillus acidophilus and avoid yeast foods.
- It is difficult to absorb vitamins because the microvilli are easily destroyed during radiation treatment. To improve absorption in the gut, take digestive enzymes and

hydrochloric acid (if a deficiency is present). This increases absorption of vitamins and minerals, allowing the body the correct nutrients to make energy.

- Vitamin B3 in its active form, (NAD) assists with energy production.
- Vitamin C and the amino acid, tyrosine improves adrenal gland function.
- Coenzyme Q10 (up to 270 mg/day during treatment) improves energy levels dramatically.
- Acetyl L Carnitine is a powerful energy stimulant, as is alpha keto gluterate
- Bee pollen, a few granules daily for 3 days, often has a marked effect on energy levels.
- Free form amino acid complexes are great for improving energy levels.
- Spirulina, barley greens, wheatgrass and chlorella are great whole food sources for providing energy.

Herbs
- Ginseng root, licorice (do not take if you have high blood pressure), gingko biloba, damiana, yerba mate, oatseed, star anise, peppermint, cayenne and gotu kola are all useful herbs for enhancing energy levels. Try to take in herbal tea form or as tinctures.
- A herbal tea made from burdock root, dandelion root and red clover promotes healing by cleansing the blood and enhancing immune system function.

Nausea/Vomiting

Nausea and vomiting are the major side effects of radiation therapy, especially if the area being treated is around the abdomen. Doctors give anti-nausea drugs like Maxalon or Zocor, but these tend to create their own nasty and energy-zapping side effects. Often nausea is caused by the body's liver trying to degrade carcinogenic substances and toxins left over from the radiation therapy.

Diet
- Try to eat small amounts of food often. Eat six small meals a day instead of three large ones. Take at least one bite of food each hour to keep food in your stomach. An empty or full stomach can cause discomfort.
- Avoid greasy, fatty or fried foods. Plain foods are better tolerated than spicy foods. Do not eat large amounts of food prior to treatment.
- Regular sips of cool, clear drinks are useful, especially if you don't feel like solid food. Drink plenty of liquids especially energy-dense vegetable juices, fruit juices, ice cubes and soups.
- Fresh salads are easy to digest.
- Barley water is also useful. Try drinking water mixed with baking soda to ease nausea. This reportedly works by neutralising stomach acids.
- Try blending your meals into a liquid form, warming and eating like soups.

Beneficial Foods
- Ginger is great for nausea. You can chew on ginger or use it in your soups or cooking.

- Mustard seeds in cooking are also useful.
- Olives help to dry the mouth and minimise excess liquid that adds to stomach queasiness.
- Crackers or dry toast in the morning is helpful if you can't face a large meal.
- Eat fresh fruits such as papaya, pineapple, apples, grapefruit, and watermelon if you feel queasy in the stomach.

Herbs
- Cinnamon sticks and cardamom seeds (about 8 seeds) are great. Use a nut or coffee grinder, place mixture in a jar and use one teaspoon in boiling water.
- Goldenseal root (1 or 2 capsules 3 to 4 times/day) is useful. Do not take for more than one week.
- Bitters formula (contains gentian, calamus, angelica, turmeric) – 1 teaspoon in 60 ml of water, sipped over 20 minutes aids nausea.
- Cloves taken as an infusion or take 1 to 2 drops of essential oil on food or clove powder sprinkled onto food.

Herbal Teas
- There are many useful herbal teas. Ginger tea made with fresh grated ginger (1 teaspoon in boiling water) is very helpful. Other useful teas include peppermint tea, meadowsweet tea, chamomile tea, grapefruit tea (made from fresh grapefruit peel), peach tea and raspberry leaf tea (600 ml of boiled water poured over 2 rounded teaspoons of dried raspberry or chamomile leaves. Steep, strain and drink throughout the day.)

Vitamins and Nutrients
- Supplements containing slippery elm, glutamine, glucosamine, fructo-oligosaccharides, modified citrus pectin, aloe vera and pysllium husk) – take 1 teaspoon in water 3 to 4 times/day. These nutrients in combination provide quick relief from the dreaded nausea; it also helps to protect and repair the gut lining and prevents diarrhoea and constipation.

Homeopathics – Ipecac is effective.

Neuropathy (numbness and tingling)

This is a common side effect which is basically caused by poor peripheral circulation and if neuritis is involved, inflammation to a nerve. The symptoms experienced are numbness and tingling, normally in the extremities. Another similar symptom is pain in the palms of the hands and soles of the feet.

Vitamins and Nutrients
- This condition is primarily a sign of severe vitamin B6 deficiency. Adequate Vitamin B6 will reduce any pain in the palms and soles of the feet (at least 100 mg per day). Do not exceed 500 mg per day.
- Vitamin B3 is believed to alleviate symptoms.

- Inositol improves the function of the sensory nerves adding relief.
- Vitamin B5 is useful with neuritis (inflammation to a nerve).

Reproductive System Effects (to prevent infertility/sterility)

Diet
- Eat a healthy wholefoods diet rich in fruits, vegetables, adequate protein, sprouts, whole grains, nuts and seeds and fresh vegetable and fruit juices.
- Avoid nicotine, caffeine, alcohol, sugar, processed foods and fried foods – these are all harmful to the body's sex glands.
- For men, increase intake of oysters and mussels (these contain high amounts of zinc) to protect the prostate and sperm. Onion juice and honey mixed together encourages the production of sperm in men.

Vitamins and Nutrients
- Selenium is important at (400 – 800 mcg/daily). Sodium Selenite drops can be obtained from a chemist on prescription from your doctor. Deficiency of selenium leads to reduced sperm count and is linked to sterility in men and infertility in women.
- Vitamin C (2000 – 6000mg/day) is important in sperm production.
- Vitamin E (400 IU – 1000 IU/day) is needed for balanced hormone production and carries oxygen to the reproductive organs.
- Zinc at 80mg/day helps with the functioning of reproductive organs.

Herbs
- For men – Siberian ginseng (100 mg 3 times/day before 4 p.m.). Astragalus protects the immune system and aids with sperm motility.
- For women – false unicorn root and vitex in tincture (1 teaspoon 3 times/day) or royal jelly (1000 to 2000 mg/day) is helpful. Other good herbs include licorice root, dong quai, yarrow, blessed thistle and sarsaparilla.

Toxicity

Diet
- Chlorophyll inhibits the toxic effects of radiation therapy.
- Cabbage has a protective effect against the toxicity of radiation and helps to detoxify the body, due to its high indole content.
- Kelp acts as a chelating agent and protects against the toxic effects of radiation.
- Consume avocados, lemons and safflower, linseed and olive oil. Miso paste and soy sauce/tamari/shoyu protect against the toxic effects of radiation therapy.

Vitamins and Nutrients
- Glutathione, beta-carotene and vitamin E protects against the toxic effects of radiotherapy.

- Alkylglycerols (fatty acids) when consumed prior to the commencement of radio-therapy prevent some of the toxic effects of radiotherapy.
- Vitamin A (35 000 to 60 000 IU/day) minimises the toxic effects of radiation therapy.
- Coenzyme Q10 protects against the toxic effects at 90 to 270 mg/day.
- Vitamin B5 protects against radiation (200 mg before and after exposure) and B-complex vitamins.

Herbs
- Garlic supplementation limits the toxic effects of radiation therapy.
- Kampo (Juzen-taiho-to) a Chinese herb, decreases the toxicity associated with chemotherapy and radiotherapy.
- Astragalus and cat's claw are believed to protect against radiation damage and toxicity.

For a further list of natural treatments for side effects, refer to Chapter 12 'Under-standing Chemotherapy'.

Table of Natural Remedies to Speed up the Actions of Radiation Therapy

Certain vitamins, minerals and enzymes when used in conjunction with a whole foods diet can enhance the actions of radiation therapy, causing tumours to shrink much faster. Below is a table of helpful recommendations:

Table 13.1

Vitamin and Nutrient	Actions
Bioflavonoids	Reduce the side effects of radiation
Cat's claw (unicaria tomentosa)	Cat's claw is believed to reduce the severity and side-effects of radiation treatment
Chinese herbal teas	Are believed to increase the actions of radiation therapy by 40%
Coenzyme Q10	Improves oxygenation to cells and tissues. Oxygen saturated cancer cells find it difficult to survive. Co-Enzyme Q10 is a free radical scavenger and antioxidant – helps to regulate mitochondrial function.
Fish oils, omega 3 fatty acids, DHA/EPA	Improves the killing of cancer cells, prevents toxicity and side effects of radiation treatment.
Glutamine	Helps to support and speed up the actions of radiotherapy

Table 13.1

Vitamin and Nutrient	Actions
Histidine	Reduces the side effects of radiation
Lycopene (VERY IMPORTANT)	A carotenoid that protects proteins, DNA, cell membranes and low density lipoproteins from oxidation – overall it improves intercellular communication and individual cell cycles of growth, differentiation, migration and apoptosis, helps to prevent scarring and burning of the skin (must be started at least 3 weeks before treatment)
Medicinal mushrooms – e.g. shitake, reishi, maitake, ganoderma, cordyceps	Boost immune system function and are believed to relieve many of the side effects related to radiation therapy
Methionine	Reduces the side effects of radiation, protects and cleanses the liver
Niacin and nicotinamide (vitamin B3, NAD)	Improves the effectiveness of radiation treatment against tumours, reduces many of the side effects of radiation therapy
Selenium, magnesium	Reduces the side effects of radiation
SOD (Superoxidase Dismutase)	Reduces the side effects of radiation
Vitamin A and carotenes	Strong antioxidants which reduce the toxicity of radiation therapy, protects the mucous membrane linings throughout the body preventing burning and scarring
Vitamin B5, B6 and B-complex	Reduces the side effects of radiation, boosts energy
Vitamin C	People who are given vitamin C in adequate doses often only need half the normal amount of therapy, boosts energy levels, improves the efficiency of white blood cells, boosts immunity
Vitamin E	Extremely healing and protective for tissues

Ginseng, cysteine, vitamin C, vitamin E, glutamine, lycopene, SOD (superoxide dismutase) and the herbs cat's claw and Astragalus reduce and counteract the side effects of radiation therapy. Seaweed acts as a chelating agent and protects against the harmful effects of radiation by binding with the radioactive elements and then excreting these from the body.

A wholesome, natural diet rich in potassium foods also enables patients to tolerate radiation therapy much better. It is important to eat more broccoli, brussel sprouts, cabbage, cauliflower, kale, carrots, spinach, apricots, bananas, apples, brown rice, wholegrains, seeds, yogurt, apples, soy beans, tofu, tamari, miso and seaweed.

For a further list of nutrients and dosage amounts refer to Chapter 12 'Understanding Chemotherapy'.

Chapter 14

TRANSFORM YOUR HOSPITAL ENVIRONMENT

How many people dread the thought of spending time in hospital? I'm sure the majority of the population falls into this category. Unfortunately, we are not all born superhuman and there may be times in life where a visit to the hospital is unavoidable. If you do find yourself flat on your back in a hospital bed, there are ways you can make the most of this trying situation.

When we think of hospitals many of us envision an environment of white, chilly rooms, overworked medical staff and an aroma of clinical smells drifting through the hallways. It can be nerve-wracking enough having to spend time in a strange room with strange people doing foreign things to your body without having to think of the depressing environment surrounding your being.

Hospitals should be a place where people are inspired to heal in an environment of relaxing and healing colours, uplifting and soothing tunes, medical professionals with a desire to work WITH the patient, cheerful staff and an abundance of rejuvenating foods. Realistically, there are still very few hospitals that have attained this goal. Some private hospitals are slowly realising the benefits of a positive environment and are adapting methods to attain healing and inspirational surroundings. Many public hospitals are still far off the mark, although a few are slowly adapting.

I know many patients dislike the clinical smells drifting through hospital wards, such as disinfectant. Both patients and staff could derive great benefits from the simple addition of calming and healing aromatherapy oils. They would feel a greater sense of relaxation and positivity, two key elements in the healing process.

Some doctors in hospitals look at you with a superior, closed-minded attitude and often follow the old school of medicine. This air of superiority often comes when a doctor spends all day relating to people who have given up their personal power, lying flat on their backs, looking helplessly up. Many doctors fail to recognise the healing potential contained within each individual and the benefits of utilising alternative and natural therapies to stimulate the patients own natural healing responses.

How open-minded can most doctors be concerning the benefits of nutrition in healing, when they receive only a few months of nutritional training in a six year university study? I know of too many doctors who fail to work with the individual to generate their natural healing powers or fail to explain everything in detail, including side effects and possible complications, length of treatment and use of other dangerous medications.

If you are lucky enough to have been guided in the right direction towards a doctor who is open-minded, accepting and empathetic to your needs, you will no doubt experience a faster recovery and a less traumatic illness. If you are given a doctor with a self-righteous attitude who you feel vibrates very differently from your nature, seek another doctor. Believe me, it will never work, as these types of doctors will work against you, not with you and inevitably this may cause you to experience a longer recovery time. Find a medical professional that understands you and emanates natural empathy to your condition.

How to Create a Healing Hospital Environment

It is too easy for your individuality and personal worth to be lost amid the hospital routine, in the hospital organisation, by the processing of patients day after day, year after year. Some of the hospital staff are trying to do their best in a daunting situation. To expect them to change at this stage is unrealistic. So how do you deal with a hospital environment that places you in a sick, weak and helpless role?

If you do find yourself in a hospital atmosphere which is drab and dull, you can take personal responsibility by uplifting the atmosphere in your own room. There are a number of simple ways you can do this. The following are some great examples of how to decrease your hospital stay, speed up your recovery time and how to uplift your hospital surroundings.

The Beauty of Colour

Colours in their essence are healing and contain within each of their individual aspects a different healing vibration. Colours have the ability to transform emotions and provoke positive feelings and thoughts. Colour can be incorporated into your environment easily with the addition of flowers, colourful pyjamas and nightwear, brightly coloured silk scarves, paintings and artwork, and anything precious and colourful which you cherish from your home.

It would be great if nurse's uniforms were brighter and livelier, instead of the sickly pale blue, pink and white we see nurses wearing. This leaves many people with an empty and cold feeling, not very conducive to healing. Red, green and violet are considered the most ideal colours for cancer-healing. Each colour has the ability to stimulate a different healing potential. So surround yourself in beautiful, lively colours and feel the vibrations of joy and healing radiating from every magnificent colour in your hospital room. (Refer to Chapter 32 – 'Rays of Light' for a full discussion of colours and their healing effects)

Melodious Music

Classical music is believed to benefit healing and shorten the stays of hospitalised patients. Music enhances physical, emotional and biological functions. Music and other sounds pleasant to our ears contain powerful immune stimulating qualities. Take in your own CD player or tape recorder and play your favourite music and sounds. It is highly beneficial to listen to relaxing music before your operation, to calm the mind and body and bring about a sense of peace and relaxation. There are a wide variety of relaxing and inspirational tapes and CDs readily available in stores today. (Refer to Chapter 30 – Good Vibrations for more details about music).

Ancient Aromas

Smells have been used for centuries throughout ancient civilisations, to alter mental, physical and spiritual health. Aromatherapy uses essential oils obtained directly from flowers and plants to uplift the spirit and increase well-being and health. Specific oils promote different healing responses and alter the emotions and spirit in unique ways. It is a good idea to bring an oil burner into the hospital and burn four or five drops of essential oil in water with a candle oil burner, or simply use an electric oil burner that doesn't require water. Likewise, essential oils can be applied directly to the skin to enhance emotions or promote healing. Place a couple of drops on the skin with a good carrier oil. If you are having trouble sleeping, place two drops of lavender oil directly on your pillow. Other useful aromatherapy oils to use in hospital include:

- arnica – excellent for bruising;
- bergamot – uplifts the spirit, great for depression and enhances creativity;
- calendula – great for cuts, wounds and healing;
- clary sage – one of the best oils for post-operation depression;
- eucalyptus – great for colds, clearing of the chest and head if congested, and for sinus problems;
- fennel – great for indigestion, nausea and vomiting;
- lavender – relaxes the body, calms the nervous system, excellent for insomnia and great for burns if applied directly;
- peppermint – great for nausea, vomiting and provides a sedating effect;
- tea tree – a great antiseptic and disinfectant, good for cuts, tinea and fungal infections.

Food for Life

The typical hospital food is often devitalised, lifeless and lacking in life-giving nutrients. Dieticians in hospitals follow their education, providing for patients a diet that falls into the 'balanced food chart' category. Often the food served in hospitals is a combination of overcooked vegetables, red meats filled with antibiotics, jelly, sugar-filled cordials, frozen fish, white processed bread, margarine, full-fat dairy products and sugary desserts. How is a person meant to heal rapidly and efficiently on such a devitalised diet, lacking in healing life-giving nutrients? The lack of quality in hospital food that is given to patients never ceases to amaze me.

I suggest asking friends and family to bring in salads, wholemeal bread, grilled ocean fish, fresh fruits and vegetables, herbal tea bags and your own juicer. If you wish to speed up your recovery, a healthy nutrient packed diet is the major key! Don't forget the benefit of balanced nutritional supplements to add extra impact to your healing potential.

Healthy Connections

As human beings we are social creatures by nature, as well as solitary beings. We thrive on fulfilling relationships and connections with other beings including humans, plants and animals. If we are isolated and cut off from others, we tend to lose our vitality. Try to consciously open yourself to other people and express how you are really feeling – that is, if you are ready for this. Establish healthy relationships while in the hospital with other patients, staff and friends who visit you. Many nurses are wonderful listeners and caring souls who are willing to listen to your thoughts and feelings.

Don't block yourself off from the nurturing energy of human compassion and understanding. Often we try not to upset loved ones by expressing negative feelings while in hospital. I recommend the opposite. Your loved ones are most likely in a stronger position than you at the moment – let them carry some of your emotional burden. Recovery is faster if you are given a chance to express your fears and apprehensions. Get them off your chest; this is the initial step to healing. Surround yourself with caring souls who are there to encourage your healing. Remove any people who may hinder your recovery to perfect health.

Many hospitals and aged care homes are now allowing 'special dogs' with calm temperaments to enter them. What a wonderful idea, as dogs are unconditionally loving creatures with the ability to bring new life, love and nurturing into people's lives. They give a person who is ill something to look forward to and a new ray of inspiration to increase one's fighting spirit. If we have something wonderful to live for, our mind is taken away from the possibility of dying and driven towards the hope and desire of living.

Television Trauma

Television can be a great distraction. It is often placed in hospitals as a form of entertainment. It can be useful in distracting the mind from thinking about your present illness, as the attention is taken away from your physical body, slightly decreasing the pain and physical suffering. However, it also limits you from exploring the deeper purpose and cause of your cancer or other illness, which can be easily accomplished without distractions. Having cancer is an opportunity to resolve inner conflicts, emotional trauma and fears and requires attention to be able to resolve these issues and beat your cancer.

Television decreases the body's full breathing cycle and places the nervous system in a constant state of fear, excitement, anger and other jittery emotions. These feelings are fine if experienced naturally, but if overstimulated through television drama and suspense they tend to interfere with normal digestive and immune functions. Television often has a negative influence on recovery time. If you plan to watch television while in hospital, watch programs that make you laugh, add sunshine to your day and make you feel much more positive.

Drawing

Drawing pictures while in hospital is another wonderful, simple and inexpensive tool to alter your destiny in life. Drawing can be done by anyone, even people who feel that they are unable to draw. It is especially a wonderful tool for children. To create the outcome that you desire, try to draw pictures of yourself healthy and cancer-free. Alternatively, draw pictures of the white blood cells in your body defeating the cancer cells. Creating visual images of this outcome sends signals to your subconscious mind which leaves a positive imprint to set up the pathway to better health and happiness.

Breathing Exercises

Breathing exercises are great for increasing healing and directing energy to the area of the body that needs attention. A simple breathing exercise to enhance healing is as follows:

Become aware of your own breathing, of every breath in and every breath out. Try to slow your breathing down. Be aware of the air flowing through your nasal passages and into and out of your chest. Breathe only through the nose. Concentrate on slowing your breath down and taking deeper breaths each time. Don't think of anything else but your breathing.

This is such a simple exercise, yet very effective in relaxing the mind and improving oxygenation throughout the body to increase healing. If your room has windows that can be opened, then do just that; allow some fresh clean air to enter your room and fill your lungs. Unfortunately, many hospitals use air conditioners that can dehydrate you and rob you of the full benefits of clean fresh air.

Guided Fantasy

Guided fantasy is a great exercise to do while in hospital. You can memorise the following exercise yourself, or ask a friend or loved one to read it out to you. Positive and creative imagery are essential to healing, as the mind and body are eternally and electrically linked. By imprinting a positive outcome on your mind, you set up the path to a positive outcome in the body and soul.

Close your eyes. If your room is very light, place a beautiful coloured cloth or piece of material over your eyes. Visualise your breathing process – let it be free, let your breath come and go as it wants. Imagine your body becoming more and more relaxed with each exhalation.

Wiggle your body, and then stretch your toes and fingers. Yawn and stretch your entire body, then relax completely. Let your breathing become increasingly relaxed.

Imagine now, that you are lying outside on a sunny day. You are alone, the air is fresh and pure, and the sky is perfect aqua blue. The sun is warm on your skin. You feel relaxed and content. The grass around you is so green. You feel the coolness of the crisp air on your skin. You roll over and feel the grass on your face. The grass feels like soft clouds. You feel so relaxed and calm.

A gentle breeze is blowing on your face. You can feel it against your skin. Your skin feels alive and is glowing with light. You hear beautiful birds singing, the gentle croaking of a frog and the peaceful humming of crickets.

There is a magnificent waterfall in front of your eyes. You can hear the gentle trickling of the water against the rocks. You see the water running over the shiny boulders and hear the sound of trickling and dripping from the water. The water is so clear blue. It resembles a mirror.

You feel so happy inside – overflowing with happiness just like the beautiful waterfall. Happiness in the colour of golden light is beginning to flow from your heart and surrounds your body. The warmth of the sun on your skin increases the light around your body. The light makes you want to sing or hum a tune with the birds and nature around you. Your entire body is surrounded in golden light.

Everything feels so peaceful, relaxed, content and beautiful. Your heart feels alive with joy and love. You feel so much energy in your body. Your body feels so light, like you could float. Imagine yourself slowly rising up with the lightness of your body. Your body is surrounded by golden, vibrant light pouring out from your heart. It is lifting your body up into the air, slowly and gently. You can feel the breeze uplifting your body, raising you up into the beautiful blue sky. You feel completely relaxed and at ease.

With a slight movement of your hands, your body turns slightly. You have complete control over your body. You are floating, watching the rolling green fields and peaceful waterfall below. A bright coloured bird flies up beside you and sings a tune in harmony. You are floating, slowly, feeling the breeze against your skin, brushing your hair aside. Float as long as you like, through the clouds and the clear blue sky. Let the golden light carry you wherever you wish to go.

When you are ready to slowly come down, let the breeze guide you down to a cushioned area. Slowly descend, gently. You feel so happy and in control. You feel your feet gently touch the soft ground and bounce slowly up again. Again you come down, completely relaxed rolling onto the soft grass. You feel the softness of the grass on your back again. You smile and your smile lights you up inside, you are so content and happy.

You can hear the trickling of the water against the rocks and the chirping of birds. A feeling of hope, peace and inner fulfilment overwhelms you and fills your heart. Slowly and peacefully open your eyes when you are ready.

A hospital visit should be a healing and inspirational experience. By enhancing your immediate surroundings you have the power to control the direction of your healing and destiny. Having the wonderful tools of healing at your fingertips gives you the chance to become your own best doctor and to play a key role in the positive outcome of your health!

Chapter 15

EMOTIONAL OVERLOAD

Feelings and Emotions Experienced in Stages during Diagnosis, Treatment and Recovery from Cancer

When I first discovered I had cancer, I was in total disbelief. All that kept circulating through my mind was, 'That's impossible, they've made a mistake. I've always been so healthy. I couldn't possibly have cancer'. I had always associated cancer with 'sick' people or 'unlucky' people. I couldn't have been further from the truth.

As time went on and I went through different stages of my treatment, I found myself also slipping into different types of emotions. Cancer doesn't involve just one emotion, it is a rainbow of emotions all affecting us to different degrees, and at different times during our treatment and recovery.

Orthodox cancer treatment is aggressive and surgery can be mentally and physically uncomfortable. Radiation treatment and chemotherapy often causes more discomfort and pain than the initial disease. Treatment can extend over a number of weeks, months or even years and the patient is forced to deal with an array of emotional reactions caused by the treatment, as well as many physical and emotional side effects. It is difficult to convince yourself you are recovering when you feel so sick. It's hard to be so optimistic, as everyone says, when you feel much worse now than when you were first diagnosed. It seems in your mind and heart that this pain will never end. It's hard to imagine ever feeling normal again, although this is a wish you hold closest to your heart.

I hope I can help other cancer patients, their friends and family to understand the spectrum of emotions experienced in our spirited fight against cancer, how to deal with these in a positive way and direct them into the healing we so desperately need.

Shock and Disbelief

Shock is the first emotion or feeling experienced upon the realisation that you have cancer. When the doctor informs you, a coldness rushes through your body, your spine tingles and it feels like your heart is being stabbed. Part of you wants to just fade away into the darkness and disappear forever. Very little desire is felt to talk to anyone, hear anything or to make any decisions. Your mind and body goes numb. There is very little anyone can do to ease your pain.

Shock is also felt by some family members and accompanies the feeling of disbelief. It is not unusual to want to panic, as we so often associate cancer with death and running out of time. It is important not to panic. In the majority of cases you do have time to make decisions, to make changes and decide which path is best suited to your healing. It may all seem so overwhelming and daunting in the beginning, but as time passes you will adapt mechanisms and attitudes to cope with the changes. It is natural to face the possibility of death and in facing the possibility of death, we also learn to face the probability of living!

The only thing that can help at this stage is simply patience – you must wait until the feelings pass. Shock, fear and panic in any situation, whether it be news of an accident, death of a loved one or loss of something precious to us, is natural and is released from our lives in time. One thing is sure, nothing in life is permanent. As time passes, life changes and our feelings of shock, grief and disbelief also pass.

We must remember that we do not all operate on the same emotional timetable. One family member may feel the need to talk, while others may feel like becoming private or introspective. It is important to let the person who has cancer decide the right time for discussion. For the family and friends involved, love, compassion, understanding and patience are needed to help the person involved feel secure and loved. If the person realises they have plenty of support and understanding from precious loved ones, it can help bring the person out of shock faster than expected. Remember that it is a stage that all persons involved with cancer must go through. For the loved ones involved, just be patient and be there when everyone is ready to talk and open up.

Denial, Avoidance

Denial is usually the second and most common emotion felt by the cancer patient and sometimes by his or her own families. It is hard to believe it could happen to you. Once again a feeling of disbelief is followed by denial or avoidance of the situation. You may think such thoughts as, 'This is not happening to me, this is impossible, someone has made a mistake.'

We often go through life thinking we are invincible, that diseases like cancer usually happen to other people, not to someone like us. Many people believe that cancer usually affects sick, aged and stressed individuals. However this is not always the case. Go into a chemotherapy room or the cancer ward in a hospital, and look at all the babies and children and teenagers and young adults, some very healthy looking, being afflicted with cancer. How could a baby experience so much stress in their short lifetime to develop cancer? Or why is the fit athlete having chemotherapy for bone cancer?

Of course, then, it is easy to go into self-denial and protest when being informed that you have cancer. Denial is a form of human self-defence. If I deny this, then it's not true. However, at some stage you must face the fact that you have developed cancer and learn to accept your condition, to be able to encourage the healing process. Denial in its essence accompanies disbelief, which ultimately accompanies pre-determined judgments on the way things are meant to be. By releasing your conditioned judgements, you can learn to accept the fact that no one is perfect and being a human being and living in today's society, we all run the risk of developing some type of health condition.

At some point you will have to pick yourself up and try to accept your condition, and then look at where you may have slipped off the path. You can then make the necessary changes in your life to help place yourself back on the path to recovery and greater health and happiness. Open your heart to completely accepting your condition. This will allow you the opportunity to embrace your healing completely. If you remain in a state of self-denial and avoidance, it will be difficult to permanently heal your cancer. Full healing takes place when you accept responsibility for past actions, reactions and your own disease.

Blame

Blame is an inevitable emotion experienced by a high per centage of cancer patients. In today's world, we all want to blame someone or something for our lives, mistakes, tragedies and imperfections. Why do you think we have so many wars? As humans we always want to blame someone if life is not going according to plan. It is the same when a person finds out they have cancer.

It's very hard for people to accept responsibility for their own actions. This would be acknowledging that 'I am not perfect, I have made mistake'. It's much easier to pass the blame on to someone or something else, to ease our own conscience and allow someone else to bear the burden. In most cases, blame is not justified; it is just easier at the time to not accept the responsibility and consequences of past mistakes.

However, in some cases blame may be justified. If a doctor removes an organ without the patient's permission and at the time it is not necessary, then in this case it is totally understandable for a cancer patient to blame someone else for their unhappiness, as due to carelessness they must suffer. These particular types of cases occur, yet are becoming less common today as people accept responsibility for the health of their own bodies.

If a person with cancer wishes to heal, they should try to release blame and learn to accept their condition fully. Only then can healing be realised. As a fully-grown adult, you are responsible for our own actions and mistakes. Know this, accept this and learn to change your responses to situations, and blame will become a feeling of the past. Meditation, creative visualisation and positive thinking and laughter are great ways to move you through the blaming stage and into a state of acceptance.

Anger

Anger is a natural response or reaction accompanying and often following blame. If you feel someone is responsible for your condition then it is a natural human emotion to also feel angry with that person for causing your discomfort and pain. Anger is an emotion which allows you to release pent up feelings, anxieties and hurts. Anger is a healing emotion, as long as it is released in a positive way. It is definitely not beneficial to your recovery if you hold on to the feelings of anger and keep them bottled up inside. This will simply make you feel worse and leave little room for healing your condition.

Any release of emotion is healing, as it stops the hurt and pain from being contained within your heart. Anger contained within the heart eventually leads to sickness. If you feel angry about something, ask yourself, 'Is it going to help me by being angry?' If the answer is no, which it usually is, don't allow yourself to fall victim to the anger. Is it really worth the consequences to let others upset you? Why lower yourself to their level? They're not the ones getting sick, you are.

A great exercise for releasing anger can be done at home, at any time of the day. Grab a pillow, cushion, stick or something which feels comfortable in your hand. Try to do this in a large open space, where you feel no inhibitions.

Think of something or someone who makes you angry. Breathing in, raise the pillow or object above your head and on the out breath, bring the pillow down as hard as you can (without hurting yourself) against a tree, the ground, another pillow or some other supporting object. Feel all the anger and pent up emotions being released as you swing the pillow and release your breath. On the out breath it is a good idea to release the breath with a loud 'Aaahhhhh...'

If it is someone in particular you are angry at, imagine yourself hitting this person with the pillow and with every hit, that person disappearing into thin air, as you become happier and happier. With every swing and exhalation, imagine yourself feeling lighter and lighter. Laugh, have fun, enjoy yourself. Repeat over and over until you have released all of your anger and negativity and you feel happier, more relaxed and lighter.

Here is another great exercise for releasing pent-up anger. Say the following affirmation at any time of the day, as often as you like:

'I am eliminating all of the anger, in all of the roots and the deepest cause of all of this problem. I forgive you _____ and know that you are/were doing the best that you can/could.'

Withdrawal

As humans, we rarely want anyone to know about our faults. Think about when we're courting the loves of our lives; initially we rarely let out our little treasure trove of bad habits. Our partner seems perfect and vice versa, and in an instant we've got starry eyes; we're in love with most perfect person in the world. This is part of being human. We want our loved ones to know we are as close to perfect as possible, as we believe it attracts more admiration and attention, which is really a form of love. Love is what we all desire and what we all seek, from birth through to death. We forget that love is already present within our own hearts and what we should really be searching for and attaining is inner peace.

It is no wonder that when we develop a disease such as cancer, we experience the need or desire to withdraw from people we care for and society in general. Sometimes it just seems much easier to withdraw, to avoid the questions, which at this stage we may not have an answer for, or the answer we like. By withdrawing we do not have to face questions or to expose ourselves to pity – which can be humiliating for many. By slipping into our own world we do not have to admit to ourselves or to others that we are not perfect, in a world where most people are trying to act perfect.

It is difficult for those who have never had cancer to understand the complex feelings, emotions and questioning that the cancer patient experiences. Many people associate cancer with 'stressed, weak or aged' individuals. This is a total fallacy. It is another reason why people with cancer withdraw from society and loved ones, as they may become labelled in this category. A category considered imperfect. Society can be extremely judgmental and no one likes to be judged. Cancer patients find it easier to withdraw to avoid judgmental attitudes.

It's really funny how complex we have made our lives. We mentally run in circles every day, worrying what people think of us, and we often go into hiding until we are happy with the way we look, or the way we feel. This is another reason cancer patients withdraw. 'I will come back out when I look better or when my hair grows back'.

Choose wisely whom you tell your condition to, as many people are simply gossips and live for human tragedy. Share your feelings with understanding souls whom you love and trust with your heart and you are sure to feel safer and more supported in your fight against cancer. For family and friends in this situation, ensure the cancer patient knows how much you love them unconditionally, without expectations or conditions. The cancer patient needs to be reassured of your unconditional love especially during this unstable period.

Sadness – Why Me?

Sadness is an emotion that overcomes all of us, particularly women, when we discover we have cancer. Men are often taught to withhold their emotions and may not release this sadness until later. Any release of emotion is good, as it stops bad emotions from being pent-up inside.

Sadness is a natural feeling running through life. We feel sad if we lose something or someone, if we feel lost or without direction, or if we don't like the way our lives are heading. It's like a wave that washes over our souls. It's perfectly natural to feel sad if we are faced with losing part of our body, a limb or an organ, or even our hair. This is something that has always been a part of us; it's part of who we are and what makes up our characters. Of course we will feel a sense of loss or emptiness if part of who we are is taken away from us. Don't ever feel bad about mourning or feeling sad.

It is natural with cancer and cancer treatment to feel overwhelmed by this new world of uncertainties. Allow yourself and those around you to feel this sense of sadness for as long as it takes. Eventually you will come out of the darkness into the light, as nothing stays sad forever. With every action there is an equal and opposite reaction. Often sadness in life is followed by happiness. It is the law of opposites.

Try to plan activities you enjoy, set positive current and future goals for yourself, and have things to look forward to. Play with a child or puppy dog; nothing makes you feel happier than seeing a child or puppy playing innocently, or walking on the beach at sunset. Try to make the most of every moment! You should never have to justify your feelings or actions to anyone. To all loved ones involved, let the person with cancer hear your positive words, show love and express your feelings. Everyone loves a big hug! Now is a great time to let go of judgements, learn to accept, understand and love openly.

Here is an effective exercise for releasing deep sadness that you can say at any time of the day, as often as you like:

> *I am eliminating all of the sadness, in all of the roots and the deepest cause of all of this problem. I forgive you _____ and I know that you are/were doing the best that you can/could.*

Acceptance, Resolution

True acceptance is reached after experiencing a whirlpool of other emotions and feelings. Acceptance is attained when we fully learn to acknowledge our condition and realise we are responsible for all our own actions, mistakes and experiences. Acceptance is attained at different periods of time for everyone. Learning to truly accept the fact that we have cancer allows us to undertake on a journey of true healing for our soul.

Humans are similar to instruments, animals and plants – we are all adaptable. If a blossom is cut off a plant, it adapts to the changes and grows a new, stronger bud. If an animal is put into a new environment, it accepts the change and develops new senses to cope with the changes. Everything in life is adaptable, which makes us uniquely intelligent beings that fight for survival. Humans are adaptable. We have the ability to react to situations, accept the condition and make the necessary changes to ensure survival.

Accepting that we as humans are ultimately responsible for our cancer allows us to fight this disease with courage and vitality. On reaching this stage and accepting all possibilities and outcomes, we open ourselves to all methods to heal and overcome our cancer. Without acceptance, we remain in a state of denial and avoidance, deeming it impossible to reach permanent healing. Embracing your illness and understanding your condition takes you one step closer to greater health, happiness and inner peace.

Courage – Fighting Spirit

As humans we are born with an inherent courage. We possess a true fighting spirit. It is in our nature to stand up and fight bravely, and not to let life pull us down for too long.

Courage abounds in human spirit! How wonderful to be in the presence of courageous souls with the bravery to fight and overcome a disease or illness. I take my hat off to anyone who has had to go through conventional cancer treatment like surgery, radiation or chemotherapy. To even step into this treatment takes a tremendous amount of courage, willpower and determination, as the side effects experienced are extremely debilitating and uncomfortable.

No one in this world likes being uncomfortable. We are ultimately creatures of comfort. And to be willing to put yourself in this unusual position of pain and discomfort signifies your desire to live. It is part of being human. As humans we never give up; it the essence of our genetic structure to fight for survival. This is a mere fragment of the human character I will continue to admire and respect for my entire existence. We are all ultimately fighters with an innate instinct to survive not only for ourselves, but also for our loved ones. To survive through these obstacles involves a large amount of courage and strength.

If you have journeyed through the myriad of emotions experienced in your fight and you have learnt to fully embrace your illness – congratulations! You have overcome the most difficult part of your healing. You are endowed with a fighting spirit and have discovered the path to better health, inner fulfilment and well deserved happiness. Nothing can stop you now. See health, feel health and know health – perfect health is your natural state of being. Don't let this condition pull you down, use your strength and fighting spirit to beat this disease. After all you have nothing to lose and absolutely everything to gain!

Chapter 16

SHH – YOUR SECRET'S SAFE WITH ME!

Who to Tell, Who Can You Trust?

One question that may haunt us when we discover we have cancer is 'Whom should I share this personal information with?' Many people with cancer find the best choice is to share the diagnosis with close friends and family, to give them the opportunity to offer their support and understanding. Others find it easier to hide their fears and hopes rather than sharing them.

Life is an impermanent cycle of change, death and growth. With this knowledge in mind, we know that no-one lives forever. Since life is so short, we should make the most of every single moment and learn not to take the gift of living for granted. By telling loved ones, you give them the opportunity to support you and carry some of your emotional baggage for a change. I'm sure many loved ones, friends and family are in a stronger position than you are at this stage to help carry some of your burdens.

Eventually, if you plan to go through with orthodox treatment, it will be difficult to keep this news from those you love. Symptoms and side effects may begin to become apparent to those around you.

Cancer not only affects your life but it also affects those closest to you. You may feel like keeping it from those you love in the initial stages, however if you continue orthodox medical treatment you may need help from those you love, both physically and mentally to get through this difficult and exhausting time. Often, we like to keep things to ourselves to save others the stress or anxiety of worrying about us. Many people with cancer dislike pity, which unfortunately is how many people express love. We must remember everyone is different and we can't expect people to react exactly the way we want them to.

You will know from your own personal experience, the souls you can trust to keep your secrets and who is really a true and honourable friend. Ask yourself 'Why do I want this person to know?', 'Can I really trust them?' and 'How will this help me? It is important to think about yourself when you have cancer and not how other people feel. This is your time to re-evaluate your present situation, put energy into your own healing and to clear any blockages in your life.

Of course, many cancer patients find it easier to keep the details of their condition to themselves from most people, depending on the type of relationship they have with friends and loved ones. Just because someone is family, it doesn't mean they are completely understanding or empathetic to your needs. Many people realise when they develop cancer just whom they can really trust. You will certainly discover who your true and trusted friends are with a condition such as cancer.

Friends to whom you confide your condition may pretend to understand and vow to be there for you during your treatment. In the long run, this may turn out to be untrue. Some people will contact you initially with best thoughts, admirable words and well wishes, and then over time the news and good thoughts may ease off.

I find many so called 'friends' may use your illness as a way of propping up their own lives. It is human nature to judge our own life by the lives of other people. Why do you think newspapers and news programs filled with tragedy are so popular? We hate and love human tragedy. Seeing someone else's tragedy makes many souls feel better about their own lives, choices and existence. Friends who are not real will spread the news around that you are sick like wildfire, as a means of uplifting their own status and justifying their own method of living.

So think carefully about whom to share your illness with. Tell only loved ones and friends who love you unconditionally and will be there for you through ups and downs, highs and lows, tears and laughter and who have the ability to keep a secret, if you so desire. It is certainly a great time of self-discovery and you will no doubt uncover the answer to who your true and trusted friends really are.

Hush, Hush from the Doctor – What You Don't Know Won't Hurt You

You've all heard the saying, 'what you don't know, won't hurt you'. I feel this saying is all too often employed in the practice of medical doctors, especially surrounding certain aspects of cancer. This may come from the fact that many doctors actually don't know everything about cancer and refuse to admit they don't have all of the answers. It also stems from the fact that many doctors place themselves in a superior class, higher than most people. They therefore feel the normal person just wouldn't understand what they are talking about.

Understand or not, it is your moral right to be given all of the facts about your condition. Before undertaking chemotherapy I was told very little, apart from the fact it was the only solution to possibly cure my cancer and some of the possible side effects. As the treatment progressed, everything I was told in the beginning turned out to be less than ten per cent of what I really needed to know. Treatment was completely different to what I was informed it would be like, so no doubt it made me feel frustrated and helpless.

Many medical professionals simply feel that the average person with an illness does not possess the full comprehension to understand what they are talking about. Doctors may feel it is better to keep certain things from you to avoid unnecessary stress or anxiety. This should be the patient's decision, as you will ultimately have to deal with the problems at some stage, whether it is now or later.

Always seek a medical professional who treats you with respect and is empathetic to your needs. Ask them to share everything with you, including all possibilities and options. Inform them it is okay for them to ring you with results immediately and to give you full copies of every report.

Maintaining secrecy about your results and physical health, due to whatever reason, is simply not good enough. There are many open, understanding doctors out there who realise that no person is better than the next, we are all just different. And for this reason, we should all be treated equally with the same amount of respect we show towards the person who is treating us. That means if you are divulging valuable and personal information about yourself to the doctor, then you have every right to expect the doctor to divulge all of the information regarding your condition back to you.

Chapter 17

KNOWLEDGE IS THE KEY

You Have Rights!

Knowledge in its essence is self-empowerment. It provides us with a level upon which to communicate, to ask questions and seek answers. Without knowledge, we remain in a dark and ignorant position and hand our power over to those people we believe have the right to choose the direction of our lives. Knowledge of your own health condition is extremely important. If you wish to have some control over the direction of your cancer and you still want to keep your strength and self-worth, then seek answers.

I now realise there is very little information available to people with cancer, as the medical profession prefers to keep details of this a closely guarded secret. Even they understand the power of knowledge and wield this all too dangerously to their advantage. This is one of the main reasons I chose to write this book. During my fight against cancer, I found very limited information about my type of cancer and the doctors were less than happy to provide me with further details. This can make you feel extremely frustrated and helpless. Many medical professionals prefer to keep information regarding your cancer on a strictly need to know basis. For whatever reason this is chosen, try not to give in and seek your own answers, especially if the doctor you are seeing is reluctant to delve deeper for you.

One advantage of today's modern world is the advent of the internet. Here we can find a multitude of answers and it is, in most cases, totally free. At the back of the book I have listed a number of wonderful and informative websites that you may find useful in your fight against cancer.

Ask your doctor for copies of all test results and statistics about your type of cancer, and any other printed information they have available about your illness. It is advisable to ask the doctor to provide you with a photocopy from the latest MIMS concerning the side effects of your cancer treatment and drugs. (MIMS is a drug guide used by health professionals, detailing pharmaceuticals and their side effects). At least this way you can be aware of any nasty side effects or symptoms from cancer treatment. It is definitely less of a shock to be forewarned, than to wake up with some frightening symptom that you've never experienced and you were never warned about.

Control your Cancer

Discovering you have cancer or any serious illness is both a shocking and life-altering experience. It tends to stir up a whirlpool of mixed emotions that swirl around inside your head, making your normal thinking processes cloudy and unfocused.

There are so many stages we must go through to fully accept the fact that we have developed a possible life-threatening condition. We all experience these stages at different times and in varying degrees. I may feel immediate denial, whereas someone else may feel immediate anger and blame. Every person is different, which is what makes us unique and individual in our responses, reactions and healing capacity.

As soon as you hear the word cancer, it is natural to panic. Don't panic, it is not going to kill you today or tomorrow, as many people believe, and don't let anyone rush you into any decisions. Cancer can be such an overwhelming and all-consuming experience; it is easy to let others make your decisions for you about which direction is best suited to your needs, right then and there. You do have time. Take a deep breath, sit down, make every effort to relax and write down your possible options.

If you know something is going to happen, don't just watch it and let it control you – take charge and control it. Take control of the direction of your illness, your cancer and your health. For instance, if you plan to undergo chemotherapy and you know you are going to lose your hair, go out and get a beautiful short hairstyle that you may have been too afraid to try before. Or if you are aware that you are going to have an operation, take steps to build up your strength, nutritional levels and health before the operation to ensure a more rapid and successful recovery. By making the first move and controlling your destiny, you have not given your personal power away to anyone.

Letting someone else make all of your decisions about your health forces you to lose your confidence, decision-making ability, self-worth and personal strength. It can leave you feeling weak and at the mercy of the course of the illness, as preordained by those in so-called authority or more knowledgeable positions. No one is more knowledgeable about your body, than YOU! Your body is your temple; you have lived in this beautiful place since the day you were born. Ultimately you know what works best for your body, what feels great and what enhances your health, more than someone who has spent a few minutes with you on several occasions.

You may have slipped off the path a little in some way or overburdened your body, forcing it to go into a state of illness. But this is the perfect chance to re-grasp your power and natural self-healing knowledge. Find out every detail about your condition and make positive steps to walk ahead on the right path to health, happiness and self-fulfilment.

Many times we do need the expert opinions of medical professionals who have spent many years working with cancer and other chronic illnesses. It must also be understood that many doctors who work with cancer know only limited and tried treatment protocols, and many do not want to stray from this set regimen. Never hand your decision-making ability over to anyone else.

Often we have pushed our bodies to the limit and forced them to go into a state of serious collapse or illness. You have the ability to work hand-in-hand with the practitioner of your choice, whether you choose an orthodox practitioner or an alternative therapist, to discover the treatments that work best for you and to guide your body and spirit back towards better health and well-being. What a fulfilling and satisfying experience it is, to have taken part in the process of your own self-healing!

If you are worried about whom to trust when dealing with your cancer, learn to trust yourself first. Use your own intuition; let it guide you in the direction that is right for you. Listen to all avenues, all arguments and advice, seek knowledge about your condition and ask yourself whether the practitioner working with you has the ability to treat a condition such as yours and why. I cannot emphasise enough how important it is to arm yourself with knowledge, find out everything about your condition and available treatment options. If you go into this forearmed with the right information, you will maintain your self-confidence and personal power without having to feel helpless. Make sure you understand all of the good news about your cancer and that you are happy with your treatment, so you remain positive and optimistic throughout.

Taking control, even in the smallest way, enables us to learn how to master other areas of our lives. Very often when we are sick, we are caught up in a feeling of helplessness or uselessness. We need to take a part in our own healing process in order to feel useful and essential in life. All too often we give this power away and block ourselves from feeling pride in our accomplishments, our achievements and in our mastery over our health.

Having cancer is a turning mark in one's life. It is an opportunity to grasp change in a positive and life-transforming way, to release hurts, past traumas and long standing resentments. It enables you to take charge of your life and to ride on life's back like a wild tiger. Life is a daring adventure, giving us opportunities to change and grow. We often only get one chance. By taking an active role, no matter how small, in your own healing you open the doors to health, happiness and contentment. What a beautiful and ever-changing experience life can be! Seize this opportunity to take part in your own healing process and watch the miracle and magic of life unfold.

Chapter 18

NATURAL VS ORTHODOX – PROS AND CONS

O rthodox and natural medicines both have their place in healing and in society. All too often doctors bag natural therapists as being 'quacks' and natural therapists bag doctors as being cruel and aggressive in treatment. Often doctors show little respect towards natural therapists and many natural therapists show little respect towards doctors. This lack of respect is very disappointing, as so much can be gained from each other's medicine and forms of treatment. Both have an extremely important place in healing.

Modern surgery is remarkable and extends life to many souls who before the advent of medical technology were condemned to an early death. The new techniques and advances in transplant surgery, brain surgery and heart surgery have improved the quality and length of life for many people. Surgeons are amazing people with incredible skills to repair damage and to recreate healthy working functions of organs and body tissues. However, surgery can be quite invasive and uses man-made drugs to treat side effects, and in many cases attempts to patch up the symptoms rather than deal with the cause of the problem.

Likewise, natural medicine plays an equally important role in healing and health. Natural therapy is designed to treat the individual as a whole and to solve the causative problem, rather than to patch up the symptoms. Natural medicine is equally good in preventing and treating symptoms. It is usually non-invasive and uses gentle, natural methods to restore the health of the individual. Forms of natural therapy include nutrition, naturopathy, vitamins, herbs, homeopathy, acupuncture, Chinese medicine, Ayurvedic medicine, Tibetan medicine, aromatherapy, reflexology, iridology and many more. Natural medicine has been used in all cultures for thousands of years. Orthodox medicine is a relatively new form of medicine, being developed originally from the art of natural medicine.

Orthodox medicine definitely has a prominent place in healing. Any taint to the medical profession's reputation has been received because of errors in surgery, removal of healthy body organs and the overuse of pharmaceuticals by general practitioners to treat patients. It is common knowledge that some doctors receive expensive bonuses and incentives from pharmaceutical companies for selling large amounts of certain types of drugs. With this carrot in front of their faces, many doctors prescribe medical drugs in excess without proper investigation and reason. Doctors are human beings like you and me and are therefore not perfect, and prone to making mistakes.

Unfortunately, doctors are not in a good position to make mistakes or errors as they are dealing with people's lives. They are rarely held liable for any errors in treatment, as patients naturally baulk at the time and expense of legal action. When being treated medically, you are placing a enormous amount of trust and faith in your doctor.

Natural medicine is entirely different. It has been around for thousands of years in nearly every culture in the world. The American Indians have used shamanic healing and herbs to heal since the first existence of life. The Chinese have traditionally used Chinese medicine and acupuncture, the Indians in Asia incorporated Ayurvedic medicine to rebalance the individual since their culture began, and the Africans and Australian Aborigines are known for natural medicine and healing.

Natural medicine is used to heal the actual cause of the problem and prevent it from reoccurring in the future. It is a process of re-educating the individual to heal himself or herself by maintaining a healthy diet, mind and spiritual body. Of course, there are also unskilled and unqualified natural healers out there who have given this ancient method of healing a bad reputation. These healers may work primarily from a position of financial gain lacking the true empathy to heal individuals in accordance with nature. However, these healers are few and far between. The majority of natural healers are caring, passionate, empathetic and highly skilled souls.

Combining both orthodox and natural therapies in cancer treatment can for many, speed up the healing process dramatically. It is sad that so many people, in both the medical and natural field, remain ignorant of the benefits of each other's therapy. We have lost the essence of healing. It is not about the doctors and the natural therapists and whose therapy is better than the other. Nor is it about a practitioner's pride of 'who is more right'. It is about the individual and restoring balance and health to the person as a whole.

If the egos of both natural and orthodox practitioners were to be set aside, and the financial incentives to 'prove' the other is wrong were eliminated, we could remember what the true essence of healing is about. True healing comes from the soul and understanding the cause of the problem, and working to solve the problem, not to patch it up. It involves spending time with the patient (longer than 10 minutes), attentively listening to their problems and using the best healing methods possible, whether they be natural or orthodox or both, to solve the problem and bring about a healthy state of equilibrium and balance to the patient. If only more practitioners could open up their hearts to the immense healing potential contained within each other's amazing therapies, I'm sure there would be less illness in this world today.

Chapter 19

MIND MEDICINE

Positivity is the Link

A positive mental attitude is the real key to optimal health and beating cancer. Overcoming cancer begins by taking personal responsibility for your own mental state, your life, your current situation and your health. It has been proven time and again that your everyday thoughts and emotions largely determine your level of health and the quality of your life.

Life is full of chaotic and crazy events that are beyond our control. One thing we do have control over is our reactions and responses. We have the ability to respond to situations positively, rather than to react to situations negatively. Our attitude goes a long way in determining how we view and respond to the challenges that life throws at us. You will be much happier, healthier and more successful in life if you learn to adopt a positive mental attitude than if you have a negative, pessimistic outlook on life.

I know many people believe it's easier said than done. Once again, we always have choices. You can choose to be happy or choose to be sad, you can choose to respond or choose to react and likewise, you can mentally choose to be positive or choose to be negative. Always remember that a positive remark or reaction always outshines a negative comment. The choice to be more positive doesn't happen all at once. It happens by degrees, subtle changes accumulating step by step.

Emotions and Cancer

A person's mood and attitude has a tremendous bearing on the function of their immune system. It has now been significantly proven that the emotions of anxiety and chronic stress negatively affect the function of our immune system and lower our body's immune resistance, leaving it open to developing cancer.

Other negative emotions such as depression, repressed hostility, resentment, anger, feelings of helplessness and grief also weaken the immune system and enhance the development of illness, cancer and tumours. It has been proven in countless studies that the loss of a spouse, one of the deepest emotional grieving periods in one's life, causes a depressed immune system and opens the body to an array of illnesses, including cancer.

In the past, stress, also known as the 'fight and flight' response, was automatically developed by humans as a method of survival in a 'wild, primitive world'. When faced with danger during battles, man's metabolism would increase and his senses would become more acute and alert, allowing him to survive in perilous situations. In those days, stress was short lived and once the danger was past, the body readapted and returned to normal.

The difference in today's crazy world is that we don't have the occasional caveman chasing us around with a club but, rather, a continuous onslaught of daily stressful situations to cope with. Rather than being able to release the stress and relax, our bodies stay in 'stress mode', constantly on edge. No wonder health has declined so rapidly in today's society and the occurrence of more serious health conditions such as cancer, high blood pressure, insomnia, strokes, heart attacks, chronic depression, nervous twitches and ulcers have become an almost normal and accepted part of life.

It would be fantastic if we could all just move to the country and build a tepee up on a mountain top to escape our stressful society. However, for most people this is definitely not an option. The key to maintaining optimal health in today's fast-paced society lies in natural relaxation techniques and stress reduction. Now, this doesn't mean quick fixes either, such as smoking, drinking five cups of coffee a day, grabbing a sweet or a chocolate for a quick energy burst or excessive eating. It may make us feel better while we are doing these things but in the long run, they place added stress on the body and will actually make us feel worse as time goes by. A good example of this is bingeing on sugar. While it might give us a temporary boost of energy, it also depletes valuable B vitamins. This can lead to our nervous system weakening, which leads to more susceptability to stress, a weaker immune system and thus opening the doorway to sickness, and more chronic conditions, such as cancer.

So what is the answer? To release our negativity and emotional stress we need to learn holistic relaxation techniques such as yoga, deep breathing, tai chi, positive affirmations, meditation, laughter, exercise and a healthy, nutrient rich diet. By giving your body these beautiful gifts you will not only treat the immediate effects of stress but you will also make your body and mind stronger and more able to cope with the pressures in your everyday life. A stress-free mind that is free from negative emotions will ensure that you remain healthy and cancer-free.

At the other end of the scale, positive emotions such as love, playfulness, bliss, joy, contentment and self-mastery seem to have a beneficial effect on good health and promote healing. It is believed that laughter can heal many chronic conditions including cancer. When we are happy and optimistic, our immune system functions much better. In addition, guided imagery, hypnosis, positive affirmations and meditative states all enhance our immune system and our ability to cope with stress.

When we are stressed, our body increases its production and release of adrenal hormones including cortisol, cortisone and adrenaline, to cause internal bodily changes that allow us to cope with stress. ACTH (adrenocorticotropic hormone) is released from the pituitary gland and thymosin (a group of thyroid hormones) is also released to increase our coping mechanisms.

If our body is continuously bombarded with these 'stress hormones', white blood cell formation and function is inhibited and our thymus gland (the 'maestro' gland of the immune system) shrinks. Stress can also decrease lymphocyte count, specifically natural killer cells ('the front-line soldiers of the immune army') and T helper cells ('the commanders of the immune army'), and reduce the body's ability to produce interferon. This is an obvious suppression of the body's immune system, leaving a person open to illness and cancer.

Blocking negative emotions isn't the answer to preventing illness and cancer. Inhibiting emotions will not make them go away, it simply drives them into more subtle and usually more destructive avenues of expression later. Holding on to your emotions, especially negative emotions, is like sealing a volcano that is waiting to explode. The lava has to go somewhere and more often than not it flows to one specific area of the body, creating illness there.

As human beings, we carry inside ourselves an array of emotions and feelings. This is part of who we are, what we are born with. If we inhibit our emotions from direct expression (many men are taught to hide their true emotions), we may cause more serious health problems to arise. Many people block the expression of their anger, turning it back onto themselves rather than letting the anger go out in a clean, quick release towards the person or situation that provoked the emotion. Once the anger is blocked and turned inward, serious health imbalances can result. Many heart attack patients are the victims of inhibited anger.

Emotions developed in humans because of their survival value. We need every single one of the emotions that we are born with. Negative emotions lead to sickness when we block them and allow them to literally eat us up inside. The mind and the body function together as a biochemical whole. It is thought cancer cells suffer from isolation of a positive flow of energy and metabolism. If this is the case, then people with cancer have pulled their consciousness away from the cancerous growth. When the mind pulls away from this part of the body, it is termed avoidance.

The area of the body being ignored is possibly part of a deep hurt or pain. Those most prone to developing cancer are often people with a high anxiety/low love acceptance profile and those who tend to steer clear of cancer are people with a low anxiety/high love-acceptance profile. It is no wonder cancer is so rampant in today's world, with an increase in anxiety due to higher stress levels and a decrease in loving relationships and self-acceptance.

If you do have cancer, ask yourself, 'What is really the source of the anxiety I am feeling inside? What am I afraid of deep down? What am I trying to destroy inside myself? What or who is hurting me or causing me pain?' 'Where is the cancer located in my body and what emotion is associated with this body area?' Answer these questions honestly and perhaps they will reveal the emotional manifestation of your illness.

To enhance the healing process from an emotional viewpoint you need to stop judging yourself and start accepting yourself for who you are. No one is perfect. We are all struggling to survive, we are all hoping to be accepted for who we are and we are all souls looking for true love, balance and eternal peace. If you learn to understand that every human being is ultimately driven by the same goal, 'acceptance and love' and try to release any judgements or expectations of who you think you are meant to be – then you can really learn to accept and love yourself exactly for who you are, not for what you want to become or for what others think of you.

The Harmful Effects of Stress

Table 19.1

Our Natural Response to Stress	Short-Term Benefit to Allow the Body to Cope with Stress	Long-Term Effects on the Human Body from Continual Stress
A heightening of our body's senses	Pupils dilate to see better at night time, better hearing, touch, smell and taste (to get the body ready for trouble)	'Burnt out' from over-stimulation, chronic fatigue, low ATP production that weakens cells leaving the body open to illness and cancer.
Cortisone and Cortisol Production and Release	Protects us from allergic reactions, causes bodily changes to allow us to cope with stress	Damages and weakens the immune system, leaving us more open to disease and cancer, inhibits antibody production, depression
Digestive tract shuts down	Blood is re-directed away from digestion to muscles and heart for increased strength	Dry mouth, digestive problems, weight gain, bloating, cramps, diarrhoea or constipation, toxicity
Fast, deeper breathing	More oxygen to the muscles for added strength	Aggravates breathing problems and increases damage done by smoking, possibly leading to lung cancer, may cause sleeping problems, snoring, respiratory problems
Increased adrenaline production and release	Quick metabolism of proteins, fats and carbohydrates to provide a quick energy source	Excretion of amino acids, potassium and phosphorous, lowered calcium storage, anxiety, fast heartbeat, insomnia, fears, phobias, nervousness, panic attacks, high blood pressure
Increased blood cholesterol	Is used as a fuel to make adrenal hormones that are used in response to stress	Hardening of arteries, heart attacks, prostate problems, impotence, hypertension, circulatory and memory problems
Increased blood sugar and insulin	Quick energy boost to run and survive	Diabetes, hypoglycaemia, obesity, carbohydrate and sugar cravings
Increased endorphins	A natural painkiller to assist during stress and in case of injury	Chronic headaches, backaches, lowered pain threshold, suppression of the immune system

Table 19.1 *continued*

Our Natural Response to Stress	Short-Term Benefit to Allow the Body to Cope with Stress	Long-Term Effects on the Human Body from Continual Stress
Increased thyroid hormones	Speeds up the metabolism for extra energy needed in an emergency, increases the body's resistance to stress	Shaky nerves, weight loss (or in some people weight gain), insomnia, exhaustion, endocrine imbalances
Increased production and release of norepinephrine	Stimulates the release of hormones to give the thymus gland the correct instructions	Schizophrenia, depression
Low hydrochloric acid levels in the stomach	A shutting down of digestive functions to put energy into internal survival 'fight and flight' mechanisms	Digestive problems, poor absorption of foods, reduced calcium absorption leading to osteoporosis, weak bones and teeth, lowered immune status
Lowered production of sex hormones	Decreased ability to conceive children	Premature ejaculation and impotence (men) and decreased ability to orgasm (women), diminished sex drive, infertility
Rapid heartbeat	More blood to muscles and lungs for added strength	High blood pressure leading to heart attacks and strokes, palpitations, irregular heartbeat
Skin goose bumps and sweats	Increases sensitivity to touch, cool down body during stress	Perspiration problems and body odour
Thicker blood	Better ability to carry more oxygen and fuel to muscles, stops bleeding	Strokes, thrombosis (blood clots), heart attacks, circulatory problems

Seven Easy Steps to Beat Stress

1. *Share the Baggage* – Do not take on everything yourself. Try to offload some of your responsibilities so that you can find some time to relax.
2. *Eliminate Boredom* – If we are bored, our minds begin to create niggling fears and anxieties. Don't wait for something exciting to happen in your life, seek out challenges and adventures to add some spice to your life.
3. *Self Esteem Tricks* – Do happy, exciting things to uplift your confidence. If you are lacking in self-esteem take positive steps to change those areas of your life that need adjusting. Surround yourself with positive people. Write down a list of all of your wonderful qualities.

4. *Plan and Organise* – If we are disorganised, we become stressed. Sit down, plan and only take on as much work as you can cope with.
5. *Take a Break* – Take some time out for yourself for relaxation. Don't keep putting off that holiday.
6. *Sleep and Eat well* – Sleep rejuvenates the body and mind and helps to alleviate stress. Likewise, a healthy nutrient packed diet increases the body's ability to cope with stress much more effectively.
7. *You are most Important* – It is not important to please everyone or to make others feel proud of you. What is important is pleasing yourself first, without harming others. If you can create inner happiness and peace, then this self-fulfilment and happiness will flow over into other areas of your life.

Emotions and Their Effect on Our Physical Body

Asian and other ancient cultures have believed for centuries that negative and even positive emotions, if over-expressed or overemphasised in one's life, will manifest in the body as illness. The chart below shows the positive and negative emotion of each organ and how an overbalance of either of these emotions may affect that organ.

Table 19.2

Organ	Positive Emotion	Negative Emotion	Over-expression of Either Emotion can cause:
Bones	Feeling balanced and structured in life	Feeling unbalanced, lacking direction and structure	Bone cancer and other bone problems
Brain	Open to change, correct beliefs, adaptability, acceptance	Set in ways, refusing to change old patterns, incorrect beliefs that may have been passed down through generations	Brain tumours, psychological problems, schizophrenia
Breasts	Freedom, allowing others their freedom, feeling safe and protected	Over-mothering, over-protection of others, forgetting about self, controlling others	Breast cancer and other problems with breasts, including cysts, lumps and pain
Cervix/ vagina	Self-approval, appreciating own unique sexuality	Anger at lover, sexual guilt, self-punishment	Cancer of the cervix or vagina, cervical dysplasia, vaginitis and other related problems
Gallbladder	Good decision making ability, releasing the past	Sarcastic, indecisive, bitter, hard thoughts	Gallstones and other gallbladder problems.

Table 19.2 *continued*

Organ	Positive Emotion	Negative Emotion	Over-expression of Either Emotion can cause:
Heart	Joy, expression of love and gratitude to others, materialism	Lack of joy, serious, stressed, long term emotional issues, overly materialistic	Heart problems, heart disease and heart attack
Kidneys	Feeling safe, secure and protected, courage	Fear, lack of money, feeling insecure, unprotected	Kidney cancer and other related kidney problems
Liver	Love and peace, happy, reacting positively	Anger, irritable, nagging, nit-picker	Liver cancer, liver problems
Lungs, respiratory organs	Peace, accepting life and situations, freedom, happiness	Grief, depression, feeling suppressed, desire to get something off your chest, sadness, worry	Lung problems, lung cancer, asthma, bronchitis
Ovaries	Creativity, happy with own femininity and sexual attraction, happy with life	Extreme sadness and old hurts, loss of feelings of femininity and attraction, lack of creativity and expression	Ovarian cancer, ovarian cysts and other problems with ovaries
Prostate, testicles	Feeling strong in your masculinity, fighting spirit	Sexual pressure, guilt, fears of ageing, resignation	Prostate or testicular cancer and problems
Spleen	Self-approval, grounded, secure and protected	Obsessions, unbalanced, scattery	Blood related problems, spleen problems
Stomach/ bowel	Relaxed, able to assimilate new ideas, accepting change	Fear of new, anxiety, something in the past is eating away at you.	Stomach and bowel cancer, digestive problems
Throat, Larynx	Self-expression, expressing how you really feel.	Lack of expression, scared to say how you really feel.	Cancers of the throat, mouth, sore throat
Uterus	Feeling creative, loved and feeling useful as a woman	No creativity, feeling unloved and worthless as a woman	Cancer of the uterus or endometrium

The Mind-Body Link

The mind and the body are inseparable. Improving your level of mental fitness and emotional health will directly and positively benefit your body. Modern medicine defines illness on a purely physical level and aims to find the most suitable pharmaceutical drug or surgical procedure to provide temporary relief from health symptoms. Many orthodox doctors refuse to recognise the integral link between our emotional state and health.

A direct relationship exists between the mind/consciousness, the brain/nervous system and the immune system. By observing changes in our body's immune system in connection with various stresses in our lives, emotional states and personalities, an undeniable link has been adopted between our mind and emotions, what we feel and think on a daily basis and how we react to situations and changes in our environment. Our thought patterns and reactions to stress have a profound effect on the overall health of our internal body systems and general health. Shamans, medicine men and natural healers have known this for centuries and have based their natural methods of healing on this premise. By treating the mind, the spirit and the body as a whole, long-term wellness is attained rather than short-term relief of symptoms.

How Changes in Our Emotions Affect the Function of Our Immune System and Lead to Cancer

Cells in the body's immune system contain receptor sites on their membranes for neurotransmitters or neuropeptides, which are secreted by the brain. Neurotransmitters may be considered the 'chemical mediators of emotion'. Your immune system knows when you are scared, depressed, angry, in love, happy or lonely and hence weakens or strengthens immune functions in accordance with these changes in your emotions.

When we become stressed, the pituitary gland (a major, regulatory gland located in the brain) increases its production of adrenocorticotropic hormone (ACTH), which in turn causes the release of the hormones cortisol, cortisone and adrenaline. These 'stress hormones' are secreted in order to alter body functions to allow us to cope with stress more effectively.

If these 'stress hormones' are produced in excess due to continual stress, they cause a suppression of our body's immune system by decreasing the function and efficiency of white blood cells (our body's disease fighters), thereby suppressing our body's immune responses. At the same time, these 'stress hormones' alter our emotions causing depression, anxiety, insomnia and nervousness which makes us feel more stressed thereby weakening immunity further. So stress, our emotions and our immune responses are inextricably linked.

The immune system is our body's most important ally in fighting disease. If we continually stress our body's immune system with negative emotions, we open the doors to weakened immunity, sickness and eventually cancer. Our body's immune system not only receives messages from the brain on our emotional state, but it can also relay information back to the brain regarding our emotional state. If we remain positive and balanced emotionally, our immune system also remains positive and balanced physically allowing us to maintain optimal levels of health and happiness.

It would be naive to think that we could remain happy and positive twenty-four hours a day, every day. In today's world this is not the reasonable answer to maintaining optimal health and high immunity levels. The key lies in finding a 'balance' in our lives. That means that we should try to remain as positive as possible, learn good techniques in dealing with negativity and stress and try not to ignore our precious time for relaxation, exercise, hobbies, healthy eating and beautiful connections. By doing this we nourish our body, mind and soul, which ultimately nourishes our immune system in its vital role of disease and cancer prevention.

Ten Steps to a Positive Attitude

Below are 10 easy steps used to develop and maintain a positive mental attitude and outlook on life. These can be incorporated easily into your everyday life improving your health, well-being and contentment.

1. Become an Optimist – Be Aware of Your Everyday Dialogue and Conversations with Others

The first step to developing a more positive attitude and outlook on life is to become an optimist (positive thinker), rather than a pessimist (negative thinker). As human beings we are inherently optimists by nature. An optimistic outlook on life allows us to succeed in achieving our goals, creates better levels of health and happiness and prevents illness. Optimism is a vital friend in our fight against cancer and disease.

The first way to begin your optimistic path is to be aware of your speech patterns. See if you can go a whole day without saying something negative or derogatory. Every day we engage in conversation at home, work and in society. Not only is it important to be aware of our internal self-talk, it is also necessary to become aware of what we say to others. Our everyday conversation also has an effect on our lives, our self-image, relationships and mental attitude. Any type of talk or thought leaves an imprint on our subconscious mind and will ultimately lead towards fulfilment or lack of fulfilment of our life's dreams.

Become aware of what you say and try to say positive comments and words. If you catch yourself saying a negative phrase, turn the negativity around by saying a positive phrase or making a positive comment. Think positive thoughts, perform positive actions and avoid negativity in every form. Try to say at least one positive, honest comment to another being every day and watch the magic unfold in your life.

2. Be Aware of Your Internal Self-talk

As humans, a constant dialogue of words occurs daily within our minds. This self-talk or mental chatter makes an impression on our subconscious mind. In order to develop a more positive mental attitude it is important to guard against negative self-talk. Become aware of your self-talk and consciously work to imprint positive self-talk and comments on your subconscious mind. A powerful tool in creating positive internal self-talk is to use affirmations. If you catch yourself saying negative comments in your mind, imagine yourself crossing this out with a pen and writing inside your mind the opposite positive comment. A positive always outweighs a negative every time. Consciously think positive thoughts and your positive thoughts will become your reality.

3. Use Positive Affirmations and Phrases Daily

An affirmation is a statement with an emotional intensity. Affirmations leave a mark on our subconscious mind to create a healthy, positive self-image and enhance positive changes in our lives. Affirmations enable us to fulfil our desires and attain success, happiness and inner fulfilment. By achieving our goals through setting and fulfilling affirmations, our self-confidence is increased, attaining a positive mental attitude (read on for a list of life-transforming affirmations). Try writing down positive affirmations on a piece of pink or yellow paper. Fold this piece of paper eight times and place this under your pillow. Within no time, your inner wishes and dreams will manifest right before your eyes!

4. Set Positive Short Term and Long Term Goals

Motivated, successful people have written hundreds of books on the benefits of goal setting. Setting goals enables us to attain our short and long term desires. Achieving goals enables you to feel better about who you are and the better you feel about yourself, the more likely you are to reach your goals.

Always state or write down the goal in positive terms and never use any negative terms in the goal. Always try to make your goal attainable and achievable. Be specific and certain about your goal. The clearer it is, the more likely it is you will reach it – be precise and exact about what you want. Always state the goal in the present or past tense. In order to achieve your goal, you have to believe you have already attained it.

Try to balance your goals between your physical, mental and emotional needs, rather than purely financial needs. Many people tend to write only work-orientated goals. Try to work out which areas of your life have received the least attention ie relationships, personal growth or health. Set goals to fill in these missing gaps in your life and watch the happiness unfold. See and feel yourself having already achieved your goal and success will naturally be yours for the taking.

5. Practise Creative Imagery

Positive visualisation or creative imagery is a powerful tool in creating health, wellbeing, happiness and success. In terms of ideal health, you must picture yourself with perfect health if you truly wish to attain this state. You can use visualisation in all areas of your life, but particularly in creating better health levels. Creative visualisation is a unique and simple tool in helping to overcome cancer. Some of the most prominent research on the power of positive visualisation involves enhancing the immune system in the treatment of cancer. Be creative and have fun with your visualisations and you will soon find yourself experiencing your dreams in real life. Dreaming is a powerful and inspirational means to self-healing and fulfilment.

One of the easiest ways to achieve your desires, whether it be ideal health or a better state of mind, is by using your favourite photographs. Place these pictures of yourself looking full of vitality, health and youthfulness beside your bed, in your office and home. These ideal images are transformative and leave a positive imprint on your subconscious mind to create the positive changes that you desire.

6. Laugh Heartily and Often

It has been proven that laughter enhances the body's immune system and improves general health and well-being. Research indicates that laughter enhances blood flow to the body's extremities and improves cardiovascular function. Laughter actively causes the release of endorphins and other mood elevating and pain killing chemicals. It likewise improves the transfer of oxygen and nutrients to internal organs. Here are some simple tips to create more laughter in your life:

- Watch comedy shows and movies on television. Go and see a comedy movie with a friend or even by yourself.
- Listen to comedy tapes in your car while driving.
- Play with children and animals.
- Learn to laugh at yourself – try not to take life too seriously.
- Learn jokes. Play games. Humour and laughter make life enjoyable and fun.
- Do fun things – go out and immerse yourself in exciting and fun activities.
- Read the comics or funny magazines.
- If you feel depressed, jump up and down and shake yourself out of this space.
- Have FUN! FUN! FUN!

7. Surround Yourself with Positive People

Life is full of struggles and trials, joys and new experiences. There are all types of people in this world, dealing with their problems in different ways. Knowing this, to keep your natural happiness, positivity and joy in life, it is wise to surround yourself in positive, light-hearted people.

Happy, positive souls can lighten your life and brighten your day. Negative, pessimistic people can bring you down and fill you with foreboding and unhappiness. Likewise many negative people do not like happy, successful people and will often say nasty things to make themselves feel better about their lives. I know which people I prefer to be around – definitely positive people. Family, friends and colleagues are a prominent part of our lives for so many of our waking hours. If these loved ones are negative, it won't be too long before you're brought down to their level. Our everyday moods are partly a reflection of the moods of the people that we surround ourselves with. So it is important to make sure that the people you surround yourself with are joyful, optimistic and positive in nature.

8. Keep the Playfulness and Joy in Your Life

Life is too short to be serious. We have such a limited time in this world, so why waste a single minute? Every single day, a beautiful and completely different sunrise and sunset blesses our presence. How many sunrises and sunsets do you miss? So often we become caught up in the demands and stresses of life and we forget the magic of the world right under our noses.

Children and puppies have so much fun, absorbed in every moment! We can learn a great lesson from these little wonders of life. Keep your inner child alive and have fun, enjoy yourself, take part in activities that make you happy. Keeping a playful attitude is a definite way to maintain a positive mental state.

9. Reward Yourself with Treats

Everyone loves to receive a gift or present. You deserve a treat for achieving your goals and having the courage to follow your dreams. It's a great sense of satisfaction and fulfilment to have attained a goal, no matter how small, so reward yourself for this achievement. Dogs get treats for performing tricks, many children receive money or presents for getting good marks at school, a sportsperson receives a medal for performing well – so you should receive a gift for attaining one of your goals. No matter how old we get, we all deserve recognition. Be proud of yourself!

10. Take Time Out for Yourself

In today's fast-paced world it can be quite a challenge to avoid the 'rat race' of work appointments, social commitments, family obligations and meeting deadlines. To maintain a positive attitude, you must never forget about yourself and your relaxation time. By putting aside ten minutes every day to sit down and contemplate or even meditate, the mind has time to assimilate your experiences and the physical body has time to rejuvenate and restore its delicate functions.

Without this time, your mind actually becomes a 'whirlwind' of crazy, jumbled thoughts and your body's immune system begins to suffer the consequences of non-recovery time. Ten minutes of meditation or relaxation daily will provide the 'key' to optimal wellness and positive transformation in every facet of your life.

Important Point!

How much time do you spend working? For most people it can be anywhere from 35 to 70 hours a week. That's a fair amount of time out of your life every week. Now what if you are working these hours and you don't like your job? Do you think you will be able to keep a positive attitude while doing something you dislike? It's very unlikely. If you do not like your work and you have dreams to do something else, never give up on your dream. If you are going to put 70 hours into doing something you don't like, why not put 70 hours into something you do like?

By striving for this your work life can become a pleasure, allowing you to bring the happiness and positivity home to your loved ones and family. If you are unhappy in your work life, no doubt you will bring this discontentment home to those you love and other areas of your life will begin to suffer. Dreams are attainable at any age; you just have to have the willpower and desire to try. Positive affirmations, goal setting and creative imagery are great ways to begin.

Ten Easy Rules for Making Each Day a Wonderful Day

1. Think beautiful thoughts from the moment you wake and watch them happen.
2. Be patient with irritating or annoying people.
3. Do something special for yourself – shout yourself a treat!

4. Express gratitude to others, especially your loved ones. It doesn't take much effort to thank someone that you care for.
5. Reach out and touch someone who needs comfort or support.
6. Focus intently on each moment.
7. Learn from your mistakes.
8. Write down your gripes or negative comments and put these away in a box.
9. Take a moment each day to look at nature, especially a tree or flower that you haven't noticed before.
10. SMILE and LAUGH!

Positive Affirmations

Positive affirmations make an impression on our subconscious minds to create a healthy, optimistic self-image, to bring about positive changes in our lives and to fulfil desires. Always have fun with affirmations, both when creating them and saying them. They can be written down, spoken out loud or said in your mind throughout the day. Follow these simple guidelines:

- Always phrase an affirmation in the present tense. Imagine that it has already come to fruition or that it has already occurred. That is, visualise having already attained your desired goal.
- Write down balanced goals and affirmations that provide not only personal meaning but pleasure.
- Imagine yourself really feeling what you are currently affirming.
- Always phrase the affirmation as a positive statement. Do not use the words 'not' or 'never' or 'can't' or 'cannot' or 'no'.
- Try to really feel the positive feelings and emotions that are generated by the affirmation.
- Keep the affirmation simple, short and sweet, but full of feeling and intensity. Be concrete and specific about what you desire.
- Be creative and have fun.
- Make the affirmation personal and relative to you and full of meaning.
- Don't expect these changes to occur instantly. Allow yourself time for these special gifts to unfold.
- Always have fun!

Below are some wonderful, positive affirmations, which can be used to increase levels of health and to help beat cancer. Try making your own affirmations and remember, always have fun with them.

- *I am growing healthier and healthier every day.*
- *I am full of vitality, health and energy.*
- *I am a radiant being, glowing with health.*
- *I am growing stronger and stronger every day.*
- *I am perfectly healthy and full of light.*
- *My cells are regenerating and rejuvenating every day.*
- *Cancer is now a distant memory.*

- *I am blessed with an abundance of energy.*
- *Love, joy and happiness flow through me with every heartbeat.*
- *I love life and life loves me.*
- *I am thankful to God for all of my Good Fortune.*
- *YES I CAN! I KNOW I CAN!*
- *I am full of health, life and overwhelming happiness.*
- *Good health and balance are my natural states of being.*
- *I am growing emotionally and spiritually, through the creative power of my thoughts.*
- *I direct my thoughts toward experiences of growth and expansion.*
- *I am radiating cheerfulness, joy and good health.*
- *I feel uplifted and encouraged.*
- *I fill my heart with peaceful courage.*
- *I am deeply relaxed and at ease.*
- *I am emotionally strong, unaffected by the emotional pull of others.*
- *I feel alive with vital energy.*
- *I know the source of universal love and healing within me.*
- *I am inspired to create practical realisation of my heartfelt dreams.*
- *I experience cleansing on all levels of my being.*
- *I cleanse myself of any toxicity and disharmonious energy.*
- *I feel clean, pure and harmonious.*
- *I feel my unity with all of life in a universe of abundance.*
- *I respond to life with understanding and compassion.*
- *I feel soothed in my mind and body.*
- *I accept the self-healing power within me.*
- *I receive nourishment from the life energy around and within me.*
- *I am a centre of knowing.*
- *I feel strong and energetic*
- *I am open to spiritual and psychic awareness.*
- *I am a unique and radiant individual.*
- *I am overflowing with health and happiness.*
- *I am protected from harm by the strength of my Inner Light.*
- *I am at peace within.*
- *I am creating a harmonious life by my thoughts and actions.*
- *I forgive others for past hurt.*
- *I release all feelings of blame and bitterness.*
- *COOL, CLEAR, CALM – This is one of my favourite affirmations and may be said at any time of the day or night. The simple use of these positive words enhances your subconscious mind with a feeling of peace and inner calm.*

Two of the best books available that contain affirmations are Louise Haye's 'You Can Heal your Life' and Shakti Gawain's 'The Power of Creative Visualization'.

Mood-altering Flowers – the Australian Bush Flower Remedies

Indigenous people have used flower essences all over the world for centuries. The Australian Aborigines have always used flower essences to restore emotional balance, as did the ancient Egyptians and African tribes. They were also extremely popular in the Middle Ages. Paracelsus in the fifteenth century wrote in scriptures how he collected dew from flowering plants and diluted it to treat emotional imbalances. Much of this natural healing knowledge has sadly been lost, although in some parts of the world healers and tribesmen have retained these skills.

Flower essences are used as catalysts to help unlock your full creative potential, attain emotional, spiritual, mental and physical balance, resolve negative beliefs and bring about a condition of harmony. Flower essences help to promote healing by releasing negative emotions and thought patterns. They enhance one's soul with positive feelings that are already inherent in our essence. When this occurs, negative beliefs and thoughts that may have caused or enhanced your illness are dissolved and balance is restored. Flower essences can assist in resolving distress and drama in one's life. They are also beneficial in maintaining positive attitudes and thought patterns necessary in overcoming cancer and other illnesses.

Australian plants possess an amazing strength, resilience and unique beauty, similar to the Australian landscape. There is abundant wisdom and timeless knowledge contained within nature and combined with the magnificent power of the land, this lends creation to the Australian Bush Flower Remedies. These remedies are useful for clearing emotional blocks that may stop a person from getting in touch with their true self and life purpose. They help to give clarity to one's life purpose yet also offer courage and strength to follow one's goals and dreams.

I have been using the Australian Bush Flower Remedies in my practice for many years. I am constantly amazed at the positive transformation power shown by the Bush Flower Remedies. Using flower essences will enhance your creativity, enthusiasm, confidence, strength and positive healing powers.

Table of Australian Bush Flower Remedies for Health and Happiness

Table 19.3

Flower Remedy	Negative Emotion	Positive Outcome	Comments
Banksia Robur or Swamp Banksia	Disheartened, lethargic, frustrated, low in energy	Enjoyment of life, enthusiasm, interest in life, higher energy levels	Treats temporary loss of drive and enthusiasm due to burnout, disappointment or frustration – for people who are normally very dynamic

Table 19.3 *continued*

Flower Remedy	Negative Emotion	Positive Outcome	Comments
Bauhinia	Resistance to change, rigidity, reluctance, hesitation to change	Acceptance, open mindedness, embracing new concepts and ideas	Great for older people who are very set in their ways
Billy Goat Plum	Shame, physical loathing, inability to accept physical self, self-disgust	Sexual pleasure and enjoyment, acceptance of self and one's physical body, open-mindedness	If you feel revolted and dirty about sex and feel unclean after. Feelings of revulsion about your own body.
Black Eyed Susan	Impatience, over-committed, constant striving	Ability to turn inward and be still, slowing down, inner peace	If you are continually rushing around and your life is overflowing with commitments, this helps you to slow down, find calmness and peace
Boronia	Obsessive thoughts, pining, broken hearted	Clarity, serenity, creative visualisation	Helps to resolve obsessions and leads to clarity and focus – enhances your focus for creative visualisation
Bottle Brush	Overwhelmed by major life changes	Serenity and calm, ability to cope and move on	Helps you to move through major life changes – is often only needed for one week
Bush Iris	Fear of death, physical excess, atheism, avarice, materialism	Awakening of spirituality, acceptance of death as a transition state, clearing blocks in trust centre	Opens your heart to spirituality, great for meditation
Crowea	Continual worrying, out of balance	Peace and calm, balances and centres the individual, clarity of one's feelings	This is great for worry and distress – this purple flower has five petals and five relates to emotional integration.
Dagger Hakea	Resentment, bitterness towards close family, friends, lovers	Forgiveness, open expression of feelings	For anyone who feels bitterness, resentment or holds grudges – this is an important step to self-healing

Table 19.3 *continued*

Flower Remedy	Negative Emotion	Positive Outcome	Comments
Dog Rose	Fearful, shy, insecure, niggling fears, nervous with other people	Confidence, belief in self-courage, ability to embrace life fully	Helps to overcome fears and increases the flow of vital force, quality of life and self-esteem
Fringed Violet	Damage to aura, distress, shock, grief, poor recuperation since trauma or shock	Removal of effects of recent or old distressing events, heals damaged aura	Acts to protect a person's psychic aura and remove effects of stressful events
Kapok Bush	Apathy, resignation, discouraged, half-hearted	Willingness, application, persistence, perception	If you are thinking about giving up on your treatment, use Kapok Bush to bring your outcome to fruition
Little Flannel Flower	Denial of the 'child' within, seriousness in children, grimness in adults	Carefree, playfulness, spontaneous joy	Great for people who are feeling sombre and serious – enhances playfulness, natural joy and spontaneity
Macrocarpa	Drained, jaded, worn out, low immunity	Renewed enthusiasm, inner strength and endurance, vitality, energy	This essence is great to overcome the draining effects of cancer treatment
Mountain Devil	Hatred, suspiciousness, holding grudges, anger	Unconditional love, happiness, forgiveness, healthy boundaries	Helps to deal with feelings of hatred, anger, jealousy and blocks to expressing love – great for suspicious people
Old Man Banksia	Weary, disheartened, frustrated, low energy	Enjoyment of life, renews enthusiasm, interest in life, energy	Brings a spark into those people's lives that are heavy and burdened
Paw Paw	Overwhelmed, unable to resolve problems, burdened by decisions	Good problem solving, assimilation of new ideas, calmness, clarity	Great for helping to solve problems – acts on the intuitive processes to provide solutions
Peach Flower Tea Tree	Mood swings, lack of commitment to follow through projects, easily bored	Ability to complete projects, take responsibility for one's health, emotional balance	This essence helps to develop stability, consistency, drive and commitment – great if you're considering giving up treatment

Table 19.3 *continued*

Flower Remedy	Negative Emotion	Positive Outcome	Comments
She Oak	Female imbalance, inability to conceive for non-physical reasons	Emotionally open to conceive, female balance, hormonal balance	Beneficial in overcoming imbalances and bringing about a sense of well being in females – the fruit of this tree is similar in size to a woman's ovary
Southern Cross	Feeling like a victim, complaining, bitter	Personal power, positiveness, taking responsibility	Great for people who feel they are victims, life is hard on them or they have been hard done by – helps to accept responsibility for actions
Spinifex	Sense of being a victim to illness, physical ailments	Empowers one through emotional understanding of illness, physical healing	For those who believe they have no control over their illness
Sturt's Desert Pea	Emotional pain, deep hurt, sadness	**Letting go, triggers healthy grieving, releases deep held grief and sadness**	**Treats deep hurts and sorrows – can bring about amazing changes in your life**
Sunshine Wattle	Stuck in the past, expectation of a grim future, struggling	Optimism, acceptance of the beauty and joy in the present, open to a bright future.	For people who have had a difficult time in their past and wish to feel excitement, optimism and happiness in the present
Tall Yellow Top	Alienation, loneliness, isolation	Sense of belonging, ability to reach out, acceptance of self and others	Needs to be used for 6 to 8 weeks without a break – beneficial for those who feel no connection or belonging with family, work, country etc.
Waratah	Hopelessness, inability to respond to a crisis	Courage, tenacity, strong faith, enhancement of survival skills, adaptability	For those in utter despair, gives strength and courage to get through a crisis

Table 19.3 *continued*

Flower Remedy	Negative Emotion	Positive Outcome	Comments
Wild Potato Bush	Weighed down, feeling encumbered, heavy	Freedom, ability to move on in life, renews enthusiasm	These people may feel burdened with their physical body – helps with feelings of physical restriction and limitation

Information supplied by the Australian Flower Remedy Society (founder – Ian White – Naturopath/Homeopath). The columns that are highlighted in bold refer to extremely good essences to use for cancer and cancer treatment.

Emotional Healing – Bach Flower Remedies

Bach Flower Remedies were discovered by the English physician, Edward Bach. His flower remedies, 38 in total, were discovered well over 50 years ago and are still widely used throughout the world today in the healing of many emotional problems. Edward Bach used essences from English plants and shrubs to restore vitality to the sick and ailing, so that the diseased person could overcome their worry, fear, depression or other emotional distress and restore health.

Bach flower remedies are prescribed according to the person's state of mind. A disharmonious state of mind limits and prevents the recovery of physical health and is, in many cases, primarily the cause of sickness and disease.

The remedies are prepared from the flowers of wild English plants, bushes or trees. A state of mental imbalance and distress depletes an individual's vitality, weakens the body's immune system and prevents a person from overcoming cancer. When emotional peace and harmony is restored in the mind, health and strength will return to the body.

Negative states of the mind which will lead to disease include, fear, uncertainty, insufficient interest in present circumstances, jealousy, hate, despondency or despair, over sensitivity to influences and ideas, loneliness and over-care for the welfare of others. Flower essences are completely safe to use and will not affect the use of any other type of medicine. These remedies are designed to raise your vibrations, uplift your spirits and give you the power to bring about your own healing. After all, you are your own best doctor!

Table of Bach Flower Remedies for Health and Happiness

Bach flower remedies (see Table 19.4) are most effective if used in conjunction with affirmations.

Table 19.4

Remedy	Negative aspects of the personality	Behavioural symptoms	Characteristic expressions	Positive outcomes
Centaury	Over-anxious to please, weak-willed, easily exploited, docile, timid, shy, lacks individuality, easily dominated, good nature taken for granted	Easily tired, lacks vitality, often pale and languid, dark rings under eyes, shoulder and back problems – may manifest illness to avoid saying 'no'	A 'yes' man always in agreement. Doormats, looks like a victim, head bowed, eyes cast down	Personal strength – still quiet and gentle, but maintains individuality knowing when to give and when to say NO; confident, not exploited by others
Elm	Temporary feelings of inadequacy, overwhelmed by responsibility, tired from temporarily being over burdened, feelings of not being able to cope or continue	Strong and fast, broad back and upright posture, solemn, serious looks confident, may suffer chronic stress and extreme exhaustion	For those in positions of importance who have others dependent on their decisions	Confident, self-assured, capable, able to take on great responsibility, knowing help will always be there when needed
Gorse	Utter hopelessness, great despair, belief that no change is possible, resigned, loss of will to improve the situation, soul depression, feels an inherited condition means suffering all life	Incurable, terminal or genetic illnesses, dark around the eyes, sallow complexion, hopeless expression, sits head in hands	'What's the point?' 'What's the use?' 'I know it will do no good, there's no point in trying,' beyond tears	Hope after a long series of failed setbacks, faith and certainty in overcoming difficulties, gives fight and strength, lifts the soul
Hornbeam	Weariness, temporary state of tiredness, mental or physical fatigue, doubts own strength to cope, general lassitude, wakes feeling tired	Yawning, sighing, sleepy, bored, desire to lie in bed in the morning, acute fever with temporary exhaustion	'I'm so tired', 'I've no energy', 'I'm too tired to think properly'	Energy, certainty, strength, fortifies mentally and physically, encourages effort, helps believe in own ability and strength, even if the task is formidable

Oak	Incessant effort, plodding on, struggling and persevering against all odds, not giving in but despondency and despair through lack of progress, brave without loss of hope, shattered when strength suddenly goes	Strong, rigid in body, head held high, chest raised, tight lips, heart problems, nervous breakdowns and collapse	'I must be strong', 'I won't give in', 'I must keep going at all costs'	Courage – able to fight against the odds without losing hope and despairing, persevering, reliable, strong and stable
Olive	Exhaustion after long-term stress and suffering, total fatigue – mind and body drained of strength, mental fatigue, weakness, lack of interest, unhappiness, no pleasure in life, too tired to eat, no vitality	Needs a lot of sleep, crying, sighing, anguish shows on face, facial and shoulder tension, crying and collapsing after effort, over-reacting to pain	'I feel utterly exhausted', 'I'm so exhausted, I can't carry on another minute'	Strengthening with peace of mind, calmness, becomes interested in life, vital and strong, trusts life and gives strength to help overcome difficulties.
Pine	Guilt, self-reproach, blames self, feels unworthy, constantly apologising, sets high standards for themselves, feels undeserving of love, despondent, takes blame for mistakes of others	Headaches, Tiredness, Clinging, eyes downcast, hands covering mouth, suicidal	'I'm sorry', 'No, its my fault', 'I'm stupid, aren't I', 'If only I'd...', 'I feel worthless', 'I could have done better'	Realisation of self-worth, perseverance, self-assurance, ability to take responsibility, does not dwell on past mistakes
Star of Bethlehem	After-effects of Trauma – shock, sorrow, grief, numbness, refuses to be consoled, withdrawal, despondency, delayed shock, past or present; for all kinds of shock	Use before and after surgery, and for symptoms such as shaky coldness, rigidity of body, concussion, dilated pupils	For the accident or shock victim who says 'I'm alright,' then falls apart shortly after	Re-integration, calmness and clarity, ability to move on without being affected by the distress of the past – picking up the pieces

Table 19.4 continued

Remedy	Negative aspects of the personality	Behavioural symptoms	Characteristic expressions	Positive outcomes
Wild Rose	Apathy, resignation, gloom, lack of ambition, of vitality, interest and effort, cannot be bothered, loss of will to fight back, resist change, willing to give up struggle, inner collapse	Weakness, weariness, dull, pale, passive, accepting smile on face, monotonous voice, slumped shoulders, early senility	'It's inevitable', 'Well, its bound to happen', 'Well, that's life', 'I can't be bothered'	Involvement, vitality, lively interest in life, enjoyment of friends, happy, involved, enjoys making an effort
Willow	Resentment, bitterness and self pitying, feels victim of fate, focuses on negative side, complaining, unresolved suffering, irritable, sulky, loss of interest in life, blames others	Frowning, tense, eyes narrowed, chin thrust forward, migraines, backache	'It's not fair', 'It's not my fault', 'Why me, why is this happening to me?' 'poor me' attitude	Optimism, understanding and recognition of own responsibilities, ceases blaming others – takes responsibility for own fate

Laugh Away the Tears

Laughter is one of my favourite areas to explore! When I was growing up I was famous in my neighbourhood for my infectious giggle that charmed those around me to join in with fits of laughter. Now that I think about it, I'm not quite sure if they were laughing with me or at me. Never mind, at least my laughter could provoke others to laugh, and that's a good thing. As you grow up, you get so caught up in the seriousness of life that you forget the wonder and child-like innocence of laughter and it seems to flow less spontaneously than when you were a child.

Laughter is one of the easiest and most important methods used to enhance healing and well-being. Giggling for whatever reason uplifts the spirit and soul, and provides an array of positive health benefits and rejuvenating qualities.

Regular laughter vibrates the entire body and sends joyous sounds to the rest of the world. The joy and humour provoked by laugher relieves boredom, tension, guilt, depression and anger. Laughter is light-hearted; it frees depression and resentment from the heart! It is impossible to be depressed when you are laughing. Laughter stimulates the brain to produce hormones that trigger the release of endorphins. Endorphins are natural opiates or happy chemicals that decrease pain and discomfort and make you feel great.

To overcome cancer it is important to love who and what you are, and to love what you do. Laugh at yourself and at silly situations in everyday life and nothing can ever touch you or affect your health. Life is temporary anyway; everything changes, life and its events are not permanent, this is the only thing which is guaranteed. So why worry, when you can laugh? Norman Cousins is a man who is famous for curing himself of a fatal disease with laughter. He has written books on the healing properties and uplifting benefits of laughter and I recommend reading them.

Life is fun, it can be a game, and it can be a joy! It's all up to you! The sooner you can laugh at your problems, the faster you will be able to let them go. You will feel lighter, happier and full of joy. Laughing spontaneously and having fun in life will take many years off your physical and biological age. In fact, laughter is a major key to 'longevity'.

If your mind is filled with negative thoughts, old resentments, fears, anger, sadness and pain, then there is no room left for love and joy to flow freely and lighten your life. Laughter cannot flow freely if it is not allowed to be free and childlike. Learn to let go of negative emotions and allow the free flow of positive feelings and thoughts to emerge. Do whatever you can to make your transformational change a joy and pleasure. Have fun and laugh as much as you can. When was the last time you had a good 'belly laugh' like when you were a child? Why not today? Laugh yourself to better health, wealth and happiness!

'The Good Guys Vs the Bad Guys' – Negative Ions Vs Positive Ions

Beautiful environments tend to have a positive effect on our general health and well-being. Apart from being physically stimulating to our senses, certain environments also contain particles known as ions that can have either a beneficial or detrimental effect on our physical and emotional health, depending on the type and amount of ions circulating in the air.

Ions are electrically charged particles. They can be either positive or negative and are the result of natural radiation from the sun, earth, water, lightning and other atmospheric energy sources. Negative ions are formed when an electron becomes attached to an oxygen molecule. They have the ability to refresh and revitalise the air. Positive ions have the opposite effect, making you feel tired and dull.

The effects of cosmic rays, solar radiation and radioactive substances in soil such as radon and thoron, all produce ions directly or by striking the molecules of atmosphere and gas, causing them to lose or gain electrons and thus the molecules become positive or negative. Natural air sprays and waterfalls in particular generate negative ion production (the 'good guys').

Both positive and negative ions can exist together in the air because they are separated by a large number of molecules. Ions have an effect on physical, pathological and emotional processes. Biologically, ions can affect the stimulation of endocrine glands, the production of enzymes, neuro-hormones on the brain, hormone balance in the body, circulation and micro-organisms.

Negative ions stimulate the growth of plants. They have a beneficial effect on reproduction and a beneficial effect in the treatment of diseases commonly caused from air that is positively ionized, such as hot dry winds. Think back to how you feel on certain days. Imagine a hot, northerly wind blowing through your town. Does this ever make you feel irritable or anxious? This is because this wind is blowing in positive ions (the 'bad guys').

Now imagine a fresh, cool, south-easterly wind blowing into your town from across the expansive ocean. This wind is blowing in the negative ions (the 'good guys'). This is why this type of weather makes you feel energised, fresh and alive. The weather can have a positive or negative effect on our emotions and physical health depending on what type of energy or ions it is offering us.

The paving of streets, air conditioned or heated homes or offices, and air trapped in well insulated buildings all inhibit or destroy negative ions. Negative ions (the good guys) have the following beneficial effects:

- A small amount of ozone is produced, cleansing the environment.
- Enhanced physical, emotional and mental well-being.
- Increased general health, improved appetite, better circulation and a more peaceful sleep is attained.
- An improved, strong antibiotic effect and enhanced tissue repair.
- Pain relief.
- Happier and more balanced emotions
- Clearer thinking and motivation and increased positivity
- An overall balanced effect on our internal body processes

Feng shui, the ancient Chinese art of balancing your environment and surroundings, uses negative ion energy to create a positive, flowing and uplifting environment.

We tend to feel happy and more invigorated when on the beach, close to the ocean, walking in nature, in the mountains, in the snow, at a waterfall, in the desert or any other beautiful, natural place. This is largely due to the presence of negative ions in the atmosphere and a lack of positive ions.

Any environment or surrounding with negative ions has the ability to enhance healing, prevent illness and invigorate and enliven the spirit, body and emotions. No wonder so many health resorts designed to rejuvenate individuals are located near the ocean, in the mountains or close to a waterfall. Go and have a cool dip in a waterfall or a quick splash in the ocean today and feel the beautiful healing harmony of being surrounded in a negatively charged ion environment.

Chapter 20

THE IMMUNE SYSTEM AND CANCER

How Does it All Work?

The immune system is one of the most complex and amazing systems in the human body. Its primary role is to protect the body against infection and prevent the development of disease and cancer. It is designed to isolate or destroy cancerous cells, which exist in each person's body from time to time. Suppression of the body's immune system over a long period of time can result in cancerous growths.

Support and enhancement of the body's immune system is one of the most important keys in achieving resistance to disease and preventing and treating cancer. It is our first line of defence against tumour formation and cancer development.

The immune system is composed of lymphatic vessels and organs (lymph nodes, thymus, spleen, adenoids, appendix and tonsils), bone marrow, white blood cells (neutrophils, eosinophils, basophils, lymphocytes, monocytes, phagocytes), specialised cells residing in various tissues (macrophages, mast cells etc.) and specialised chemical factors. Following is a basic description of the immune system's important components:

Lymphatic System – Lymph, Lymphatic Vessels, Lymphatic Tissue and Lymph Nodes

The lymphatic system produces white blood cells that fight disease and help the body to detoxify wastes. The space in between the cells is called the interstitium and the fluid contained within these spaces is called the interstitial fluid. This fluid flows into the lymphatic vessels and becomes the lymph – the fluid that flows through the body in lymphatic vessels. Lymphatic vessels transport lymphocytes and lymph around the body and drain waste products from the tissues. The lymphatic vessels transport the lymph to the lymph nodes, which filter the lymph. The lymph nodes serve two functions:

1. They remove foreign materials from lymph fluid before it enters the blood stream.
2. They are centres for the production of immune cells, particularly lymphocytes.

The cells responsible for filtering the lymph are called macrophages. These cells engulf and destroy foreign bacteria, old red blood cells and cellular debris. The lymph nodes also contain B-lymphocytes, the white blood cells that initiate antibody production in response to disease producing organisms.

We should consider our body's lymph system as the 'rubbish removal' company. Put simply, the macrophages are the 'garbage workers' that collect and break down the wastes and employ other staff to make your internal city clean and disease free, the lymphatic vessels are the body's 'rubbish removal highways' and the lymph nodes are 'the garbage sorting dumps that remove the bad rubbish, keeps the goodies found in the rubbish and act as the hub for garbage workers (immune cells) waiting for a suitable job in the body's rubbish removal company'.

Adenoids
The adenoids are an organ of the immune system that is found at the rear of the nose. It is made up primarily of lymphatic tissue. B-Lymphocytes are stored here in preparation to attack antigens (the enemy).

Appendix
The appendix is made up mostly of lymphatic tissue and helps the immune system by beginning some defence actions.

The Thymus Gland

The thymus is the major gland or the 'maestro' of the immune system. It is one of the major sites for immune cell production. It lies just below the thyroid gland and above the heart. The thymus is responsible for the production of T-lymphocytes and for providing the commands to these cells regarding which enemies to attack. The thymus gland releases several hormones that are responsible for regulating many immune functions. A low level of thymic hormones in the blood is associated with depressed immunity. Thymic hormone levels are low in people with cancer. The thymus gland tends to shrink as we age and in response to nutrient deficiencies.

The Spleen

The spleen is roughly the size of a clenched fist. It is responsible for producing white blood cells, engulfing and destroying bacteria and cellular debris, destroying worn-out red blood cells and platelets, for coordinating the interaction between macrophages, antibodies, T-Lymphocytes and B-Lymphocytes and acting as a blood reservoir. The spleen also releases many potent immune system-enhancing compounds.

White Blood Cells (WBCs) – Lymphocytes

There are several types of white blood cells. WBCs defend the body's health. It has 2 main lines of defense, T-cells and B-cells. The function of WBCs are listed below:

Neutrophils
These cells can act as phagocytes activating phagocytosis – engulf and destroy bacteria, tumour cells and dead cell matter. Important in preventing bacterial infection. They

are stored in the bone marrow and make up 65 per cent of the body's white blood cells.

Eosinophils and Basophils

These cells secrete histamine and other inflammatory compounds designed to break down antigen-antibody complexes, but they also promote allergic mechanisms.

Lymphocytes

There are several types of lymphocytes. Lymphocytes help our body to defend against disease. These include T cells, B cells and natural killer cells. T Cells are the major component of cell-mediated immunity. Cell-mediated immunity refers to immune mechanisms not controlled by antibodies. It is important in the resistance of infection. T cells attack cancer cells and viruses. There are different types of T cells including helper T cells, suppressor T cells and cytotoxic T cells.

Helper T Cells

Helper T cells are the commanders of the immune army, which help other white blood cells to function and rouse other defender cells into motion. **Suppressor T cells** inhibit white blood cell functions in order to prevent overproduction thereby maintaining the immune system's delicate balance and **cytotoxic T cells** are the soldiers of the immune army who attack and destroy foreign tissue and cancer cells.

B Cells

Produce antibodies, large protein molecules that bind to antigens (molecules the body recognises as foreign). The antibody ultimately destroys the infectious organism or tumour cell.

Natural Killer Cells (NK)

Natural killer cells destroy cells that have become cancerous or infected with viruses. They are the body's first line of defence against cancer development. They act independently and do not need to be stimulated into action. People with cancer often have very low levels of natural killer cells in their blood.

Monocytes

These are the garbage collectors of the body. They change to macrophages and act as phagocytes. Monocytes trigger many immune responses and clean up cellular debris after infection. They have the ability to engulf and ingest infecting microbes, tumour cells, foreign debris and any other matter that needs recycling.

Special Tissue Cells

Macrophages

These large cells, found in the liver, spleen and lymph, engulf foreign particles and protect against invasion by micro-organisms and damage to the lymphatic system. Macrophages are the 'clever gobblers of the immune army'. They engulf a foreign agent and highlight their antibodies so the helper T cell can quickly identify the invaders. After marking the enemy cell, macrophages release lymphokines (interferon, interleukin-3 and 1) that attract more macrophages and WBCs to eliminate the invading threat.

Mast Cells

These are basophils that reside mainly along blood vessels and release histamine in response to allergic reactions.

Platelets

In addition to their role in clotting, platelets attract white blood cells to sites of injury.

Specialised Serum Factors/Lymphokines/Monokines

Interferon, interleukin 2 and complement fractions enhance the immune system, produced by white blood cells. These serum factors activate white blood cells to destroy cancer cells and viruses. Complement fractions are produced in the liver and involved in the final destruction of viruses, bacteria, immune complexes and cancer cells.

Antibodies

Antibodies or serum proteins known as immunoglobulins (Ig) serve as the primary cellular secretions of the humoral branch of the immune system. These B cell lymphocytes fall into the following categories:

IgG –   main serum protein, coats micro-organisms leaving them open to destruction.
IgA –   found in secretions such as milk, saliva and tears. Stops localised infections from spreading.
IgM –   Initial immune response to foreign invaders.
IgE –   These bind tightly to mast cells and basophils and are involved in allergic reactions.

Weak Links in the Immune System

Our body's immune system regularly battles foreign invaders and cancerous cells everyday, isolating or destroying these toxins so that they can do no harm. However, the immune system can become weak or depressed due to a number of dietary, psychological, environmental and physical factors. This can ultimately set up the pathway for the growth of cancer, as cancer not only requires abnormal cells to exist, it also needs the right environment, 'a suppression of the body's immune system' to grow. Factors that may suppress immunity include:

Diet

Nutrient deficiency is without question the most frequent cause of a depressed immune system. Lack of protein has a severe effect on cell-mediated immunity. Adequate protein is optimal for good immune system function. A high sugar intake decreases the ability of white blood cells to destroy foreign particles. Excess sugar, fat and calories as well as singular or multiple nutritional deficiencies all have a marked effect on our immune system. Zinc, in particular, is an extremely important mineral needed for strong immunity and a deficiency of this mineral will present in the form of lowered immunity.

Man-made Electromagnetic Frequencies

Computer terminals, power lines, video terminals, electric blankets, electric razors and waterbed heaters all have a depressive effect on the body's immune system.

Emotional State

When we are depressed, lonely, sad or grieving, our immune system also becomes depressed. The more significant the emotion is and how deeply we feel this indicates how strongly the immune system becomes affected. The link between the body and mind should never be underestimated.

Lack of Exercise

Exercise has been shown to cause a variety of improved immune functions and health benefits.

Obesity

The white blood cells of overweight people are less capable of destroying bacteria viruses and tumour cells.

Smoking, Alcohol and Other Stimulants

Alcohol decreases the function and efficiency of white blood cells and natural killer cell activity, particularly after direct consumption. Regular high intake of alcohol has a depressive effect on the body's immune system and increases the risk of cancer. Nicotine and other stimulants such as caffeine and recreational drugs weaken the body's immune system. Marijuana and amphetamine use diminishes macrophage and natural killer cell activity and impairs interferon production and cytotoxic T cells.

Stress

Stress has perhaps the greatest negative influence on the body's immune system. It has the ability to reduce lymphocyte production, diminish lymphocyte count, reduces the body's ability to produce interferon and decreases macrophage function. Secretions of adrenaline and cortisol from the body's adrenal glands affect many functions, including the ability of macrophages to scavenge lipids from arteries. They also decrease production of the antibody IgA, necessary in building the body's resistance to infections.

Stress can result from negative events like divorce, marital separation, death or illness of a family member, trouble at work and other reasons. Stress can also result from positive events like marriage, retirement, pregnancy, a new family member, career change, graduation from school and vacations. The degree of change in one's life – whether negative or positive – and how we deal with this seems to determine the level of stress we feel and the degree of our susceptibility to illness.

***

Other factors which may decrease immune system function include a lack of sleep, lack of sunlight, long-term living in air-conditioning and central heating, lack of exercise and excessive exercise, lack of fresh air and a low fluid intake.

Supporting the Immune System

Supporting the immune system is critical to good health. Here are some suggestions to boost immune system function and prevent cancer and other illnesses:

Acupuncture
Enhances many immune functions and may increase the number of T cells, lympho-cytes, natural killer cell activity, B cells and phagocytic activity. It also has a very harmonising effect on emotional and physical well-being.

Balanced Emotional State
The most important factor that stimulates and supports our body's immune function is a positive and balanced emotional state. This can be attained through a number of methods including playing with pets or children, laughing, having fun, doing what you love, skilled relaxation, positive affirmations, visualisations or imagery, giving yourself a treat, getting adequate rest and exercise, achieving goals and enjoying life.

Diet
Diet is a very important tool in supporting the health of the body's immune system. Avoid foods rich in sugar, white flour products, artificial and processed foods, satu-rated fats, caffeine, nicotine, excessive red meat intake and full fat dairy products. These devitalised foods rob the body of valuable and key nutrients required for optimal immune system function.

Try to eat more immune system-stimulating foods such as onions, garlic, ginger, bitter melon, whole grains, legumes, fish, salmon, tuna, mackerel, sardines, nuts and seeds, sprouts, dark green leafy vegetables and fruits. Eat plenty of orange, yellow and green vegetables to enhance immune system responses. Eat adequate levels of protein to maintain good immune system function and tissue repair. Variety is the key to obtaining adequate levels of life-giving nutrients from foods.

Environment
Living in clean environments with good fresh air circulation is important to health. Beautiful environments like the beach, ocean, waterfalls, mountains and deserts have high amounts of negative ions in the air, which promote a healthy immune system function and uplift emotions.

Exercise
The immune system is greatly influenced by regular exercise. The endorphins and enkephalins released by exercise make you feel wonderful and uplifted. Remember that excessive exercise can have the reverse effect and diminish immune response.

Fasting/Cleansing

Regular detoxification increases immune response, gives the immune system a chance to repair, heals damage and prolongs life. Fasting rapidly builds lost energy levels.

Herbal Medicines and Neutraceuticals

A number of herbs stimulate the immune system in a variety of ways. These include pau d'arco, echinacea, ginsengs, licorice root, burdock root, astragalus, osha, mistletoe, lomatium and many others. Their benefits include macrophage stimulation, increased phagocytosis, increased natural killer cell counts, increased interferon and increased lymphocyte production.

Neutraceuticals are a new range of healing medicines such as lactoferrin, glucans, alkyglycerols (human milk, shark liver oil), shark cartilage, bovine cartilage and transfer factors. These are natural products that are powerful immune system boosters derived from nature.

Homeopathy

Homeopathy can be used effectively in the treatment of immune depression and emotional rebalancing. It is a subtle, yet very powerful healing modality.

Hydrotherapy

Alternating hot and cold showers or applications of hot and cold compresses mobilise white blood cells to effectively combat localised infection. Hydrotherapy stimulates general resistance and vitality. There are many different forms of hydrotherapy that can be used.

Laughter

Try to cultivate a good sense of humour, have fun and laugh often. Laughter has an anti-stress effect on the body. It can lower serum cortisol and adrenaline, and ease the body's stress response and preserve immune function. Smile and laugh more often.

Magnetic Induction Therapy

Using magnetic induction devices at the correct low frequencies benefits the health of the entire body. Magnetic Field Therapy has a positive effect on cancer, emotional illnesses and immune system deficiency. (Refer to Chapter 31 – Magnetism).

Medicinal Mushrooms

Shitake, reishi, maitake, cordyceps and ganoderma to name a few mushrooms, have the ability to stimulate the production of interferon and white blood cells and provide many other positive immune system effects. These ancient medicinal mushrooms are extremely powerful immune system boosters.

Nutrients

Specific nutrients are very important in maintaining adequate functioning of all levels of the immune system. If one single nutrient is lacking in the body, the immune function can dramatically become depressed. It is important to maintain good levels of beta-carotene, vitamin A, vitamin C, vitamin E, zinc, vitamin B6 and other antioxidants. Coenzyme Q10, lipoic acid, N. Acetyl cysteine, germanium, selenium and bioflavonoids have immune system-boosting effects.

Antioxidants are vital for maintaining optimal immune system function as they act to prevent free radical damage to immune cells and the thymus gland. Recent clinical trials have found that antioxidants can significantly improve immune response, including increasing the activation of cells involved in tumour immunity.

Lactobacillus Bulgarius, a common bacterial culture from yogurt, has been used to stimulate T-lymphocyte production and anti-tumour activity of macrophages, thereby enhancing the function of the immune system.

Ozone Therapy
Supersaturating oxygen in the blood oxidizes foreign agents, improving immunity. Liquid oxygen is available from health food stores.

Pets
The human/animal bond is emotional in nature. Given that emotions and neurotransmitters are linked, our pets may help to maintain or enhance our immune system's strength. Pets teach us the magic of 'unconditional love' and provide us with a wonderful stress release. If we are stress-free emotionally, we remain stress-free physically. After all, we can talk to our pets all day long and get all of our worries off our mind. Can you think of an simpler way to release your stresses and improve your physical health?

Relaxation/Meditation
Meditation or placing ourselves in a relaxed state brings about a sense of calm, peace and serenity, and hence has a positive effect on immune function. Visualising positive outcomes and good health sets up a plan for the subconscious mind to carry out these desires and wishes.

Sleep
Get adequate sleep. The hours slept before midnight are twice as beneficial as the hours slept after midnight. Go to bed early. Sleep is a revitalising nutrient that enhances immune system function and provides resistance to infections.

Sunlight
Sunlight is extremely important in enhancing immune system function and having a positive effect on moods and emotions.

Thymus Gland Tapping
Tapping or gently pounding on your thymus gland daily stimulates the release of white blood cells and improves thymus gland health and function.

Touching and Being Touched
As humans we need to feel accepted and loved. Touch in whatever form, whether it be a kiss, a hug, a gentle touch or holding hands, enhances the psychoneurological phenomena that support immune system function.

Table of Immune Enhancement Nutrients

Vitamin and mineral supplements can play a significant role in maintenance and support of immune function. The following table shows a list of important vitamin and mineral supplements.

Table 20.1

Nutrient	Action
Betacarotene – 15 – 30 mg/day	Stimulates the production and number of immune cells such as B, T, lymphocytes and natural killer cells, increases the size of the body's thymus gland
Bioflavonoids – 250 – 500mg/day	Bioflavonoids are good scavengers of free radicals, they stabilize mast cells, they can dampen inflammatory responses and they decrease leukotriene formation
Biotin – 500 mcg/day	Biotin deficiency also affects the immune system by decreased number and reduced function of white blood cells
Calcium 600 – 1000mg/day	Has been shown to improve immune function
Co-enzyme Q10 – 100 – 300mg/day	Acts as a cellular antioxidant, protects cells from oxidative stress
Essential Fatty Acids 1000 – 2000mg/day (e.g. DHA/EPA, flaxseed oil, fish oils, omega 3s	Studies on the immune T cells in cancer patients suggest that omega 3 fatty acids have beneficial affects on immune function
Folic acid – 400 to 800mcg/day	May prevent abnormal cells from becoming cancerous
Glutathione – 100mg/day Glutamine – 1 to 4 g/day	Thought to strengthen the immune system protect cells from free radicals, removes toxins and heavy metals, growth of immune system cells and aids in cell metabolism.
Iron – 10 – 20mg/day	Immune cells rely on iron to generate oxidative reactions that allow these cells to kill off bacteria and other pathogens
Lipoic acid – 100mg/day	A powerful scavenger of free radicals. It also maintains the effectiveness of vitamins C, E, CoQ10 and glutathione
Magnesium 300 – 600mg/day	Improves cellular metabolism and energy production, improves immune competence, particularly the removal of transformed cells
Manganese – 5 – 10mg/day	Protects the mitochondria from free radical damage
N. Acetyl Cysteine (NAC) – 100mg/day	Has been shown to fight bacteria, protects immune cells while they kill microbes

Table 20.1 *continued*

Nutrient	Action
Nicotinamide adenine dinucleotide (Activated B3) – 50 – 100mg/day	Directly involved in the cellular immune system by increasing the phagocytic capacity of leukocytes
Pycnogenol – 50mg/day	Contains catechins that have strong free radical fighters, also has anti-cancer effects
Pyridoxal-5-Phosphate (Vitamin B6) – 50 mg/day	Important role in cell multiplication and antibody production
Riboflavin (Vitamin B2) – 25 – 50mg/day	Is instrumental in cell respiration, helping each cell utilise oxygen
Selenium – 50mcg/day	Selenium has important relationships with betacarotene, vitamin C and E – also has immune stimulating properties and helps to protect the reproductive organs
Thiamine (Vitamin B1) – 50mg/day	Has a key role in the cellular production of energy
Thymus Extracts	Boosts and re-regulates thymus gland function
Vitamin A – 10,000 IU/day (the safest form of Vitamin A to use is beta-carotene or alpha-carotene)	Vital for the development of the body's barriers to infection, stimulates and enhances immune function
Vitamin B12 – 200 mcg/day	Vitamin B12 deficiency leads to reduced numbers of white blood cells, which causes increased susceptibility to infection
Vitamin C – 2 – 10 grams/day	Critical to immune function as it is involved in antibody production and white blood cell function and activity – vitamin C requirements increase when the body is under stress, increases the size of the thymus gland
Vitamin D – 400 IU/day	Involved in the regulation of the immune system, in particular, monocytes
Vitamin E – 400 – 800 IU/day	Protects the thymus gland and circulating white blood cells from damage – particularly important in protecting the immune system from damage during times of oxidative stress
Zinc – 45 – 80mg/day	Considered one of the most important nutrients for the immune system, as it is necessary for healthy antibody, white blood cell, thymus gland and hormone function (low zinc levels can cause the thymus gland to shrink).

Chapter 21

BACK TO OUR ORIGINS – DIET IS THE ANSWER

How Important Are Organics?

A balanced diet and moderate consumption of healthy foods without regular overeating are the most important components of a healthy diet, especially on a long-term basis. Other aspects, such as eating organically produced foods, are important in the fine tuning of our diet and perhaps to avoid conditions/diseases related to the ingestion of pesticides, and other chemicals and toxins.

Nowadays, fruits, vegetables, meats and grains are produced relatively quickly to allow for the increased demands of a growing population. To do this, most farmers use pesticides, hormones and special chemicals to speed up the overall production process, and keep their crops and livestock in the best looking condition possible. This also allows for a higher per centage of sales, but what about you as a consumer? As a consumer you may be unaware of the long-term harmful effects these chemicals may cause. Conditions such as cancer, asthma and chronic bronchitis have been linked to deadly chemicals produced from crops and meats.

Chickens are a good example of this intensive farming process. They are cruelly kept in tiny little cages and injected with large amounts of antibiotics and hormones to rapidly increase their growth rate. A little chick grows from being a baby to an oversized chicken in less than six weeks due to the use of harmful antibiotics and growth hormones placed in their feed, and injected into their bodies. Where do you think these chemicals go?

These chemicals do not evaporate into thin air. When you buy these chickens from supermarkets and chicken shops, you are exposing your children to the effects of harmful antibiotics and growth hormones. In my naturopathy practice I have been able to see the effects that excess intake of poultry has on the health of my clients. Women and men often present with conditions such as infertility, candida, emotional and hormonal imbalance, menstrual problems and other similar health conditions related to excess hormone and antibiotic intake. By simply avoiding these hormonally treated meats and using free-range poultry instead, many of my clients have returned to good health. In fact, two of my female clients who were unable to fall pregnant, conceived after simply removing hormonally treated meats from their diet and replacing these with free-range and organic produce.

It is a much safer choice in our society today to try to purchase organic produce. What this means is that the crops and meats have reached the market without the use of any chemicals. The soils have a good amount of nutrients and minerals, allowing you to get a greater value of nutrients from organic produce. Try to avoid chemical additives and chemically treated foods. Instead purchase organically grown produce, which provides ten times as much nutrition as its comparative chemically sprayed produce and allows you to avoid any harmful side effects associated with the use of pesticides, chemicals, antibiotics and growth hormones.

Cancer Dietary Guidelines

As you have read in previous chapters of this book, nutritional support is essential to feed your immune system, to beat cancer and to give you the strength to better tolerate cancer treatments. Eating a wholefoods diet composed of fresh fruits and vegetables will provide important vitamins, minerals and fibre necessary to reduce tumour size and eradicate unwanted cancer cells. Certain foods provide specific cancer-fighting biochemicals, called phytochemicals.

I found diet to be one of the most important supporting therapies available to me in my fight against cancer. Not only did it decrease my tumour size very rapidly, but also provided the right nutrients to maintain good energy levels, balanced emotions and prevented a variety of side effects caused from orthodox medical treatment. Follow the dietary recommendations listed below to prevent and conquer cancer, and to support your body's immune system:

- Remove all refined, processed and devitalised foods from your diet. For example, aged, bruised, mouldy and deep-fried foods. Remove foods with additives, colours, flavours, white flour products, low/no nutrient foods and sugar-rich foods. Be aware of the effects of certain preservatives and colourings found in foods.
- Reduce or avoid the intake of foods that contain natural carcinogens such as smoked, pickled or barbecued foods. Avoid foods that contain artificial sweeteners such as saccharin, artificial colours, nitrates and nitrites.
- Reduce or avoid fat and deep fried foods – a high intake of these foods has been linked to breast, colon, ovarian and prostate cancers. A low-fat diet is thought to slow the spread of non-melanoma skin cancers. Always use olive oil in your cooking and flaxseed oil on your salads. Use avocado instead of margarine.
- Avoid tea and coffee. Tea (over three cups/day) depletes the body of zinc and iron. Coffee (over two cups/day) depletes adrenal gland function and congests the body's liver. Use herbal teas as an alternative. Specific herbal teas used to fight cancer include red clover tea, pau d'arco tea, astragalus tea, dandelion tea, echinacea tea, essiac tea and green tea. Green tea contains polyphenols which stop the enzymes of cancer-producing substances. Chapharral tea is believed to have potent anti-tumour properties (use in moderation under professional guidance).
- Avoid alcohol, cigarette smoke and drugs.
- If you are in an occupation where you are exposed to chemicals or man-made

electromagnetic frequencies, for example, farmers working with pesticides, miners and plastic makers in factories etc. try to avoid. If you cannot leave this occupation, take plenty of antioxidants and glutathione to detoxify heavy metals.

- Try to buy organic produce. Avoid all hormonally treated meats such as poultry and beef. Try to buy free range poultry, eggs and grain fed meats.
- Avoid irradiated foods and pesticide sprayed foods.
- Do not consume peanuts, junk foods, soft drinks, salt and sugar. Instead of salt use kelp, sea salt or a natural salt substitute.
- Try to avoid most yeast foods such as Vegemite, Promite and yeast powders.
- Limit your consumption of full fat dairy products. A small amount of natural acidophilus yogurt, ricotta cheese and cottage cheese is recommended. Fermented foods that contain lactobacillus acidophilus such as yogurt are essential to good digestive health. Sauerkraut is also very good. Soy milk is beneficial as it contains a compound called genistein, which is believed to inhibit oestrogen and hormonally sensitive tumours, particularly breast tumours.
- Foods to be eaten in high amounts include broccoli, soybeans, shitake mushrooms, mung beans, red dates, lentils, olives, organic citrus peel, sesame seeds, almonds, parsley and seaweeds.
- Eat five to six small meals per day to keep blood sugar levels balanced and to allow for plenty of nutrient-rich variety in your diet.
- Eat plenty of vegetables rich in phytochemicals. Eat more garlic, collards, onions, leeks, shallots, chives, broccoli, cabbage, kale, spinach, eggplant, lettuce, mustard greens, capsicum, cauliflower and green beans. These act as antioxidants, inhibit and treat cancer, and trigger the formation of glutathione S-transferase, an important enzyme involved in protecting a cell's DNA from carcinogens. This further prevents cells from turning cancerous. Brussels sprouts contain a compound that is believed to protect against breast, lung and bowel cancer.
- Consume plenty of yellow and deep orange vegetables such as carrots, apricots, sweet potatoes, papaya, pumpkin, squash and yams. Apples, berries, brazil nuts, cantaloupes, cherries, blueberries, blackberries, tangerines, grapes, ginger, legumes (including chickpeas and red beans) and plums all help to fight cancer. Berries, particularly raspberries, protect against DNA damage. Cherries help to induce tumour cell death. Eat more bananas, avocados, pineapple, wheat germ, mango and pawpaw, which are good sources of live enzymes.
- Support a healthy digestive function by supplementing your diet with apple cider vinegar with meals or with digestive enzymes.
- Eat plenty of watermelon, tomato paste, sun-dried tomatoes, tomatoes and pink grapefruit – these foods contain lycopene to protect against breast and prostate cancers.
- Eat plenty of garlic, onions, ginger and turmeric to boost immune system function. Try to eat two to three cloves of garlic per day.
- Eat plenty of medicinal mushrooms i.e. shitake, reishi, maitake and button mushrooms. These little wonders strengthen immunity and prevent cancer.
- Eat a diet rich in grains, nuts, seeds and unpolished brown rice. Millet cereal is a good source of protein and an alkaline grain. Include oats in your diet.

- Eat 10 raw almonds a day. They contain laetrile, a substance that contains anti-cancer properties. I often eat a small handful of nuts mid-morning and mid-afternoon – containing almonds, brazils, pumpkin seeds and sunflower seeds.
- Try to drink spring or distilled water, not tap water. Eight to 10 glasses of water every day is considered optimal, as this helps to detoxify the body of harmful chemicals.
- Use blackstrap molasses, brown rice syrup, manuka honey, stevia or pure maple syrup as a natural sweetener instead of sugar.
- Eat whole wheat, sour dough, yeast-free bread or rye bread and flour, instead of white bread and white pastries. White flour products are lacking in fibre and contain limited nutritional value.
- Cook all sprouts lightly (except for alfalfa sprouts) which should be eaten raw.
- Drink plenty of juices (four to six glasses/day) particularly beet juice, carrot juice, green juices, cabbage juice, pineapple juice, lettuce juice and watermelon juice. Drink at least 100 ml of beetroot juice every morning if fighting cancer. Wheat-grass shots are highly beneficial. For a more detailed selection, refer to Part Three of this book.
- Cottage cheese mixed with flaxseed oil provides good levels of omega oils and protein. Take flaxseed meal daily – its rich lignan content reduces the effect of hormones on hormonally sensitive cancers. Take two to three tablespoons of freshly ground linseed per day or two to three tablespoons of flaxseed oil.
- Eat fish three to five times per week. The best types of fish include deep-water ocean fish such as mackerel, cod, halibut, sardines, tuna and salmon or supplement with fish oils. These contain high levels of omega-3 oils that act as natural anti-inflammatory agents and anti-cancer agents. It is important to maintain good levels of protein.
- Eat plenty of organic, dark green leafy vegetables for excellent sources of vitamins, minerals and chlorophyll to boost the body's immune system.
- If overweight aim to reduce weight. Increased weight is associated with factors that may promote cancer growth.
- Increase dietary fibre, in the form of whole grain cereals and lots of fresh fruits and vegetables, to improve colon function. Fibre-rich foods help to promote the production of butyric acid in the colon, preventing or reducing tumours in this area of the body.
- Supplementing the diet with iodine rich foods may decrease the risk of breast, ovarian and endometrial cancer. Refer to Part Three of this book for a full list of iodine-rich foods.

Cancer Clearing Diet

Upon Rising

2 glasses of lukewarm water squeezed with ½ fresh lemon or 1 to 2 teaspoons of apple cider vinegar.

If you feel like something warm in your stomach, prepare some herbal tea. Great herbal teas for the morning include lemongrass tea, chapharral tea, rosehip tea, essiac tea, red clover tea, licorice tea, burdock root tea or dandelion root tea.

Breakfast

Fresh vegetable or fruit juice.
This may include:
Carrot/quarter of beet/kale/garlic/celery
Watermelon/ginger
Apple/lemon/ginger
Carrot/kale/ginger/apple/celery
Carrot/celery/green apple
Carrot/kale/spinach/parsley and a shot of wheatgrass in every juice (if possible).
100 ml of beetroot juice can be added to any of these juices.
Remember to water juices down 50/50 with purified water.
AND
Energy breakfast mix – 2 parts oatmeal/2 parts LSA mix/1 part psyllium husks/2 parts
lecithin granules/1 part crushed pumpkin seeds/half a part slippery elm. Serve with
chopped fruit. Use either chopped dried apricots and figs, chopped banana, paw paw,
berries, apricots, a few almonds and a small amount of soymilk/skim milk/rice milk or
nut milk. Add 1 teaspoon of Manuka honey, blackstrap molasses or brown rice syrup
to flavour.
OR
Chopped fruit – choose from, papaya, pineapple, banana, apple, pear, berries, apricots
plus 4 tablespoons of natural acidophilus yogurt and 1 tablespoon of LSA mix and
1 tablespoon of organic flaxseed oil.
OR
Whole-wheat, sour dough or rye bread (yeast-free), toasted, with a thin spread of
avocado, cottage cheese/linseed oil mix, lemon juice or apple cider vinegar and natural
salt substitute.
OR
Energy/Protein Shake – refer to recipe in Part Three of this book.

Mid-morning

Any of the following:
10 almonds
Herbal tea
A piece of fruit
Fresh vegetable or fruit juice

Lunch

Fresh salad – choose from recipes in Part Three of this book. Best vegetables to use
include avocado, broccoli, brussel sprouts, cauliflower, snow peas, green beans, grated
carrot, grated beetroot, fresh sprouts, kale, spinach, lettuce, red onion, sun-dried
tomatoes, tomato, red or green capsicum, cabbage. If desired, spread with sesame
seeds, sunflower seeds, pumpkin seeds, almonds or walnuts. Dressing made from
apple cider vinegar or fresh lemon juice, chopped garlic, ginger, flaxseed oil.
AND

Choice of protein – Tempeh, tofu, grilled fish, tuna, salmon, sardines, organic chicken breast/thigh, free range eggs (no more than 3/week), grain fed or organic red meat (no more than 3 times/week) or legumes such as lentils.

Mid-afternoon
Any of the following:
A handful of figs
A herbal tea
A piece of fruit
Fresh vegetable or fruit juice

Dinner
A piece of protein such as grilled fish (salmon, tuna, mackerel, sea perch, cod), organic chicken breast/thigh, tofu, tempeh or legumes. Try to have 4 to 5 different vegetables. Good choices include pumpkin, potatoes, green beans, brussel sprouts, broccoli, cauliflower, snow peas, kale, spinach, cabbage, zucchini, parsnip, onions, garlic, ginger, turmeric.
OR
Brown rice with lightly stir-fried vegetables in olive oil and tamari.
OR
Vegetable soup or miso soup with legumes, buckwheat noodles and vegetables.

Before Bed
Herbal tea – good choices include chamomile, peppermint, echinacea, pau d'arco, dandelion, red clover, essiac, lemongrass or burdock tea.

*For more healthy cancer-fighting recipes, refer to Part Three of this book.

Chemotherapy/Radiation Therapy Diet
General Tips
If you are feeling nauseous try to blend any of the foods featured in the following diet in a food processor or blender and then drink hot or cold. It is important to keep energy and nutrition levels high while undergoing chemotherapy and radiation therapy, as nutrients are required in large amounts by the body.

If you are in the hospital for long periods, it is advisable to take your own foods. Try to make fresh salads, take in plenty of purified water, soups and fruit.

Try to drink eight glasses of water throughout the day. Pure water helps to flush toxins from the body and cleanses and protects the kidneys.

Upon Rising
Every morning drink two glasses of pure water with ½ lemon squeezed into them.
Fresh vegetable juice – any combination of the following – carrot, kale, celery, beetroot, garlic, ginger, apple, pineapple, lemon, broccoli, lettuce, wheatgrass.

Breakfast

Fresh fruit or vegetable juice.

This may include any combination of the following:

Carrot, kale, celery, beetroot,

garlic, ginger, apple, pineapple,

lemon, broccoli or lettuce

AND

Cereal made from a combination of oatbran, lecithin granules, psyllium, LSA mix (linseed, soy and almond) and millet, dried apricots, prunes, chopped figs or chopped banana. Use nut milk or soymilk on top.

OR

Grilled or baked fish, preferably mackerel, tuna, cod, sea perch, dory or salmon.

OR

Wholegrain or rye bread with a thin layer of avocado, chopped tomato, sprouts and lemon juice for flavouring.

OR

Energy/protein shake

Mid-Morning

Any of the following:

Vegetable juice diluted half/half with pure water.

Fruit for a snack if you feel hungry.

Herbal teas including echinacea, red clover, chamomile, essiac tea, pau d'arco, chapharral, burdock root or dandelion tea.

Lunch

Vegetable soup made with lentils, brown rice or polenta.

OR

Miso soup made with buckwheat noodles, onions, garlic and ginger.

OR

Fresh vegetable salad. Good vegetables include lettuce, carrot, capsicum, tomatoes, cherry tomatoes, celery, spinach, avocado, broccoli, green peas, green beans, and cabbage.

AND/OR

Wholemeal bread, rye bread or yeast-free pita bread. Spread avocado over the base. Add sun-dried tomatoes, lettuce, cottage cheese, grated carrot, grated beetroot and either salmon, tuna or tofu.

Mid-Afternoon

Any of the following:

Vegetable juice, diluted half/half with pure water

Fruit for a snack if you feel hungry

Herbal teas, including echinacea, essiac tea, pau d' arco tea, red clover, chamomile, dandelion tea

Dinner

One source of protein, either free-range chicken breast, turkey breast, fish (particularly cod, mackerel, salmon, tuna, halibut or sardines), tofu or tempeh, or organic red meat (no more than 3 times/week). Add this to steamed or raw vegetables. Good vegetables include broccoli, cabbage, cauliflower, green beans, carrots, pumpkin, potatoes, spinach, brussel sprouts, turnips. Choose vegetables in season and organic if possible.
OR
Fresh vegetable soup.
OR
Wild/Brown Rice with fresh vegetables and shitake mushrooms.

After Dinner

Fresh chopped fruit with natural low-fat yogurt. Good choices of fruits include apple, banana, paw paw, pineapple, berries, strawberries, kiwifruit, grapes, and melon. Add LSA mix and lecithin granules for added benefit.

Herbal teas throughout the day are very helpful.
After chemotherapy or radiation therapy stops, it is important for you to detoxify your body of the harmful carcinogenic toxins put into your body during treatment. To do this, follow an intense detoxification/purification diet as outlined in this chapter.

Soft or Pureed Diet

With chemotherapy and radiation treatment you may need to change the consistency or texture of your foods to cope with chewing or swallowing difficulties. Following are examples of a soft or pureed diet. It is important to eat regularly throughout the day to maintain good energy levels and to help your body to detoxify and heal quickly, and to prevent harmful reactions from treatment.

Foods to Enjoy

Meat/fish/poultry – in casseroles, vegetable/legume stews, soups, fish dishes. All foods can be blended in a processor. Try to buy organic meats if possible.

Nuts/legumes – blended soybeans, lentils, dried peas made into soups, casseroles, soaked almonds, soaked sunflower seeds.

Vegetables – serve mashed/steamed and blended. Good vegetables include beetroot, broccoli, brussel sprouts, turnips, radish, potatoes, cauliflower, pumpkin, carrots, peas, kale, and spinach. All vegetables can be blended in a food processor.

Cereals – breakfast porridge made from oats or millet. Alternatively, a great combination includes oatmeal, LSA mix (linseed, soy, almonds ground), slippery elm, lecithin granules and psyllium. Cut mashed banana on top and serve with hot soy milk, rice milk or nut milk.

Soups – chicken soup with the bones, fish soup, beetroot soup, vegetable soup, miso soup.

Fruit – fresh banana, pear, mango, apricots, pineapple, watermelon, papaya – stewed fruits, pureed or mashed. Stewed apples and pears are great.

Dessert – creamed brown rice, fruit, natural yogurt and natural fruit bars.

Drinks – freshly made fruit and vegetable juices, herbal teas, protein energy drinks, fruit smoothies and nut milks.

Breads/sandwiches – use flat pita breads (yeast free, gluten free), soft wholemeal bread, sour dough or rye. Use soft toppings like avocado, natural sugar-free fruit spreads, hoummus, banana, tahini etc.

Breakfast
Scrambled tofu, egg white omelette.
AND
Fresh fruit and fruit juice.
AND
Rye bread/sour dough/yeast-free wholemeal bread together with natural toppings.

Mid-morning
Any of the following:
Fruit
Pureed fruit
Fruit and vegetable juice
Fruit smoothie
Energy protein drink

Lunch
Blended fish/chicken/tofu with mashed vegetables or a fresh salad.
AND
Any selection of healthy soups.
OR
Pureed fruit or soft baked potato with cottage cheese.

Mid-afternoon
Any of the following:
Fruit pureed or blended
Nourishing drink such as energy protein drink
Herbal teas
Fresh fruit or vegetable juice

Dinner
Blended meats and gravy with mashed/blended or steamed vegetables.
OR
Vegetable and bean casserole.
AND
Some soft fruit for dessert.

Supper

Any of the following:
Herbal teas
Nourishing drink
Energy drink
Nut milks

*For more healthy recipes, refer to Part Three of this book.

Delicious and Healthy Alternatives to Sugar, Milk, Salt and Caffeine

Alternatives to sugar include:
Stevia (up to 100 times stronger than sugar, so use carefully. It is safe and calorie-free.)
Licorice root
Brown rice syrup or barley malt
Honey (raw, unprocessed honey or Manuka honey)
Blackstrap molasses
Date sugar
Maple syrup (pure)
Fruit puree or concentrate

Alternatives to milk include:
Nut milk (blended nuts in water, preferably almonds)
Soy milk
Goat's milk
Rice milk

Alternatives to salt include:
Kelp
Dried herbs – can be a mix of garlic, shallots, thyme, parsley, celery, oregano, basil, fennel, leek, sea salt.
Sea salt or rock salt
Herbamere

Alternatives to caffeine include:
Dandelion root
Herbal teas
Chicory root
Ecco
Caro
Licorice root

Table of Specific Foods for Individual Cancers

Table 21.1

Type of Cancer	Beneficial Foods	Foods to Avoid
All types of cancer	Almonds, beans, beetroot juice, brazil nuts, broccoli, brussel sprouts, cabbage, carrots, cauliflower, cherries, eggplant, figs, fish (salmon, tuna, mackerel, sardines, cod), flaxseed oil, garlic, ginger, grains, grapefruit, green apples, green peppers, green tea, leafy greens, lemons, lentils, lettuce, limes, medicinal mushrooms, mint leaves, mung beans, mustard greens, onions, papaya, parsley, raspberries, red dates, pumpkins, sesame seeds, seaweed, shallots, spinach, strawberries, sweet peppers, pineapples, tomatoes, turmeric, turnips, wheatgrass, winter squash, yogurt	Alcohol, caffeine, fats, fried and barbecued foods, foods rich in colourings, flavourings and preservatives, packaged meats containing nitrosamines, nitrates and nitrites, pesticide sprayed foods, pickled foods, smoked meats, sugar
Bladder, kidney	Brussel sprouts, cabbage, cauliflower, celery, citrus fruits, grapefruit, medicinal mushrooms including shitake, papaya, pineapple, tomatoes, watermelon	Caffeine, fats, fried foods, salt, sugar, alcohol
Breast cancer	All seeds, apples, apricots, beans, berries, broccoli, brown rice, brussel sprouts, cabbage, caraway, cauliflower, celery seeds, cherries, citrus peel, dill, garlic, medicinal mushrooms such as shitake, mint, onions, radish seeds, sesame seeds, soy products (not genetically engineered) such as tofu, tamari, tempeh, tomato, soybeans, soy flour and soy milk, yellow and orange vegetables	Caffeine, saturated fats, red meats, alcohol
Colon/ stomach cancer	Beans, broccoli, brown rice, brussel sprouts, cabbage, capsicum, cauliflower, chives, fibre-rich foods, garlic, grapefruit, onions, radish seed tea, sesame seeds, soy products, tomatoes, whole grain cereals, yogurt (acidophilus)	Alcohol, barbecued and fried foods, pickled foods, false morel mushrooms, white champignon mushrooms, red meats
Digestive tract/ oesophagus	Carrot juice, fibre-rich foods, garlic, grapefruit, green peppers, seaweed, particularly nori and kelp, tomatoes, whole grain cereals, yogurt	Alcohol, fats, junk food, pastries, white flour products, red meats

Table 21.1 *continued*

Type of Cancer	Beneficial Foods	Foods to Avoid
Lung cancer	Apricots, beetroot, broccoli, carrots, green leafy vegetables, kale, mango, miso, orange fruits and vegetables, papaya, pumpkin, spinach, sweet potato, tamari, tomatoes	Alcohol, caffeine, insecticide and sprayed foods, junk food, meat and other animal products, nicotine, salt, saturated fats, sugar, white flour
Ovarian cancer	Beans, broccoli, brussel sprouts, cabbage, cauliflower, garlic, medicinal mushrooms such as shitake, selenium-rich foods, soy products	Alcohol, caffeine, saturated fats, sugar, white flour products
Prostate cancer	All seeds, beetroot, berries, broccoli, brown rice, brussel sprouts, cabbage, cauliflower, grains, pumpkin seeds, sunflower seeds, tomatoes – including cherry and sun-dried varieties, yellow and orange vegetables such as apricots cantaloupes, carrots, pumpkin, squash	Alcohol, saturated fats such as animal fats found in red meats
Skin cancer	Blackcurrants, garlic, grapes, papaya, raspberries, rhubarb, squash, sweet potatoes, yellow and orange vegetables such as carrots, pumpkin, apricots	Alcohol, margarine, saturated fats, animal fats

The Miracle of Fasting, Detoxification and Cleansing

Over a lifetime, toxins build up in the body as the result of the pollutants in the air and soil, the chemicals in water and food and by other means. The body attempts to maintain balance by ridding itself of these toxins from the tissues and placing them into the bloodstream, causing you to experience a 'low' or 'down' cycle with symptoms such as fatigue, headaches, depression, skin problems and diarrhoea.

Fasting, cleansing or detoxification is an effective and safe method of helping the body to detoxify itself, to give bodily organs and systems a rest, to rejuvenate and to heal minor and major illnesses. Cleansing has these added benefits:

- The energy usually used for digestion is redirected towards healthy immune function, cell growth, elimination and healing of body tissues and organs.
- The immune system's workload is greatly reduced and it can concentrate on healing tumours and cancer.
- Regular cleansing prevents cancer and other serious illnesses.
- Detoxification enhances healing speed, clears and adds a sparkle to the eyes and tongue, cleanses the breath and helps you to lose excess weight and fluids.

- Tissue oxygenation is increased and white blood cells are moved more efficiently.
- Fat-stored chemicals such as drugs and pesticides are eliminated.
- Physical awareness and sensitivity to environment and surroundings is improved.
- Improves vitality and rejuvenates, helps to clear symptoms, treat disease and to prevent further problems.
- It can make you feel more productive, creative and open to subtle and spiritual energies. It helps to move your energies from the low centres of digestion and elimination up into the heart, mind and consciousness centres.

Cautions when fasting:
- Fasting on water alone can be dangerous. It releases toxins rapidly, intensifies symptoms and should only be done under supervision and care.
- If you are fasting for longer than three days, try to have someone around you to care for you and watch over you. If you have diabetes, hypoglycaemia or another chronic health problem, consult with a medical practitioner first.
- Pregnant and lactating women should never fast.

Eleven Day Purification Diet

By following this special eleven day purification diet, you will accomplish the following:

- Clean your system – rid it of all the waste matter that has contributed to sluggishness, tiredness, discomfort, pain and illness.
- Improve the organic function of the important eliminative organs, such as bowel, kidneys, liver, lungs and skin.
- Increase your vitality and energy by 100 per cent.
- Remove harmful toxins and carcinogens, and benefit chronic conditions such as cancer.
- Remove harmful by-products and toxins from orthodox cancer treatments such as radiation therapy and chemotherapy. This is to ensure that secondary cancers do not manifest in the future.

Explanation of the Purification Diet.
The body has organs especially designed for elimination of waste or toxins. These organs are the bowel, kidneys, liver, lungs and skin. It is very apparent that in today's society, because of the large amount of processed foods in the average diet, that at some time or another the function of these organs will be impeded, thus precipitating trouble. When this happens it is important for the sake of good health that the restoration of normal function proceeds as quickly as possible. A brief rest from normal food intake will aid the body in its self-regulating function and immensely improve its return to health.

Diet as Follows:
A hot epsom salts bath should be taken every night for the first week, especially on the night before the first day of cleansing. It is also essential that you have a good bowel evacuation the day or night before you begin this purification diet.

Day 1–3

Pure water and vegetable or fruit juice, preferably including:
Carrot/celery
Carrot/kale/beetroot
Carrot/apple/celery/spinach/ginger
Grape
Apple
Grapefruit
Carrot/celery/ginger
Watermelon/ginger
Or a combination of your own making.
Drink 1 glass every 3 hours, diluted 50% with pure water.

Day 4–5

Add fruits only. Fruits such as apples, pears, grapes, watermelon or sun dried fruit which has been soaked overnight are all suitable. Baked apple with stewed prunes or figs, or fresh juicy fruit when in season are also good choices.

Day 6–11

Breakfast should consist of sweet fruits only. Fruits such as melons, cantaloupe, watermelon, papaya and honeydew melon are all good. Between breakfast and lunch have any other kind of fruit.

Lunch should be a salad of 3 to 6 vegetables and 2 cups of cleansing broth. Use lots of green leafy vegetables. If hungry between meals, take fruit or fruit juices.

Dinner should consist of 2 to 3 steamed vegetables and 2 cups of cleansing broth. Fruit juice may be taken before bedtime, if desired.

Cleansing Broth Recipe

1 medium to large carrot, well washed and unpeeled
1 to 2 sticks of celery
A hand full of parsley and spinach or silverbeet
1 onion, peeled and chopped
1 tomato, chopped
1 unpeeled medium sized potato
1 litre of water

METHOD
Place all ingredients into a non-aluminium saucepan and simmer for ½ an hour. Strain and add kelp on serving.

Useful Suggestions When Following the Purification Diet

- Get as much rest and sleep as possible. The body heals and repairs faster on an elimination diet if the body is adequately rested.
- Try to drink at least eight glasses of pure water throughout the day also. Dilute all juices 50/50 with pure water.
- Do only gentle exercise like light walking, stretching, yoga, tai chi.
- Regular dry skin brushing daily is useful to help remove dead skin cells and promote detoxification through the skin.
- Epsom salts (magnesium sulphate) baths are great for cleansing, relaxation and soothing sore muscles.
- Drink as many herbal teas as you like. The best herbal teas for cleansing and boosting immune system function include dandelion tea, pau d' arco, echinacea tea, lemongrass tea, peppermint tea, red clover tea, rosehips tea, burdock, milk thistle, yellowdock herbal tea.
- If desired, you can take spirulina during the fast. Spirulina is rich in protein, vitamins and minerals and contains large amounts of chlorophyll for cleansing. There are some excellent 'green' powder combinations available including Greens plus from Orange Peel Enterprises, Nature's Secret, Earth Source Green's Plus and More by Solgar, Pro-greens from Nutricology and Kyo-Green from Wakunaga of America.

Symptoms That May Be Experienced During the Purification Diet

Fatigue, bad breath, body odour, scaly skin, skin eruptions, headaches, dizziness, irritability, anxiety, nausea, coughing, confusion, body aches, smelling stools, diarrhoea, dark urine, insomnia, mucous discharge, visual or hearing problems.

Three Day Spring Cleanse Diet

A three day spring cleanse helps the body to remove toxins, cleanses the blood and helps to restore good health and well-being.

Day One
On Rising
Warm water – 2 glasses with ½ a squeeze of lemon or lime.

Breakfast
Fresh Papaya with lime or lemon juice squeezed on top.

Mid-morning
Freshly made juice – suitable juices include carrot, beet, kale or apple and ginger.

Lunch

Fresh watermelon or grapefruit and a vegetable consommé or cleansing broth.

Mid-afternoon

Your choice of fresh apple/lemon and ginger juice, or pear and grape juice.

Dinner

Fresh pineapple and vegetable consommé.

Before retiring

Your choice of herbal tea – choose from chamomile, dandelion, red clover or peppermint.

Day Two

On Rising

Warm water – 2 glasses with a squeeze of lemon or lime juice.

Breakfast

'Morning Energizer' – carrot, celery, ginger, beet and parsley juice.

Mid-morning

Herbal tea of your choice. Good choices include dandelion, lemongrass, red clover, rosehip or peppermint.

Lunch

Fresh vegetable juice and a vegetable consommé or cleansing broth.

Mid-afternoon

Herbal tea of your choice. If you are hungry, vegetable juice or vegetable consommé.

Dinner

Fresh watermelon juice and 2 bowls of vegetable consommé.

Before Retiring

Herbal tea of your choice.

Day Three

On Rising

Warm water – 2 glasses with a squeeze of lemon or lime juice.

Breakfast

Compote of stewed apples with prunes or figs.

Mid-morning
Fresh fruit or freshly made vegetable juice.

Lunch
Salad of mixed lettuces with green beans, bell peppers and tomatoes.

Mid-afternoon
Fresh fruit or freshly made fruit juice.

Dinner
Steamed vegetables – kale, spinach, broccoli or cabbage, together with 2 bowls of vegetable soup.

Before Retiring
Your choice of herbal teas.

Useful Suggestions When Following the Spring Cleanse Diet

- It is important to drink adequate amounts of pure, filtered water while cleansing. At least eight glasses of pure water daily are necessary.
- Take a fibre supplement the day before the cleansing diet, to clean out the bowels. Colon cleansing or cleansing enemas are also useful.
- It is best to avoid taking supplements while on the cleansing diet. The only recommended supplement is vitamin C powder with bioflavonoids.
- Have an epsom salts bath every night before bed. Contains magnesium sulphate to relax muscles and aid detoxification. Use a dry skin brush and use long strokes all of your body towards your heart, before every bath.
- Make sure you relax and get plenty of sleep. Do not overdo the exercise. Light, gentle exercise such as stretching, yoga, tai chi and slow walking are very beneficial.
- The vegetable consommé recipe also known as the 'cleansing broth' featured in the Purification Diet earlier is easy to make and store, and should be drunk as often as possible throughout the day, especially if hungry. Kelp can be sprinkled on top of vegetable consommé for flavouring and extra cleansing benefits.
- An energizing shiatsu or a relaxing Swedish or aromatherapy massage is very useful while cleansing.
- Herbal teas are cleansing and rejuvenating. Good herbal teas to use include dandelion, red clover, rosehips, chamomile, lemongrass, milk thistle or peppermint.
- Symptoms you may experience while cleansing include body odour, bad breath, dizziness, fatigue, mood swings, irritability, aches and pains and other detoxification symptoms.
- Make sure you eat or drink at least six times daily to keep blood sugar levels balanced.

Chapter 22

NATURE'S HEALING FOODS

Foods from nature are rich in vitamins, minerals, enzymes and cancer-fighting nutrients. Cultures that retain a traditional, wholesome diet have little or no incidence of cancer within their native people. Cancer is prominent in cultures whose diet has strayed from natural, organic produce towards chemically sprayed, preservative and colour-enriched foods, such as those found in many Western diets.

Many natural fruits, vegetables and whole grains are uniquely abundant in cancer-preventing and cancer-fighting nutrients. Individual foods are powerfully capable of enhancing health and well-being, and repairing specific organs and body systems. A natural, wholesome diet rich in rejuvenating and life-giving foods will ensure you maintain high levels of health, vitality and may prevent the onset of a cancerous condition.

Apples

I'm sure everyone is aware of the famous saying, 'an apple a day keeps the doctor away'. The individual who coined this saying must have understood the immense health benefits contained within apples.

Apples, when eaten regularly, may help prevent cancer due to their high content of caffeic acid, ellagic acid and chlorogenic acid (three important cancer-fighting nutrients). Apples prevent the conversion of benzopyrene to carcinogens in the body. Benzopyrene is a toxic cancer-causing chemical formed as a result of food processing involving heat such as frying, barbecuing and smoking.

Ellagic acid powerfully prevents many forms of cancer by preventing polynuclear aromatic hydrocarbons (mainly found in cigarettes) and benzopyrene (carcinogenic substances) from converting normal, healthy cells into cancerous cells. The high content of caffeic acid in apples may prevent many forms of cancer. Chlorogenic acid, found within apples, prevents cell mutations involved in cancer.

The apple pulp contains a high level of fibre, known as pectin and pectic acids. Pectin travels through the intestines, absorbing water and expanding into a gooey mass. This mass is able to soften hard stools and makes them easier to pass. As it does this it also binds to toxins within the stomach and intestines, thereby helping to prevent stomach and colon cancer.

Apples are also rich in vitamin E, biotin, folic acid, vitamin A and vitamin C. Many red apples are injected with a dye to keep their luscious red colour. For safety, try to buy green apples or organically grown apples.

Beetroot

Beetroot stimulates lymphatic function and may help to prevent and reverse some forms of cancer, in particular, some forms of lung cancer. Scientific research documents a case in Hungary of a doctor who used beetroot to totally clear lung cancer from a fifty-year-old male. After six weeks of treatment the tumour disappeared completely. A similar case, also from Hungary, of a doctor who treated prostate cancer with beetroot was indicated to have totally removed the tumour after a short period. More research needs to be conducted in this area to prove the healing potential of beetroot.

Beetroot juice is a natural prophylactic and therapeutic agent. During cancer treatment, 100 ml of fresh beetroot juice should be drunk daily. Canned beetroot does not have the same medicinal effect.

Beetroot is also useful for treating constipation, fluid retention, anxiety, memory problems, gallstones, bladder problems, kidney problems and anaemia. It is famous for its ability to enhance liver function. Beetroot is rich in iron, potassium, niacin, copper and vitamin C. Folic acid, zinc, calcium, manganese and magnesium are also present in beetroot in good amounts.

Berries and Grapes

Berries are nature's little miracle-packed fruits. Many different types of berries contain anthocyanins, which are bioflavonoids with antioxidant properties. Bioflavonoids are substances that provide berries with their magnificent colours and health properties.

Grapes, blackcurrants and raspberries may reduce the risk of developing skin cancer, due to their high ellagic acid content. Grapes are thought to possess strong life extension and antioxidant properties. They contain powerful cancer-fighting polyphenols that are also found in red wine. These polyphenols are thought to reduce tumour formation and may also activate cancer cell death in breast cancer and leukaemia.

Grapes are also rich in ferulic acid, which may help to prevent many forms of cancer. One of the most famous 'cancer-clearing' diets in the world is known as the 'Grape Diet'. For six weeks or more, a person consumes all different types of grapes and nothing else, except water. Many people who have followed this diet have claimed to have cured themselves of cancer. This diet should never be undertaken without medical supervision.

It is believed people who regularly consume strawberries are less likely to develop cancer. Strawberries also inhibit the conversion of nitrates into nitrites, which then convert into the cancer-causing substance, nitrosamine. (Nitrates are carcinogenic substances found in packaged, smoked and processed meats.) An excess of nitrosamines in the body has been linked to the development of many different types of cancer including stomach, colorectal and brain tumours.

Strawberries and grapes are good sources of the phytochemicals (ellagic acid and phenethyle isothiocyanate) which may be effective in preventing and treating cancer of the oesophagus by stopping cells from becoming cancerous when exposed to a cancer-causing chemical. Generally, strawberries are highly sprayed with pesticides to keep their perfect shape and colour. When eating strawberries, try to buy organic produce and always wash thoroughly.

Berries are so rich in bioflavonoids that they are capable of protecting the health of small blood vessels and capillaries while preventing inflammation, which therefore may help to reduce the spread of cancer. Other berries like bilberries, dewberries, cranberries and blueberries are also rich in vitamin C and other health-enhancing flavonoids. Berries are also plentiful in the minerals potassium, calcium magnesium, chlorine, sulphur, silicon and iron. Most berries have a moderate fibre content as well.

Cherries

Cherries, with their rich ruby-red colour, act primarily as a tonic for the blood. Being rich in magnesium, iron, copper and manganese, they are able to promote healthy blood development. The rich content of vitamin A and vitamin C found in cherries helps to protect the body against the harmful effects of stress and toxic pollutants found in the air, making them useful in preventing cancer and illness. Cherries contain a miraculous substance which is believed to encourage the death of tumour cells.

Citrus Fruits

Citrus fruits give you a burst of energy and exert useful anti-inflammatory actions. It is important to be wary when consuming citrus fruits as many are exposed to high amounts of food irradiation to protect them against the infestation of insects. Food irradiation creates many toxic effects on the body, which can promote cancer development. Try to buy organic citrus fruits when possible. Citrus fruits are rich in fibre and vitamins A and C. Vitamin C is a potent cancer-fighting antioxidant, which helps to ward off stomach, breast, mouth, larynx, pancreas and oesophagus cancer.

Lemons, oranges, grapefruit, mandarins and limes contain strong anti-cancer compounds called limonene, which stimulate the body to produce cancer-inhibiting enzymes and help prevent some forms of cancer, particularly breast cancer. Dutch and Swedish research indicates that people who eat citrus fruit have less risk of getting cancer of the pancreas and stomach.

Grapefruits may protect against the development of cancer due to their high pectin and glutathione content. They also promote the elimination of old red blood cells from the body. In Japanese studies, grapefruit extract has been shown to stop tumour growth in animals. Grapefruit facilitates the removal of cancer-forming carcinogens within the intestines. Grapefruit contains glycyrrhizin, a compound also found in licorice, which is thought to prevent the growth of some forms of cancer and inhibit the activity of some carcinogens. Pink grapefruits are a rich source of a potent antioxidant known as lycopene. Lycopene helps to protect against breast and prostate cancer.

Lemons are an excellent source of the mineral phosphorous, required daily for repair and maintenance of the body's nervous system. Phosphorous foods aid in repairing the brain, improve memory and promote creativity. Lemons also contain high amounts of sodium, which is beneficial for elimination of wastes, cleansing of the lymphatic system and prevention of hardened arteries.

Many people believe that lemons are acidic. This is true while they are in our fruit bowl. However, when they enter your stomach they become alkaline. It is this quality that allows lemons to help maintain the correct Ph in our body and also to act as a natural, internal antiseptic. A lemon a day will keep you clean and healthy on the inside and glowing with vitality on the outside.

Cruciferous Vegetables – Broccoli, Brussel Sprouts, Cabbage, Cauliflower, Radish and Turnips

Certain vegetables from the cruciferous family have been recognised as having anti-cancer properties. These include broccoli, brussel sprouts, cabbage, cauliflower, radish, turnips, kale and bok choy. They increase the level of the enzyme aryl hydroxylase in the liver, lungs and intestines. This enzyme detoxifies many potential cancer-causing substances and blocks their action.

Broccoli, brussel sprouts, cabbage, cauliflower and turnips all contain sulphuric compounds (glucosilinates, isothiocyanates, sulforaphane and dithiolthiones), which may help to prevent many forms of cancer, kill aflotoxins and act as powerful antioxidants. Broccoli, brussel sprouts, cabbage, kale, turnips and cauliflower also contain powerful anti-cancer compounds called indoles. Indoles are very effective in fighting and preventing cancer. They play a key role in the removal of harmful female sex hormones. These sex hormones increase the risk of breast cancer.

Studies around the world have shown that people who eat large amounts of broccoli and cabbage (indole-rich foods) tend to have a decrease in harmful sex hormones in their bodies. This indicates that indole-rich foods such as broccoli and cabbage may be useful in the prevention of hormone induced breast cancer and other hormone sensitive cancers.

Broccoli has extremely strong cancer-preventing properties. Research on humans indicates broccoli is capable of preventing breast cancer due to the ability of one of its main constituents, indole-3-carbinol. It is able to increase the excretion of (oestrone)-2-hydroxyestrone, a form of oestrogen which is linked to the development of breast cancer when in excess. Broccoli contains dithiolthiones, which stimulate your body's immune system to fight cancer on its own. Broccoli also contains a potent anti-cancer compound called sulphoraphane, which has the ability to increase anti-cancer enzyme fighting systems in cells. This compound is also found in cauliflower, brussel sprouts, carrots, green onions and kale. Steaming does not destroy this anti-cancer compound.

Women who eat lots of broccoli may substantially lower their risk of developing cervical cancer. Men who smoke and eat dark green vegetables (like broccoli) often have half the lung cancer risk of smokers who don't eat this vegetable. The rich amounts of Vitamin A and beta-carotene found in broccoli have been shown to help your body ward off many types of cancer, including lung cancer.

The dreaded brussel sprouts are a child's worst nightmare. Yet brussel sprouts are unique vegetables with an amazing ability to kill the highly carcinogenic substance, aflatoxin. This is due to their high sulphurous compound – glucosilinate. Brussel sprouts are able to retard many forms of cancer, especially cancer of the colon, very effectively. In recent studies, animals that were fed brussel sprouts and were then given incredible amounts of carcinogens were far less likely to develop cancer than animals that were not fed the sprouts.

Brussel sprouts are loaded with beta-carotene and chlorophyll and eating them has been linked to low rates of stomach cancer. Studies in Greece, Norway and Japan have shown that people who eat green vegetables (particularly brussel sprouts) have the lowest incidence of cancers. They are loaded with nutrition including, vitamins A and C, folic acid, calcium, potassium, magnesium and iron. They are nearly half protein. Brussel sprouts should not be boiled, they should be lightly steamed or finely chopped and added to salads. (Geelhoed & Barilla, 1997, p 44).

Cabbage is believed to prevent several forms of cancer, particularly breast, stomach and colon cancer. In studies in Japan, Greece and America, cabbage was shown to fight off colon cancer. Cabbage helps to protect against radiation and increases the removal of toxic drugs and carcinogens, and decreases tumours caused by carcinogens. Cabbage is effective in protecting against low level radiation.

Cultures with high cabbage intake, such as Asian cultures, tend to have very low levels of breast cancer. The Japanese people have shown that individuals who eat large portions of cabbage every day have the lowest overall death rate and Greek research has indicated that adding vegetables like cabbage to your diet can reduce the risk of colon cancer by over 800 per cent.

Regular cabbage intake may suppress the growth of colon polyps, which are thought to lead to colon cancer. People who eat cabbage once a week may decrease their odds of developing colon cancer by a very large per centage. Cabbage, apart from being a rich source of chlorophyll, also contains a magical nutrient called vitamin U. Vitamin U is believed to heal and assist peptic ulcers. Cabbage also contains two cleansing minerals, chlorine and sulphur. These nutrients work hand in hand to expel wastes from the body and to keep our blood clean and healthy.

Cauliflower is very effective at preventing colon cancer. Cauliflower supplies high amounts of potassium which helps to promote healthy circulation. Its other vital nutrients include vitamin C, magnesium, chlorine, sulphur, phosphorous and silica.

Radish seeds are thought to alleviate some forms of cancer. Radish seeds, applied topically to the breast as a heated poultice are a good accessory treatment for breast cancer. Radish seeds consumed as a strong tea may decrease the incidence of stomach cancer. Radishes are a rich source of chlorine which assists in the removal of acid-mucus poisons from the body and helps to maintain a healthy and clean respiratory function.

Enzymes – Bananas, Mangoes, Papaya and Pineapples

Bananas are rich in potassium and magnesium, and help to protect against circulatory dysfunction. Potassium helps to remove poisonous wastes from the kidneys, leaving a healthy, clean bloodstream. Bananas are also rich in pectin, a water-soluble fibre that helps to prevent hypoglycaemia by balancing blood sugar levels and aids in the removal of carcinogens from the digestive tract, preventing colon cancer. Bananas are also a good source of vitamin A (health of skin and eyes), vitamin C (immunity, healing), vitamin E (healing of scars, heart protection), vitamin B1, B2, B3, B5 and vitamin B6 (required for the production of antibodies and healthy red blood cells). Do not eat bananas with sugar or bread.

Mangos are also rich in enzymes and contain high quantities of the phytochemical, bioflavonoids. Produced when the plant grabs energy from the sun, phytochemicals act as antioxidants and immune system boosters.

Pineapple and papaya contain proteolytic enzymes that help to break down foods, strengthen the immune system and aid more efficient digestive function. Pineapple also contains antioxidants and peroxidase, a substance that is believed to inhibit the growth of tumour cells. Bromelain, the proteolytic enzyme found in pineapple, is an anti-inflammatory and is believed to enhance cancer cell death.

The proteolytic enzyme in papaya or paw paw is called papain. Papain assists with protein digestion and acts as an anti-inflammatory. Papaya leaves have long been used as an effective remedy in the treatment of cancer. Boil pawpaw or papaya leaves for 40 minutes, strain and drink the water. Cultures throughout Asia, especially Thailand, eat very large amounts of green papaya (very rich in enzymes) grated into a salad. It is called som tum or papaya pokpok. Thai and Asian people exhibit very low levels of stomach cancer, which may be due to their high intake of green papaya. Asian people believe a papaya a day will revitalise your entire system and allow for a healthy digestive function.

Figs

Research has indicated figs can shrink tumours involved in various cancers. Research on humans suggests figs are capable of shrinking tumours by an average of 39 per cent and can induce remissions in 55 per cent of cancer sufferers (Hyperhealth CD, 1995). The main active ingredient found in figs and fig extracts is benzaldehyde.

Figs may counteract and treat many of the side effects associated with chemotherapy and radiation treatment. One nasty side effect of cancer therapy is lassitude (lack of energy) and damage to the mucosal lining of the mouth, throat and digestive tract. Figs contain demulcents, substances that soothe irritated mucous membranes in the mouth, throat and respiratory system. This little fruit is rich in potassium, iron, copper, calcium, sodium, phosphorous, magnesium and B complex vitamins. If you want to put some pep you're your step, eat a small handful of figs. Their rich fructose content is able to boost energy levels.

Flaxseed/Linseed Oil

Flaxseed oil or linseed oil is the only diet oil permitted in the orthomolecular treatment of cancer patients. Flaxseeds are extremely rich in both alpha-linolenic acid and linoleic acid, magnesium, zinc, B vitamins, potassium and fibre. Flaxseed oil may alleviate the side effects and inhibit the further development of many forms of cancer.

Adding flaxseed to the diet is able to increase the body's production of energy, thereby improving stamina. It is able to improve liver function, prevents atherosclerosis and asthma, alleviates depression, assists dry and flaky skin and accelerates the healing of bruises.

Flaxseed oil or flaxseeds may help to prevent the development of cancer in the small intestine and may be a major component in anti-tumour activity. It is believed to prevent breast cancer, prostate cancer, hormone-induced cancers and metastases.

It maintains the flexibility of red blood cells, prevents fatty degeneration in the liver, lowers cholesterol and triglyceride levels and strengthens brain activity.

Flaxseed oil is a phytoestrogen (a plant containing estrogen-like qualities) that has been proven to protect against heart disease and certain types of cancers. Flaxseed oil combined with a protein, like cottage cheese, stimulates the oxygenation processes in the body harming dangerous cancer cells. This miracle medicine can be incorporated easily into your daily diet. Try using flaxseed oil as a substitute for butter or making up a delicious salad dressing – refer to the recipe section in Part Three of this book.

Green Beans

Green beans are excellent for the heart, providing fibre, protein and complex carbohydrates. They are very rich in high powered anti-cancer agents called phytochemicals and protease inhibitors. Beans stimulate colon bacteria to give off volatile short chain fatty acids, which decrease the 'bad' cholesterol, lower blood pressure and decrease the risk of developing colon cancer.

Green beans are a rich source of vitamin A. Vitamin A is an antioxidant that protects against free radical damage, protects the body against infections and promotes healthy skin and clear eyesight. Fresh green beans also supply vitamin E, vitamin C, B vitamins, folic acid, iron, magnesium, calcium and manganese. Lightly steam beans or eat them raw, add to a salad to receive the full nutritional benefits from this magical green medicine.

Juices and Juice Therapy

Freshly made juices are nourishing, living foods in liquid form, providing the body with a rich assortment of vitamins, minerals and abundant enzymes. Raw juices require minimal digestion and can be assimilated by the body very easily.

Juice therapy is a method of detoxifying and cleansing the body of unwanted chemicals, wastes and toxins and supplying beneficial nutrients needed to fight cancer. Fresh juices provide a superior vehicle by which unusually high quantities and concentrations of the food's life force can be consumed. Fresh juices supply the body with a rich assortment of cancer-fighting vitamins and minerals.

Raw juices are not recommended as the sole form of cancer therapy. They are however natural, safe and well-tried, and have returned many people in the world back to good health. When raw juices are unlocked from plants, pure and vital liquids of great healing power are released and their infinitely gentle action can coax our bodies back to normality. Raw juices have none of the dangerous side effects associated with potent medical drugs, yet they can eliminate health problems arising from many of the deficiencies created from the hustle and bustle of today's fast-paced world and nutrient-deficient foods. Commercial fruit juices are less therapeutic than freshly squeezed juices, as many brands contain sugar, preservatives and other undesirable ingredients.

It is advisable to try to drink anywhere from four to six wholesome juices throughout the day while fighting cancer, to maintain good blood sugar levels. Regular intake of juices after beating cancer will help to prevent the growth of tumours in the future. It is important to drink the juice within 15 minutes of making it, to ensure you utilise the full benefit of live enzymes contained within the plants, fruits and vegetables. If you plan to drink juices on a regular basis try to buy organic produce, free from fertilisers and pesticides.

Juice therapy can be used in a number of different ways. By eliminating solid foods for a few days and drinking energy packed juices for two to three days, you will give your body a chance to detoxify body wastes and direct its energy towards healing the diseased cells. If juice therapy is undertaken for a longer period, under supervision, the body is given a chance to heal more chronic conditions.

Juices should be watered down 50-50 with spring or distilled water.

Single juice fasts have been undertaken to fight certain types of cancer. One well-known juice therapy diet is the Grape Diet. This diet uses only grapes in season, juiced and drunk every day for one month. It enables the body to rid itself of more chronic conditions. This diet should only be undertaken with supervision by a health professional.

Only light gentle exercise, such as light walking, yoga, stretching, meditation or tai chi should be performed on any juice fast. Continue to drink pure natural drinking water throughout the day and drink juices regularly to maintain blood sugar levels.

Protein powders or supplements, chlorophyll powders, barley grass, wheatgrass powder, beetroot powder or other nutrient packed energy powders can be added to juices for extra energy and revitalising effects. Add one to two tablespoons of flaxseed oil to any juice to enhance the curative effects of juice therapy in cancer treatment.

The healing benefits of juices used in cancer prevention and cancer therapy should never be underestimated. Juice therapy is a powerful tool in beating and preventing cancer, and other serious illnesses.

Kale, Spinach, Watercress

All dark green leafy vegetables are excellent sources of vitamins, minerals and chlorophyll that are able to boost the immune system. In Singapore, people who eat high amounts of kale tend to have a low incidence of lung cancer. Kale is a rich source of beta-carotene and chlorophyll, two of the best cancer-fighting substances found in food.

People who eat spinach (and other foods rich in beta-carotene) have a lower chance of developing lung cancer than people who don't eat these foods. Spinach can block the formation of nitrosamines, one of the most potent cancer causing chemicals. Spinach is rich in ferulic acid, an enzyme inhibitor that may assist in the prevention of many forms of cancer. Its other cancer-inhibiting compounds include histidine and beta-carotene. The potent nutrient mix found in spinach is able to enhance elimination of impurities from the body. Spinach, due to its abundant iron, cobalt, manganese, calcium and copper content, is able to act as a blood building vegetable. It is also high in fibre, vitamins A and C, potassium, magnesium, chlorophyll and zinc.

Watercress is rich in glucosilinate, a sulphuric compound useful for blocking the formation of many forms of cancer, killing dangerous cancer-causing aflatoxins and acting as a strong antioxidant. Watercress is particularly high in vitamin A and calcium. It contains over 5000mg of vitamin A per 100g of watercress. Regular use of watercress will enhance immune system function and protect against the invasion of harmful cancer causing substances. It also contains vitamin C and B vitamins, biotin, iodine, potassium, iron and magnesium. Watercress is a pure vegetable, supplying amazing health-giving properties.

Kiwifruit

Kiwifruit are rich in enzymes, vitamin C and potassium, and contain cancer-inhibiting properties. Kiwifruit contains dietary proteolytic enzymes, which aid in the digestion of proteins and have strong cancer-fighting potential.

Nightshade Family – Capsicum, Eggplant, Potatoes and Tomatoes

Capsicum or green peppers are rich in phytochemicals and tend to decrease the incidence of stomach cancer. This little vegetable is extremely rich in vitamin C and bioflavonoids (Vitamin P). Vitamin P is essential for the absorption of vitamin C, making capsicum better in value than a vitamin C tablet. Capsicum is an optimal provider of living nutrients including iodine and vitamin A.

Eggplant may help prevent cancer by counteracting possible cancer agents found in the diet. Eggplant contains gallic acid, which prevents many carcinogens from causing chromosome mutations in cells.

Potatoes may prevent cell mutations that lead to cancer, due to their chlorogenic acid content. A regular intake of potatoes is believed to prevent several types of cancer. Ensure that you do not consume green potatoes and be careful how you cook potatoes. Potatoes should be cooked with the skin on to ensure that the potassium and other essential nutrients are not lost in the cooking process. Potatoes are a good source of magnesium, sulphur, silicon, iodine and chlorine. Being a starchy food, they are able to provide an abundance of energy. Potato juice is an age-old treatment for liver cancer.

Tomatoes are believed to prevent several forms of cancer, particularly stomach, lung and breast cancer. Two phytochemicals in tomatoes (p-coumaric and chlorogenic acid) prevent the formation of cancer-causing digestive nitrosamines. Tomatoes also stimulate the growth or regeneration of liver tissue. Strawberries, grapes, carrots, green peppers and other fruits and vegetables are also rich in these cancer-fighting substances. Tomatoes are believed to significantly decrease the risk of developing bladder and prostate cancer. In addition, tomatoes contain another cancer fighting substance called lycopene. Lycopene is a potent antioxidant that reduces the risk of cancer of the oesophagus, stomach, prostate, colon and rectum. Lycopene helps to guard against the toxic effects of radiation therapy, especially burning of tissues.

The lycopene content in tomatoes is dramatically increased in products such as tomato paste, sun-dried tomatoes and tomato powder. The rich intake of tomato products in Mediterranean counties may be the prime reason why their native people have a lower incidence of prostate cancer and related problems.

Onion Family – Garlic, Leeks, Chives and Onions

Garlic is an amazing food, commonly known as nature's antibiotic. Garlic may prevent several forms of cancer. Extensive research indicates kyolic garlic increases the infiltration of natural killer lymphocytes into cancerous sites, decreases the tumour mass and destroys cancer cells. The most effective form is injected directly into the tumour. However, oral forms are also very effective.

Garlic may also inhibit the growth of breast cancer cells, protect against skin cancer and decrease the incidence of colon cancer, due to its high diallyl sulphide content. Garlic provides protection against oesophagus cancer and is toxic to Burkitt's lymphoma cells (due to ajeone's ability to inhibit Epstein-Barr virus). Garlic prevents the conversion of dietary nitrites into cancer-causing nitrosamines, even more effectively than vitamin C. In 1952 Russian scientists found that garlic was a potent tumour fighter and has a strong ability to boost the body's immune system. For more information on garlic, refer to Chapter 27, The Ancient Magic of Herbal Remedies.

Leeks and chives are members of the onion family that are also believed to prevent the onset of colon cancer. They supply abundant amounts of minerals and good levels of B vitamins. The sulphur and chlorine content of leeks promotes cleansing of the bloodstream and lymphatic system.

Onions contain good amounts of silica, necessary for healthy blood circulation and to prevent mental fatigue. Scientific research has shown that onion extract can destroy tumour cells in test tubes and can arrest tumour growth in rats when tumour cells are implanted into them. Red onions are an excellent source of copper. Copper enhances iron absorption in the body and is believed to be a cancer-fighting mineral.

Seaweeds and Sea Vegetables

The vegetables that come from the sea are some of the most nutrient-rich foods we have. They are particularly high in iodine, calcium, potassium and iron, and some are very high in protein. Since these plants are constantly bathed in the mineral-rich ocean waters, they have a regular supply of nutrients. Most sea vegetables contain algin, a fibre molecule that binds minerals. Sea vegetables have been known to bind lead and mercury, and help excrete them from the body. For more information, refer to Chapter 23 – Gifts from Mother Nature'.

Seeds

Research has shown that cultures that consume large amounts of seeds have a decreased risk of developing several forms of cancer. A high seed intake can decrease the risk of breast, colon and prostate cancer. Many seeds contain antioxidant and protective compounds including oligosaccharides, fatty acids, lithium and molybdenum. Fenugreek seeds and flaxseeds are believed to prevent colon cancer and many other forms of cancer.

Sesame seeds contain potent antioxidants, including sesaminol and laetrile. Sesame seeds and flaxseeds are rich in lignan, a phyto-oestroegen which prevents many forms of harmful oestrogen-induced cancers, including breast and colon cancer.

Pumpkin seeds are best known for their concentrations of zinc and their use in the treatment and prevention of male prostate problems.

Soy Products

Soy products are protein packed sources of energy that are widely incorporated into Asian diets, particularly the Japanese diet. The high intake of soy protein in the diet is believed to contribute to Japan's low rate of breast cancer. In fact, societies with a high consumption of soybeans and soybean products, especially the fermented variety, exhibit only 25 per cent of the incidence of breast cancer, compared to populations in Western countries.

Soybeans are rich in phyto-oestrogens, particularly lignan. Lignan blocks oestrogen receptors within the body preventing the toxic effects of excessive oestrogens. The high content of lignans and isoflavonoids in soybeans and soy products are believed to be responsible for this cancer-inhibiting ability. Soybeans also contain genistein, an isoflavonoid that inhibits the growth of cancer cells by preventing the growth and formation of blood vessels that feed them.

Tofu, made from a combination of soybeans coagulated with a sea water extract called Nigari, is rich in bioflavonoids. Bioflavonoids help to lower cholesterol levels and protect against cancer.

Miso, a paste made from soybeans, is believed a valuable aid in reducing the incidence of stomach cancer. Stomach cancer in Japanese women has decreased by over 30 per cent perhaps due to a high intake of miso soup and other soy based products. Miso facilitates the chelation of the toxic chemical residues of tobacco smoking, including nicotine, from the body. Miso improves the function of the intestines and digestive system, and protects against the toxic effects of radiation. It is a useful addition to the diet during radiation treatment. Miso also contains anti-carcinogenic compounds, which neutralise Benzopyrone, a known cancer-causing agent.

Soymilk is made from soaking soybeans in water; grinding and draining the cream-coloured liquid out. Soymilk is rich in lignans, a phyto-oestrogen that prevents colon and breast cancer, and cancers caused by excessive oestrogen.

Tamari or shoyu, commonly referred to in Western countries as soy sauce, is believed to prevent stomach cancer and facilitate the elimination of toxic residues of tobacco smoking, including nicotine from the body. Perhaps this is the reason why Japanese people, who smoke so many cigarettes, have a much lower rate of lung cancer than Western societies.

Sprouts

The Chinese discovered the potential of sprouted foods over 3000 years ago and now, with modern methods of food analysis, their wisdom is being recognised by the rest of the world. Sprouting is a natural process; the seed is transformed from a state of latent energy into a completely living form with the assistance of water and air. As the seed begins to sprout, those elements contained in it are used to provide energy. The nutrient quality and digestion of the seed, grains and legumes is improved.

Sprouted seeds are one of the best sources of 'live enzymes'. Enzymes are the catalysts for all living development. There are very few foods in this world which are able to supply the amount of enzymes found in sprouts. They also supply an excellent source of certain B vitamins, vitamin C, vitamin E, vitamin G, vitamin K, vitamin U and amino acids.

Alfalfa is probably the most common sprout known to man. Alfalfa means 'best food'. Alfalfa contains an abundance of alkaline minerals, as well as protein, vitamin C, B group vitamins and traces of vitamin B12. It also contains at least eight known enzymes that enhance healthy digestion and provide new life to body cells.

Wholegrains and Legumes

Barley, oats, rye and wheat contain high amounts of lignan. Lignan blocks harmful oestrogens, and may prevent hormone-induced cancers such as breast and colon cancer.

Grains, such as brown rice, buckwheat and barley contain an immense array of health benefits. Phytic acid, found in all grains, binds to the mineral iron and prevents it from causing free-radical damage that leads to cancer. Grains are rich in the amino acid arginine, which is a potent cancer-fighting nutrient.

Barley helps prevent some forms of cancer (due to protease inhibitors, which suppress the action of various carcinogens in the intestinal tract). Brown rice may decrease the incidence of breast, colon and prostate cancer. Wheat bran, although quite harsh on the digestive tract in its raw form, is believed to decrease the incidence of colon cancer.

Legumes are rich in protease inhibitors which help to prevent cancer by counteracting toxins within the intestines.

Wine

Wine, especially red wine is believed to prevent carcinogens from causing dangerous chromosome mutations that lead to the onset of cancer. This is due to the high gallic acid content found in red wine. However, it should be drunk in extreme moderation as alcohol is also known to be carcinogenic itself.

Wonders of the Kitchen – Cinnamon and Parsley

Cinnamon contains cinnamic acid, a polyphenol. Cinnamic acid may reduce the incidence of cancer caused by several synthetic food additives. Cinnamon suppresses some forms of detrimental bacteria and inhibits the growth of yeasts and moulds. It inhibits the growth of aflatoxin, a deadly cancer-forming substance. Chemotherapy and radiation treatment causes the growth of Candida, and cinnamon helps to treat and suppress these yeast growths.

Parsley is a common herb that is extremely easy to grow. Parsley is thought to prevent some forms of cancer, due to its histidine content. It is also claimed to lower the carcinogenic potential of fried foods. It is a very rich source of vitamin C, a powerful antioxidant and cancer preventative.

Yellow and Orange Fruits and Vegetables

Yellow and orange vegetables contain many cancer-fighting properties.

Apricots are useful in preventing lung and skin cancer, possibly due to their high beta-carotene content – dried apricots contain more beta-carotene than the whole fruit. When buying dried apricots, look for low sulphur or sulphur-free apricots. Apricot seeds contain a substance called laetrile that is believed to contain strong cancer-fighting properties.

Carrots are loaded with beta-carotene, which may lower the incidence of a variety of cancers and prevents the formation of cancer in the later stages. They are particularly useful in preventing colon cancer. In extensive studies, carrots were shown to reduce the lung cancer risk of smokers, reduce the risk of cancer in ex-smokers and reduce the risk of lung cancer to non-smokers exposed to cigarette smoke.

Carrots and pumpkin contain large amounts of alpha-carotenes. Alpha-carotenes protect against liver cancer and are 10 times more effective in protecting against skin and lung cancer than beta-carotene. Carrots, apricots, pumpkin, papaya, mangoes, peaches and sweet potatoes are high in beta-carotene and this makes them very effective in enhancing the immune system by stimulating the activity of T lymphocytes (T-Lymphocytes are the 'commanders of the immune army').

Yogurt

Russian biologist Ilich Metchnikoff asserted that the secret to the longest living people in the world, the Bulgarians, was their high intake of yogurt. Recently, research in France has shown that women who eat yogurt (with live yogurt cultures) are less likely to develop breast cancer than women who don't eat yogurt. Studies in Japan, Italy, Switzerland and Poland indicate those who eat yogurt show less incidence of disease and infection as a whole. Yogurt helps to lower the risk of cancer by boosting the body's immune system and defending against disease. It is an essential aid in the prevention of stomach and colon cancer.

Lactobacillus Bulgaricus, a common bacterial culture for yogurt, has a particular strain (LV-51) that has been used in Europe for cancer treatment and immune fortification. LV-51 is found to stimulate leukocyte production, T lymphocyte production and anti-tumour activity of macrophages.

Chapter 23

GIFTS FROM MOTHER NATURE – NUTRITIONAL SUPPLEMENTS

Barley Grass or Green Barley Powder

A much talked about green powder in the world today is barley grass. This is a food supplement taken from barley before the grain has developed. It is claimed to be a powerful immune system stimulant, an antioxidant, a good source of chlorophyll and possibly a preventative for cancer, diabetes and many other ailments.

Barley grass helps to boost energy levels. The chlorophyll found in barley grass assists the oxygen carrying capacity of the blood. It is a rich source of vitamins, minerals, amino acids, chlorophyll, beta-carotene, SOD and live enzymes, which literally makes this green powder a living, healing food. SOD found in barley grass helps the body to detoxify chemicals and foreign substances, thereby helping to prevent the onset of disease and cancer.

One of the unique qualities of barley grass is its ability to protect the fibroblasts in the lung cells from the damaging effects of radiation and other cancer-causing substances. However, barley grass must be taken on a regular basis before exposure to these toxins in order for this protection to occur.

In my practice as a naturopath, I am privileged to hear of the most wonderful real-life stories of self-healing from cancer patients. I know of one man who removed a cancerous tumour in his knee and pelvis by consuming large amounts of barley grass and chlorophyll in addition to a pure, organic whole foods diet. He had previously tried conventional medicine but to no avail. After only a few months of using nature cure remedies such as these he re-visited his doctor for follow-up tests. There were no signs of the tumour present in his body, much to the surprise of his doctor.

This is one real-life account and I am sure there are many more. However, what may work for one person may not work for another, as humans we are all completely different in our genetics, personalities and physical characteristics. To find an ideal program to suit your specific needs, it is always best to consult with a caring, professional and experienced health practitioner.

Bee Pollen

Bee pollen is a powder-like material produced by the anthers of flowering plants and gathered by bees. Bees collect this powder, moisten it with nectar and pack it into 'pollen baskets' or sacs on their backs. Then they hand over their precious load to the 'nurse bees'. This pollen is then made into royal jelly, to feed the young developing bee larvae. It is composed of 10 to 25 per cent protein and also contains 18 amino acids, 28 minerals, 11 enzymes and 14 fatty acids, as well as B complex vitamins, vitamin C, carotene, calcium, copper, iron, magnesium, potassium, manganese, sodium, plant sterols and simple sugars. Many health promoters now advertise bee pollen as a 'perfect food'.

Bee pollen has anti-microbial and antibiotic properties. It is useful for combating cancer, pollution, radiation, fatigue, depression and colon disorders. It also has a strengthening and stimulating effect on the body's immune system. Bee pollen is believed to prevent cancer and may reduce the possibility of tumours if taken regularly. Research indicates that beekeepers as a whole display lower rates of cancer compared to other occupations studied.

The Chinese have used bee pollen for centuries to prevent prostate enlargement, slow down the ageing process, reduce radiation sickness in cancer patients and to boost endurance and strength. Scientists are only just beginning to unlock the amazing disease-prevention properties found within this unique pollen.

Some people can be allergic to bee pollen. It is best to try a small amount first and determine if a rash, wheezing or any other signs of discomfort occur. If allergic symptoms occur, discontinue use.

Bryostatins

Bryostatins are ocean invertebrates called Bugulaneritina (sea mats or corallines). Scientists have isolated a chemical from bryostatins called lactones. Lactones boost immunity through interleukin-2 and T-type white blood cells. They are believed to inhibit the growth of cancerous cells, especially leukaemia. Bryostatins decrease cell growth and spread in some forms of cancer.

Chlorophyll

Chlorophyll is an effective blood builder, cleansing agent, a natural antibiotic and is also able to chelate heavy metals and toxins from the body. Chlorophyll is the substance that makes plants green and is responsible for photosynthesis. Chlorophyll is a rich source of beta-carotene, folic acid, vitamin K (needed for blood clotting) and enzymes. The molecular structure of chlorophyll resembles that of haemoglobin, the oxygen-carrying protein of red blood cells.

The key difference between haemoglobin and chlorophyll is the metallic atom in the middle of each molecule of human haemoglobin is iron and the metallic atom in the middle of chlorophyll is magnesium. Blue-green algae, spirulina, chlorella wheat grass, parsley, barley grass, broccoli and dark green leafy vegetables are rich sources of chlorophyll.

The active ingredient in chlorophyll, chlorophyllin is known to have strong anti-muta-genic, anti-tumour and antioxidant properties. Research carried out at the National Institute of Occupational Safety and Health (NIOSH), in the United States, tested a variety of complex, cancer-causing substances. These included fried beef, shredded pork, red wine, cigarette smoke, tobacco snuff, chewing tobacco, airborne particles, coal, dust and diesel emission particles. Chlorophyllin stopped mutations in eight out of 10 of these tests. (Ong et al., 1986:173, p 111–15) In 1991, scientists at the Center for Health Sciences and Toxicology, in the United States tested chlorophyllin against one of the most potent carcinogens known, aflatoxin. Results showed that chlorophyllin almost completely inhibited the mutagenicity of this carcinogen. (Warner et al., 1991: 262:25–30) This makes chlorophyll useful in the prevention of many different types of cancer.

Chlorophyll has a soothing and healing effect on the mucosal lining and it has been used for skin ulcers, as a blood builder for anaemia, and to help detoxify the liver and kidneys.

Colostrum and Lactoferrin

Colostrum, generally obtained from a cow, is the 'first food' derived from the first letdown of milk following birth. When a mother first gives birth, her milk is rich in immunoglobulins and other life-supporting nutrients, including protein. The nutrients are passed on to her child through this special substance.

Colostrum is a unique combination of immunoglobulins, specific antibodies and immune enhancers designed to protect the child against viruses, bacteria and allergens. Together with acidophilus probiotic bacteria, colostrum kick-starts the immune system in the gut and helps to prevent gastro-intestinal infections.

Most of the present research on colostrum has been performed on bovine colostrum. To obtain pure colostrum, the cows must be grain-fed and free to roam in pesticide-free pastures. Hence most of the high quality colostrum available today is obtained from New Zealand cows. Try to be aware of the source of your colostrum when purchasing this product to ensure that it has been obtained from grain-fed healthy cows.

Colostrum contains some very beneficial immunoglobulins. These include IgG which stimulates phagocytosis to neutralise toxins, IgA which helps to reduce bacterial and viral infections, IgM which enhances phagocytosis against micro-organisms and IgD which stimulates B cells to produce antibodies and to reduce allergic reactions. Colostrum also contains lactoferrin, interleukin, an immune system stimulant, and oligosaccharides, a promoter of healthy microflora in the gut and live enzymes.

With these essential ingredients, colostrum may prove to be an extremely beneficial 'live food' in cancer prevention and treatment. At present, companies are isolating some unique ingredients from colostrum and making some amazing claims as to its positive benefits with cancer treatment and chemotherapy. More research needs to be performed on colostrum; its ingredients could turn out to be a miraculous healing living food.

Lactoferrin is a human protein found mainly in external secretions such as breast milk, tears and in secondary granules of neutrophils. It is a relatively new supplement that has generated interest due to a number of articles touting its benefit in application to cancer therapy. One of my previous colleagues who had been a doctor and a natural therapist for over 30 years regularly used lactoferrin as part of his natural cancer-fighting program for his clients. The success in his clinic was overwhelming.

Lactoferrin is a substance that belongs to a family of chemicals known as cytokines. Cytokines are responsible for co-ordinating the human cellular immune response that protects us from infections, cancers and tumours. A deficiency of cytokines can lead to a suppressed immune system and an excess of these can cause an over-active immune response. Lactoferrin works by regulating the cellular immune response on several different levels.

In a healthy person, lactoferrin is the first line of defence that protects body openings such as the eyes, mouth, nose and other orifices from infections. Secondly, it binds to iron to prevent pathogens and tumours from using the iron for reproduction and growth. When a healthy body is presented with a tumour or infection, lactoferrin is produced rapidly near the infection or tumour. It then binds with iron and renders it unavailable to the bacteria or tumour, causing a malnutrition situation and starving the bacteria or tumour. In theory, if a tumour is starved of its food supply, it is unable to grow and may begin to shrink.

Lactoferrin improves the immune response. It should not be used on its own, but rather as a supportive therapy in the treatment of severe immune deficiency conditions such as those seen with cancer. It is also thought to stop the replication of certain viruses, including HIV and some of the herpes family of viruses.

So where does lactoferrin come from? Lactoferrin is derived from bovine colostrum, the first fluid that comes out of the breast after a baby is born. From the first day to three days after birth, the mother produces a fluid that is not milk, but rather a mixture of immunoglobulins and about 15 to 20 per cent lactoferrin. Most sources are extracted from cow's colostrum, which is purified and free from allergic reactions.

Generally 200 to 400mg per day before bed is taken to improve immune deficiency states. It should always be purchased from a reputable source and taken under advice from your health care professional. (Ref: Singleton & Sainsbury, 1996. Brock, 1995, p417–419. Swart et al, 1996. p 769–75.)

Fatty Acids

The body needs fat. Fatty acids are necessary for health and those that cannot be made by the body are called essential fatty acids (EFAs). Essential fatty acids reduce blood pressure, improve the condition of skin and hair, lower cholesterol and triglyceride levels and reduce the risk of blood clot formation. EFAs are found in high concentrations in the brain and are needed for normal development and functioning of the brain. They aid in the transmission of nerve impulses. Every living cell in the body needs essential fatty acids. They are essential for rebuilding and producing new cells.

Essential fatty acids are also involved in the manufacture of prostaglandin substances which play a role in a number of body functions, including hormone synthesis, immune support, regulation of our response to pain and inflammation, blood vessel constriction and other heart and lung functions.

There are two basic categories of essential fatty acids, omega-3 and omega-6. Omega-3 essential fatty acids include alpha-linolenic acid (ALA) found in vegetable oils such as hemp seed oil, flax seed oil and canola oil and eicosapentaenoic acid (EPA) and docosahexaenoic acid (DHA) found in deepwater fish and fish oils such as mackerel, sardines, herring, halibut, salmon and tuna. Omega-6 essential fatty acids include gamma-linolenic acid (GLA) found in borage seed oil, evening primrose oil and other similar plant oils and linolenic acid (LA), found in various vegetable oils. Our body needs all of these essential fatty acids in the correct amounts to maintain ideal health and to prevent health conditions such as cancer.

The results of various studies throughout the world indicate that the level of dietary fat intake and the type of fatty acids consumed influence cancer risk and disease progression. A balance needs to be maintained between omega-3 intake and omega-6 intake. Very high intakes of omega-6 fatty acids seem to increase the risk of cancer, whereas moderate intakes of omega-6 and high intakes of omega-3 fatty acids may provide protection against cancer. Polyunsaturated omega-6 fatty acids in large amounts may stimulate tumour growth and metastasis, whereas long chain omega-3 fatty acids tend to have the reverse effect.

Breast Cancer and Fatty Acids
It is believed that a low level of omega-6 fatty acids may be linked to tumours spreading to other tissues. It is also thought that omega-3 fatty acids may inhibit breast cancer development, depending on the amount of omega-6 fatty acids in the diet.

Colon Cancer and Fatty Acids
Omega-3 fatty acids may help to prevent and inhibit colon cancer. Research has shown that fish consumption is associated with protection against the later stages of colorectal cancer.

Prostate Cancer and Fatty Acids
Dietary intake of essential fatty acids may play a role in prostate cancer cell growth. Studies have demonstrated that men whose dietary intake is low in omega-6 fatty acids (alpha linolenic acid) and high in saturated fats have a higher incidence of prostate cancer.

Table of Fats and Oils
Table 23.1

Saturated Fats	Monounsaturated Oils	Polyunsaturated Oils	Omega -6 Oils	Omega-3 Oils
Beef	Olive oil	Soybean	Soybean	Flaxseed
Pork	Canola oil	Safflower	Safflower	Soybean
Lamb	Almond oil	Sunflower	Sunflower	Canola
Poultry		Corn	Wheat germ	Pumpkin
Milk		Sesame	Sesame	Walnut
Butter				Fish oils
Cheese				
Yogurt				

Fibre

Fibre is a much-needed component in the human diet. It is extremely useful in preventing disturbances of the intestine and digestive system, including cancer of the colon, rectum and diverticulitis or ulcerative colitis. With the advent of the low fibre Westernised diet, cancer of the colon has become one of the biggest killers amongst people of all ages. Fibre has an amazing ability to remove toxins/carcinogens from the digestive tract, thereby preventing many forms of cancer caused by a build-up of toxins. Fibre is also good for removing certain toxic metals from the body, and is able to remove fats, thereby decreasing the occurrence of breast cancer.

Other functions of fibre include helping to regulate the rate of sugar entering the bloodstream, lowering blood fat levels, preventing the absorption of toxic heavy metals and fats, and controlling weight. There are many different types of fibre including bran, cellulose, gum, hemicellulose, lignin, mucilage and pectin. Each form has its own function. Rice bran, a form of fibre, possesses potent anti-tumour activities and has an ability to stimulate the body's immune system. Cellulose found in apples, beets, brazil nuts, broccoli, carrots, celery, green beans, lima beans, pears, peas and wholegrains helps to remove cancer-causing substances from the colon.

Pectin found in cabbage, apples, bananas, beets, carrots, citrus fruits, okra and dried peas, may reduce the side effects of radiation therapy, chemotherapy and remove unwanted toxins and metals. Hemicelluose, found in apples, bananas, beets, cabbage, green leafy vegetables, pears, peppers and wholegrain cereals may help to prevent colon cancer and to control carcinogens in the intestinal tract. The best way to obtain adequate fibre is to eat plenty of wholegrains and fresh fruits and vegetables.

Fish Oils (EPA/DHA)

Fish oils hit the health industry in the '90s with amazing force. They are beneficial in preventing arthritis, heart disease and cancer. Fish oils are rich in omega-3 fatty acids such as eicosapentaenoic acid (EPA). EPA is believed to inhibit the growth and metastasis of some forms of cancer, such as pancreatic cancer. Fish rich in EPA includes salmon, tuna, mackerel, herring oil, cod, haddock, swordfish, halibut, sardines, eel and trout.

The diet of the Inuit (Eskimos) is rich in fish oils, as is the Japanese diet. Both cultures show a low incidence of breast and colon cancer. A high fish intake is thought to decrease the risk of breast cancer and the development of many types of cancer.

Shark liver oil was discovered in 1922. It contains compounds known as alkyl-glycerols, which are also found in breast milk and bone marrow. These are active substances that provide breast fed babies with protection against infections until their own immunity is developed. Alkyglycerols have been studied as a possible treatment for childhood leukaemia and as a key to reversing cervical cancer in women.

Shark liver oil facilitates the elimination of toxic minerals from the body. It has the ability to also remove toxic organic forms of mercury and may be beneficial in the treatment and prevention of cancer. For more information on shark liver oil, refer to the entry later in this chapter.

Fructo-oligo-saccharides (FOS)

These promote the growth and activity of friendly bacteria in the gut. A naturally occurring compound found in fruits and vegetables, FOS are non-caloric substances that are not broken down by the digestive tract. It passes through us easily, inhibiting the growth of 'the baddies' and enhancing the growth of healthy organisms like bifidobacteria. A healthy immunity within the digestive system helps to prevent the formation of many types of cancer.

Genistein – Phyto-oestrogens

One of the most powerful and fascinating of plant ingredients available today is genistein, a plant hormone in soybeans that has been found to profoundly influence our hormone cycles and health. Soy contains phyto-oestrogens, or weak plant oestrogens such as genistein. The power in these phyto-oestrogens lies in their gentleness and their remarkable ability to adapt to your body's particular needs.

Phyto-oestrogens latch on to the same receptor sites as oestrogen in your body and may help prevent hormonally linked cancers. Like a light switch, they can both turn on oestrogenic effects and turn them off, depending on what your body needs.

Soy protein is believed to reduce the frequency of menstrual cycles by increasing the length of the follicular phase. This may play a role in decreasing one's risk of developing breast cancer. Phyto-oestrogens such as genistein could be a safer alternative to using tamoxifen in the treatment of breast cancer. Studies on animals have indicated that genistein may also reduce the risk of skin cancer.

Finally, genistein can help prevent excessive new blood vessel growth. Cancerous tumours grow by creating a rich network of new blood vessels. By inhibiting this ability, genistein may slow cancer down.

Green Tea

A simple, tasty and age-old beverage, green tea has potent health-enhancing flavonoids. Green tea seems to protect against several cancers and heart disease. This is good news, since after water, tea is the most popular beverage in the world.

Black tea is dried, crushed, fermented and then dried again. Green teas are not crushed and oxidized; instead they are steamed, then rolled and dried. A cup of green tea contains about 400 milligrams of polyphenols, which are highly beneficial to our health. One of these polyphenols, known as EGCG (epigallocatechin gallate), is a potent antioxidant.

The flavonoids (substances that act like antioxidants) and polyphenols found in green tea may decrease one's risk of developing many types of cancer including oesophageal cancer, sarcomas and stomach cancer. Green tea decreases a person's risk of forming polyp-like growths in the lower colon that can lead to colorectal cancer.

Green tea is believed to block the formation of carcinogenic substances such as nitrosamines and it promotes detoxification of harmful agents such as heavy metals and excess oestrogen. Studies show that green tea drinkers have a reduced risk of colorectal and pancreatic cancer. Its active ingredients uniquely boost the body's immune system, protecting against disease and cancer formation. It also helps to promote weight loss, prevents tooth decay, lowers cholesterol levels and encourages healthy heart function.

Indoles

Indoles are strong antioxidants found in cabbage, kale, turnips, cauliflower, broccoli and brussel sprouts. Indoles activate the benzaldehyde enzyme system, an internal body system which decreases and breaks down harmful female sex hormones. These hormones can increase the risk of certain types of breast cancer and other hormone-related cancers.

Indoles may also decrease the development of prostate tumours and tumours caused by carcinogens. Indoles also retard the ability of ingested or inhaled polynuclear aromatic hydrocarbons (PAHs– found in cigarettes, car exhaust fumes and smoke generated from poor cooking methods) to convert to cancer-causing substances within the liver. This, therefore, may prevent the development of many forms of cancer caused from a high ingestion of PAH. Apart from indoles, selenium, vitamin C and vitamin E also help to prevent this process.

Lactobacilli

Lactobacilli are strains of friendly bacteria that assist in creating healthy intestinal flora. Lactobacillus acidophilus is the most widely known and the most extensively researched of all healthy bacteria. L. acidophilus is the most abundant bacterium in the small intestines and probably the most effective.

Lactobacillus acidophilus assists in the digestion of proteins, has antifungal properties and aids digestion and the absorption of nutrients. L. Acidophilus helps to detoxify harmful toxins. It is found in yogurt and other cultured milk products. Its main function is in maintaining the overall health of the body's digestive system and it is also believed to prevent the onset of colon cancer. L. Acidophilus decreases the conversion of primary bile acids to secondary bile acids, which may lead to colon cancer.

Lactobacillus bifidus is also present in the intestinal flora and helps to establish a healthy environment for the manufacture of B vitamins and vitamin K. By promoting the proper digestion of foods, healthy flora prevents constipation and gas, which can lead to colon cancer. It helps to eliminate toxic waste products from the intestine and is therefore very beneficial in preventing cancer.

Lecithin

Lecithin is found throughout our entire body. The protective sheaths surrounding the brain are composed of lecithin, as are our cell membranes and muscles and nerve cells. Lecithin is a lipid that is needed by every living cell in the human body. Lecithin consists mostly of the B vitamin choline and also contains high amounts of linoleic acid and inositol. Lecithin helps to promote higher energy levels, repairs liver damage, protects against cardiovascular disease, improves brain function and enables fats such as cholesterol to be dispersed in water and removed from the body.

Most lecithin is derived from soybeans. Egg yolks also contain large amounts of lecithin. Other sources of lecithin include fish, legumes, wheat germ and grains, organ meats, lean meats, brewer's yeast and nuts. Unbleached lecithin granules can be added to breakfast cereal or smoothies on a daily basis.

Lignans

Lignans (present in flaxseed) have been shown to reduce hormone sensitive cancers (breast, prostatic cancers) by binding unconjugated sex hormones. They also inhibit the enzyme involved in the synthesis of sex hormones, thereby reducing tumour exposure to various sex hormones.

Medicinal Mushrooms

Since ancient times, medicinal mushrooms have been used by populations around the world for their incredible healing properties. Oriental people believe mushrooms enhance longevity, promote well being and prevent illness and disease. Medicinal mushrooms, such as shitake, reishi, maitake and ganoderma stimulate the production of interferon hence strengthening the body's immune system. It is believed over 50 varieties of mushrooms that have anti-carcinogenic effects exist.

Many of the health promoting components from mushrooms (lectins, polysaccharides, glucans and lentinan) are today being removed to make anti-cancer drugs and anti-infectious agents for use by the medical profession. It is much healthier, cheaper and advantageous to include these miracle-packed fungi as a regular part of your healthy diet.

Cordyceps

Cordyceps sinensis or caterpillar mushroom is a famous Chinese mushroom that promotes phagocytosis and is believed to be a powerful lymphocyte regulator as it increases helper T-cells (commanders of the immune army), Interleukin-2 (activates white blood cells to destroy cancer cells and viruses) and phagocytic activity (the engulfing and digesting of cell debris and bacteria) in lymphocyte suppressed patients.

Enoki and Karawatake

Enoki is a white, stringy Japanese mushroom that is believed to protect against some forms of cancer. It is also beneficial in strengthening the body's immune system.

Karawatake mushroom, another Japanese mushroom, may prevent many forms of cancer due to its high PSK content.

Kombucha

Kombucha has been used throughout Asia and Russia for centuries. It is often referred to throughout the world as 'The Champagne of Life', 'Gift of Life from the Sea', 'Champion of Longevity' and in China as the 'Divine Che'.

A 'tea' is made by fermenting the mushroom for one week in a mixture of water, sugar and green or black tea, with apple cider vinegar or previously made tea added to it. Kept in this mixture, the mushroom reproduces, and the 'daughter mushrooms' can then be used to produce more tea. Kombucha tea contains many different nutrients and other health-promoting substances. It is a natural energy booster and detoxifier, and may also help to slow the natural ageing process and fight cancer, AIDS and multiple sclerosis.

Biochemists ascribe many of Kombucha's therapeutic effects to 1-lactic acid and glucuronic acid. Lactic acid is also found in fermented foods such as sauerkraut and yogurt. Lactic acid activates cell respiration, increases oxygen in the blood and thus increases energy. It also balances blood pH (in acidity) and mildly stimulates liver function. Lactic acid is lacking in the connective tissue of cancer patients and its presence in large amounts inhibits the development of cancer.

Glucuronic acid plays a significant role in the removal of metabolic waste, toxins, chemicals and drugs, as well as the regulation of lactic acid metabolism. Kombucha tea is not a cure-all. However, it has generated amazing testimonials of improved health and well-being from all corners of the globe.

Maitake

Maitake is another Japanese mushroom recognised throughout the world for its amazing healing properties. Maitake mushrooms stimulate the body's immune system by activating macrophages, natural killer cells and cytotoxic T-cells, thereby inhibiting tumour growth. The major active ingredient responsible for healing is Beta 1.6 Glucan. It is capable of suppressing many viruses and improving and stimulating various aspects of the immune system.

Maitake not only helps to prevent cancer, but is also considered useful for the actual treatment of cancer. Maitake assists in lowering blood pressure, enhances weight loss and helps with the treatment of AIDS. It is therapeutically effective and well absorbed when consumed orally.

Reishi

Reishi, also known as ling-zhi or soul mushrooms, have been popular for at least 2000 years in the Far East. The Chinese believe this unique wood-decomposing fungus promotes eternal youth and longevity.

Reishi mushrooms are a traditional medicinal substance that aids the body in resistance against a wide range of physical, biological and environmental stresses. They protect against some forms of cancer and stimulate the function of the immune system by acting as antioxidants. The mushrooms are believed to have anti-tumour properties, inhibiting tumour growth and aids in building resistance to disease. They are also useful in the treatment of fatigue, viral infections, allergies, bronchial asthma, high cholesterol, high blood pressure and dizziness.

Reishi have strong antioxidant properties with the ability to scavenge free radicals in blood plasma. Studies carried out in Japan have confirmed reishi may be capable of arresting metastatic cancer. The Japanese cancer society has found reishi effective against sarcomas. The active ingredient responsible for this are polysaccharides, mainly ganoderic acid.

Reishi mushrooms are considered the most valuable medicine in the orient, far outweighing even ginseng. The mystical qualities are attributed to their rarity – only two to three mushrooms are found for every 10,000 dead plum or hemlock logs. They are documented way back in 56 BC as having the most extensive and effective healing powers.

Shitake

Shitake is a Japanese mushroom with amazing health-promoting properties. Shitake contains a polysaccharide called lentinan (lentinula) that strengthens the immune system by increasing T cell function. Lentinan is a polysaccharide with strong immune-stimulatory functions and anti-tumour actions. Lentinan is believed to suppress the growth and spread of some forms of breast, colon and stomach cancer. It is therefore able to increase the lifespan of people with colon, prostate, stomach and breast cancer by preventing its spread.

Shitake mushrooms also contain 18 amino acids, seven of which are essential amino acids. They are very rich in B vitamins, especially B1, B2 and B3. When sun-dried they contain high amounts of vitamin D. Their effectiveness in treating cancer has been reported in various studies in Japan, suggesting that shitake can retard even very advanced cancers.

Laboratory research suggests that one of the active ingredients in shitake, lentinan, enhances the effectiveness of the immune system by increasing the activity of macrophages, T-helper cells and other white blood cells (Feher et al., 1989, p 55–62). Positive results have also been seen in human studies involving people with stomach cancer (Tagachi, 1987, p 333–49), gastrointestinal tumours (Maekawa et al., 1990, p 137–40), cervical cancer (Shimizu et al., 1990: 37-44) and breast cancer (Kosaka et al. 1987, p 516–22). KS-2, a peptidomannan found in shitake is another ingredient that is thought to be highly effective in one's fight against cancer.

White Jelly Fungus and Xloud

The white jelly fungus mushroom is thought to protect against cancer. The xloud mushroom effectively fights cancer due to its high kureha content. Scientific research indicates kureha, a polysaccharide, is beneficial in the treatment of cancer.

Modified Citrus Pectin

A new and interesting cancer fighter is known as modified citrus pectin (MCP) – a soluble component of plant fibre derived from the peel and pulp of citrus fruits such as oranges and tangerines. Ordinary pectin is a complex carbohydrate found in most plants. Ordinary pectin is not absorbed into the bloodstream because of its long molecular chain. Modified citrus pectin is a carbohydrate which can be broken down to a shorter molecular chain and hence enter the blood steam.

MCP may work by preventing cancer cells from metastasising, which occurs when malignant cells spread throughout the body, first detaching themselves from the original tumour and, like seeds blown on the wind, travelling through the bloodstream until they find another site on which to tough down and begin dividing and multiplying.

Metastasis is the gravest danger a cancer patient can face. If a tumour were simply to stay where it originated, it might cause some local damage but it could be removed surgically with few, if any, complications. Studies suggest that MCP may work like a special bait that attracts migrating cancer cells and renders them harmless. It is thought to help reduce metastasis in melanoma patients.

It appears that MCP attracts cancer cells and binds with them before they get a chance to fasten themselves to healthy cells. Cancer cells contain a substance called galactin. Galactin looks for its counterpart, galactose which is found in many cells. MCP is particularly high in galactose and thus it can attract cancer cells, bind to them and then render them harmless. Cancer cells don't appear to 'care' whether they are binding to MCP or a human cell, because they are simply 'hungry' and on the hunt for galactose.

Proanthocyandins and Pycogenol

Proanthocyandins, also known as oligomeric proanthocyandins are flavin bioflavonoids. They are naturally occurring substances found in a variety of foods and plants. Clinical tests indicate they are 50 times more potent than vitamin E and 20 times more potent than vitamin C in terms of bioavailable antioxidant activity. They strengthen and repair connective tissue and contain strong anti-inflammatory actions. The two main sources of proanthocyandins are pine bark extract (pycogenol) and grape seed extract.

Pycogenol is a patented antioxidant blend of various bioflavonoids, including proanthocyandins. It is extracted from the maritime pine tree, native to France, and can also be extracted from grape seeds. Ferulic acid, found in pycogenol is believed to prevent many forms of cancer. Gallic acid is also found in pycogenol and prevents many carcinogens from inducing chromosome mutations. Pycogenol protects capillaries from attack by free radicals and protects the cell membranes of red blood cells and helps to keep them flexible. Pycogenol possesses strong anti-inflammatory properties.

Bioflavonoids, catechins and proanthocyandins all possess strong anti-cancer properties.

Probiotics

Probiotics have proved, in thousands of studies, to be indispensable in keeping us healthy by cleansing our intestines of excess pathogens, thus preventing allergies, yeast infections, diarrhoea, gas, bloating, digestive problems and disease.

Resveratrol

Another important flavonoid, made from the skin of grapes, is resveratrol. It is a relatively newly discovered compound that is believed to be the active ingredient in grape skin and red wine. It is a flavonoid that seems to protect the heart and also has been found to inhibit cancer formation. It is also thought that resveratrol is responsible for the low incidence of breast and prostatic cancers among vegetarians and Orientals respectively (Rodrigue et al. 2001, p 500-07). Rather than try to consume these flavonoids in the form of wine – and risk the adverse health effects of alcohol – I recommend resveratrol supplements to patients.

Royal Jelly

Nature and its beautiful creatures are a source of amazement and contains all of our answers to create healing remedies. Royal Jelly, the thick white pharyngeal gland secretion of the nurse bees, which is fed to the Queen Bee, is believed to prevent and treat leukaemia. The amazing size, fertility and life span of the queen bee is attributed to its dietary food source, royal jelly. It is also believed to prevent other forms of cancer due to its high free radical fatty acid content. Royal jelly is rich in B vitamins, especially vitamin B1, B3 and B5.

Royal jelly enhances energy levels, relieves body aches and pains, boosts adrenal gland function and prevents fatigue. It has been toted in different cultures around the world as a 'youth tonic'. There has been some evidence suggesting that royal jelly has anti-tumour activity. More research is presently being conducted in this area.

Sea Vegetables

Sea vegetables are gifts from the ocean, containing abundant vitamins, minerals, polysaccharides and a rich source of iodine. Iodine has a balancing effect on the body's thyroid gland, increasing general metabolism.

Kelp is a group of seaweeds with a distinct seaweed odour and salty, fishy taste. Kelp is a particularly rich source of iodine. In Japanese studies there has been shown to be a direct correlation between kelp consumption and the prevention of breast cancer. It is believed the fibre content, and particularly the algin content, is largely responsible, as well as through the stimulation of the cancer fighting T-cells thereby strengthening the immune system.

Kelp also helps to protect against heavy metals and ionizing radiation by binding in the intestinal tract and preventing their absorption. Kelp contains compounds that decrease the absorption of radioactive metallic ions like strontium, radioactive strontium 90, lead, mercury, cadmium, and barium. Kelp and other seaweeds are great to incorporate into the diet, to help protect against the toxic effects of radiation treatment, chemotherapy, x-rays and CT scans.

Alginate, a substance found primarily in kelp, pacific brown kelp and bladderwrack, enhances immune system function by stimulating T-cells. Alginate is able to dilute potent carcinogens in the intestine and binds to bile acids in the small intestine, enhancing their elimination and therefore decreasing the risk of cancer.

The sea plant wakame is known to counteract the toxic effects of nicotine. Wakame may help to prevent lung cancer and other forms of cancer by stopping the growth of tumours and inhibiting chemical carcinogenesis. Wakame is a strong immune system stimulant. Laminara, a high fibre sea plant also seems to play a large role in the prevention of breast cancer.

Studies on the sea plant *Dunaliella bardawil* found that it may inhibit spontaneous breast cancers. This may be largely due to its high beta-carotene content, antioxidant properties and its ability to stabilize our body chemistry.

Dulse and kelp powders can be used instead of salt and added to most dishes. Dulse leaves can be soaked, then added to grain dishes, salads and soups. Kombu, wakame and nori can be added to soups. Nori is the dark leafy seaweed used to make sushi. Hijiki and arame should be soaked, then sautéed and simmered. They can be used in grain or vegetable dishes and salads. Kelp, wakame and bladderwrack contain a cancer-fighting mucopolysaccharide, called fucoidan. Fucoidan stimulates the immune system and prevents cancer by retarding the growth of tumours and inhibiting chemical carcinogens.

Shark Cartilage

The tough, elastic material that makes up the skeleton of the shark is dried and pulverised (finely powdered) to make this food supplement. Shark cartilage contains a number of active components, the most important of which is a type of protein that acts as an angiogenesis inhibitor – that is, it acts to suppress the development of new blood vessels. This makes it valuable in fighting a number of disorders. Many cancerous tumours, for instance, are able to grow only because they induce the body to develop new networks of blood vessels to supply them with nutrients. Shark cartilage suppresses this process, so that tumours are deprived of their source of nourishment and often tumours begin to shrink.

Sharks are one of the only creatures in the world that are not susceptible to developing cancer. This interesting point has led to further research being performed on sharks to understand why they are not prone to tumour development. Research performed in Boston discovered that a tumour will stop growing when it reaches two millimetres in size, unless it has sufficient blood supply. From this stage, new blood vessels begin to form to feed the tumour and it enlarges. Shark cartilage contains no blood vessels and actually contains a protein that inhibits the development of blood vessels thereby starving the tumour of its supplies.

Shark cartilage also contains high amounts of calcium (16%) and phosphorous (8%) and muco-polysaccharides that act to stimulate the body's immune system.

The recommended daily intake is anywhere from 2500mg/day to 6000mg/day. Shark cartilage is generally not recommended for children or used during pregnancy or lactation without professional advice.

Shark Liver Oil – Alkylglycerols

Originally discovered in 1922, shark liver oil extract contains compounds called alkylglycerols that are also found in breast milk, the liver and spleen, and in bone marrow. These are active substances that provide breast fed babies with protection against infections until their own immunity is developed. Alkyglycerols have been studied as a possible treatment for childhood leukaemia and as a likely key to reversing cervical cancer in women. They are able to increase antibodies in the body through the building of certain types of white blood cells. This in turn has a boosting effect on the body's immune system.

Shark liver oil facilitates the elimination of toxic minerals from the body. It has the ability to also remove toxic organic forms of mercury and may be beneficial in the treatment and prevention of cancer. It may also be useful for people undergoing radiation therapy, as it prevents leukopenia (lack of white blood cells). If taken before radiation therapy, shark liver oil may help to control abnormal cell reproduction. In the 1990s, John Hopkins University discovered another healing ingredient in shark liver oil known as squalamine. Squalamine is effective against many yeast, bacterial and fungal infections, and offers promise to immune compromised persons such as cancer patients. These ancient creatures of the ocean may hold the secret to improved health and longevity for mankind.

Spirulina

Spirulina is a form of micro-algae rich in vitamins, minerals, chlorophyll and protein. It has been recognised the world over as a valuable whole food source. Spirulina contains concentrations of nutrients unlike any other single grain, herb or plant. It contains gamma-linolenic acid (GLA), linoleic and arachidonic acids, vitamin B12 (needed for healthy red blood cells), iron, a high level of protein, essential amino acids, the nucleic acids RNA and DNA, chlorophyll and phyococyanin (a blue pigment only found in blue-green algae). This pigment is believed a key compound in deterring and treating liver cancer.

Spirulina is a naturally digestible food which aids in protecting the immune system, cholesterol reduction and in mineral absorption. It supplies all the necessary nutrients to cleanse and heal the body, while reducing the appetite. Its high protein content helps to stabilise blood sugar levels, so it can be useful for blood sugar conditions and for fasting. Spirulina also boosts energy levels, preventing the debilitating fatigue caused by cancer and cancer treatment.

Spirulina is one of the richest sources of chlorophyll, which is essential in the treatment of cancer by enhancing oxygen transport to cancerous cells. It is a brilliant food supplement to use while cleansing as spirulina removes deadly toxins from the body and provides good levels of protein, vitamins, minerals and other life-giving nutrients.

Wheatgrass

Wheatgrass is a nutritional food that was made popular by Dr Ann Wigmore, an educator and founder of the Hippocrates Health Institute in Boston. Wheatgrass is an energy-packed food containing an immense array of over 100 vitamins, minerals, chlorophyll, laetrile and other trace elements. According to Dr Wigmore, one pound of fresh wheatgrass (just over 500 grams) is equal in nutritional value to nearly 25 pounds (12 kilograms) of the best vegetables.

Wheatgrass therapy combined with a wholefoods diet helps to eliminate cancerous growths and helps many other disorders. It is also very rich in chlorophyll, making it a potent antioxidant. Wheatgrass is able to increase the health of the immune system, lower blood pressure, detoxify the liver and act as a powerful kidney tonic. Wheatgrass juice is able to draw toxins from the colon, liver and kidneys, causing their elimination and ridding the body of the toxic effects of pollution.

Cancer cells cannot grow and exist in the presence of oxygen. Wheatgrass contains high amounts of chlorophyll which oxygenates the body's cells, causing death to cancer cells. Many cancerous cell mutations begin in an environment of oxygen deprivation. No wonder cancer is more prevalent in busy, polluted cities. Wheatgrass improves blood circulation, nourishing body cells and enhancing the carrying of oxygen to body cells.

Various enzymes and amino acids present in wheatgrass deactivate the cancer-causing effects of benzyprene, the dangerous carcinogen found in charcoal broiled meats and smoked fish. Wheatgrass juice prevents chromosome damage, a step the cell undergoes in becoming cancerous. Wheatgrass is a miraculous food that may have the ability to destroy cancerous tumours without the toxic effects of chemotherapy and cancer drugs.

A special juicer is needed to extract the juice from wheatgrass. Fortunately, it can now be obtained fresh from many juice bars and cafes.

Chapter 24

VITALITY PLUS – VITAMIN SUPPLEMENTS

The amazing healing potential contained within vitamins is often underestimated, especially in their advantageous use against cancer. There is nothing more beneficial than the incorporation of specific vitamins, minerals and antioxidants into your daily lifestyle in suitable amounts. Vitamins can boost the body's immune system, decrease tumour size, prevent further cancer production, increase energy levels and improve the metabolic functions of various body systems.

Vitamins are essential to life. They contribute to good health by regulating metabolic processes and assisting biochemical processes that release energy from digested food. Vitamins function as coenzymes helping in a range of metabolic reactions within our body. They are simply helpers in metabolism – essential to growth, vitality and health and are helpful in digestion, elimination and resistance to disease. Deficiencies can lead to a variety of disorders and general health problems, according to which vitamin is lacking in the diet.

For many decades, orthodox medical practitioners have played down and even denied the healing benefits contained within vitamins for the treatment of disease and the maintenance of good health. It is only in recent years that the use of vitamins in the prevention and treatment of disease is becoming more widely accepted within the medical profession.

During my fight against cancer, I used powerful vitamin and mineral supplements as a major part of my healing along with a wholesome diet, fresh juices, herbal teas, meditation, yoga and a small amount of orthodox treatment. During this period, if I ceased taking vitamin supplements, my energy levels dropped dramatically and the side effects experienced with chemotherapy treatment increased.

With a disease such as cancer, the body's levels of cancer fighting nutrients are depleted and often diet alone does not rebalance these rapidly enough. Our body requires extra amounts of vitamins including antioxidants like vitamin E, vitamin A, vitamin C, selenium, zinc and other specific nutrients. Aggressive orthodox treatment such as surgery, chemotherapy, or radiation therapy tends to deplete these vitamins even further.

There is a lot of evidence to suggest that insufficient amounts of antioxidants can increase the risk of cancer. In groups of people who have low levels of these nutrients, the cancer rates are higher. Antioxidants neutralise metabolic products, including free radicals, prevent carcinogens from attacking DNA and cell membranes, inhibit chromosome aberrations, suppress actions of cancer promoters and induce regression of pre-cancerous lesions.

It is ridiculous to deny the amazing healing potential contained within vitamins, minerals, enzymes, amino acids and other nutrients rich in life-force. To deny the healing power of vital nutrients is a crime against the human race.

'Let your food be your medicine and your medicine be your food' was a belief of the great physician Hippocrates from the fifth century BC. All those years ago, he understood the amazing healing power of vitamins contained within foods and today researchers and scientists around the world are re-confirming his findings.

B-complex Vitamins

B-complex vitamins are the catalytic 'spark plugs' of our body. They function as co-enzymes to catalyse many biochemical reactions and work as a 'team' to restore natural body functions. B vitamins help provide energy by acting with enzymes to convert carbohydrates to glucose and are also important in fat and protein metabolism.

B vitamins are all water-soluble and are not stored very well in the body. Thus, they are needed daily to support the many functions they carry out. Deficiencies of one or more B vitamins may occur fairly easily, especially during times of fasting, weight-loss, stress, or with diets that include substantial amounts of refined and processed food, white flour products, caffeine, oral contraceptive use, tobacco, sugar or alcohol.

B-complex vitamins are important in the general maintenance of health and good immune system function. It is believed they help to enhance the effects of chemotherapy and to decrease side effects associated with chemotherapy.

B-complex vitamins are useful in restoring nutritional status to underweight or malnourished cancer patients. They are excellent for improving energy levels and preventing fatigue associated with cancer treatment.

B-complex vitamins are extremely important for the normal functioning of the nervous system and are often helpful in bringing relaxation to individuals who are stressed, nervous, depressed or fatigued. Glowing skin, hair and eyes are influenced by B vitamins, as is the optimal functioning of our body's liver.

Good sources of B complex vitamins include brewer's yeast, brown rice, germ and bran of cereal grains, legumes, torula yeast, nuts and seeds.

Vitamin B1 – Thiamine

Vitamin B1 helps to prevent cancer by detoxifying various carcinogenic chemicals from the body. Thiamine stimulates the body's immune system and facilitates the formation of red blood cells. Being a powerful antioxidant, it counteracts the toxic effects of alcohol and acetaldehyde, and is able to detoxify some of the carcinogenic (harmful) compounds found in tobacco smoke.

Vitamin B1 improves the appetite, increases circulation, reduces nausea, prevents constipation and is essential for the production of energy – five major side effects of cancer treatment.

Good sources of vitamin B1 include germ and bran of wheat, rice husks and the outer portion of grains, brewer's yeast, blackstrap molasses, brown rice, nuts, soybeans, millet and lentils. Milled grains and rice, such as white flour and white rice, lose much of their vitamin B1, so choose grains and rice that are not as highly processed. Of all of the fruits, avocado is the highest source of vitamin B1.

Vitamin B2 – Riboflavin

Vitamin B2, or riboflavin, is an antioxidant which enhances cellular respiration. Vitamin B2 is necessary for red blood cell formation, antibody production and healthy cell growth. Together with vitamin A, it maintains and improves the mucous membranes in the digestive tract.

Vitamin B2 functions as the precursor or building block for two coenzymes that are important in energy production. Riboflavin is also instrumental in cellular respiration, helping each cell utilise oxygen most efficiently. Riboflavin helps with the absorption of iron and vitamin B6. Riboflavin may be effective in preventing cancer of the oesophagus.

One uncommon side effect of cancer treatment is eye problems such as burning eyes, excessive tearing and poor vision. Riboflavin helps to prevent and treat these unusual symptoms.

The most important food source of riboflavin is milk. One of the pigments in milk, lactoflavin, is the milk form of riboflavin. Other good sources include organ meats, whole or enriched grains and vegetables, torula yeast, brewer's yeast, almonds, wheat germ, legumes, avocados, yogurt, dulse and nuts. Oily fish such as mackerel, trout, eel, and herring have substantial levels of riboflavin. Nori seaweed is another good source of riboflavin. Other foods with moderate amounts of riboflavin are dark leafy green vegetables, such as asparagus, broccoli, and spinach, as well as mushrooms and avocados.

Vitamin B3 – Nicotinamide, Niacin

Vitamin B3 is essential in maintaining good blood circulation, dilating blood vessels and energy production. It also enhances the effectiveness of chemotherapy treatment by tripling the time chemotherapy drugs stay in the bloodstream. Vitamin B3 decreases the toxicity of the commonly used chemotherapy medication, Cisplatin. It increases anti-tumour activity and vitamin B3 and aspirin given with radiation therapy increases the body's anti-tumour resistance.

Vitamin B3 also enhances the effectiveness of the cancer drug L-pam. It doubles the effectiveness of the drug if given by injection, one hour before L-pam.

During malignancy or cell proliferation, the cancer cell metabolises glucose anaerobically (without oxygen) rather than aerobically (with oxygen). This results in an energy deficiency. Vitamin B3 partly solves this problem and thus reduces cancer growth and spread, by normalising cancer cell energetics.

Only moderate amounts of vitamin B3 occur in foods as pure niacin; other niacin is converted from the amino acid tryptophan. The best sources of vitamin B3 are liver and other organ meats, poultry, fish and peanuts, all of which have both niacin and tryptophan. Yeast, dried beans, and peas, wheat germ, avocados, dates, figs, and prunes are good sources of niacin.

Vitamin B6 – Pyridoxine

Vitamin B6 is involved in a majority of the body's functions. It acts as a cofactor in several hundred different biochemical reactions in nearly every part of the body. It is necessary for the production of hydrochloric acid, the absorption of fats and protein, maintains sodium/potassium balance (preventing fluid retention) and promotes red blood cell formation. It is also important for energy production, for proper functioning of the brain, formation of haemoglobin and for optimal immune function and antibody production.

Vitamin B6 plays a role in cancer immunity and aids in the prevention of arteriosclerosis. It is needed for the synthesis of nucleic acids RNA and DNA that contain the genetic instructions for the reproduction of all cells, and for normal cellular growth. It can trigger the production of other substances, stopping cancer growth. It may help to prevent lung cancer and skin cancer. Women with cervical cancer are thought to have very low levels of Vitamin B6 in their bodies.

Vitamin B6 deficiency may increase susceptibility to virus induced tumour growth. Survival time may be increased in people with cervical carcinoma, Stage Two endometrial carcinoma and Stage Two bladder cancer and breast cancer when supplemented with pyridoxine. A long-term deficiency of Vitamin B6 is thought to contribute to a depressed immune system as this vitamin is integral in the production of immune system cells.

Good sources of vitamin B6 include brewer's yeast, fish, chicken, spinach, sunflower seeds, walnuts, wheatgerm, peas, carrots, halibut, wholegrains, liver and vegetables.

Bioflavonoids and Quercitin

Bioflavonoids or flavonoids, also known as vitamin P, consist of citrin, quercetin, hesperidin and rutin. They are brightly coloured substances essential in maintaining the integrity of small blood vessels and capillaries. They are powerful antioxidants and anti-inflammatory agents. Bioflavonoids also remove toxic copper from the body. They are helpful in the absorption of vitamin C and protect it from oxidation, thereby improving and prolonging its functioning. The main function of bioflavonoids is to provide synergy in the utilisation of vitamin C.

Vitamin P was first discovered by Dr Albert Szent-Gyorgyi, who found it within the white of the rind in citrus fruit. The letter 'P' for vitamin P stands for permeability factor. This was given to this group of nutrients because they improve the capillary lining's permeability and integrity – that is, the passage of oxygen, carbon dioxide and nutrients through the capillary wall.

Bioflavonoids are responsible for the colours of many fruits and vegetables, and are found also in grains, nuts, leaves and flowers. Studies suggest their value in the treatment of a number of disorders. They are considered one of the most common biological constituents in plants. They have a gentle, beneficial action on numerous physiological processes in the body and benefit the heart, blood vessels, liver, immune system, connective tissue, adrenal glands, kidneys, musculature and nervous system.

Flavonoids improve the strength of capillaries, help to stabilise blood sugar levels and prevent the onset of infections.

Quercetin is a flavonoid occurring naturally in various fruits, nuts, seeds, flowers, barks and leaves. It is best known as an anti-allergy, anti-inflammatory nutrient, and it is able to stabilise mast cell membranes and prevent the release of histamine and other inflammatory agents.

Quercetin is an antioxidant and can inhibit the inflammatory processes so often involved in cancer and tumour development. It also inhibits leukotrienes (inflammatory agents 1000 times more powerful than histamine), hyaluronidase (collagen destroying enzymes) and lysosomal enzymes (promoters of localised inflammation).

Quercetin and other flavonoids derived from fruits and vegetables have long been considered important substances to help prevent cancer. New laboratory studies are suggesting that this belief may be accurate. Quercetin and other flavonoids have been shown in test tube studies to inhibit the growth of cancer cells, including those from breast, colon and lung cancers.

Some studies suggest that quercetin improves pain and other symptoms in men with chronic prostatitis (inflammation of the prostate). In addition, studies indicate that quercetin may inhibit the growth of prostate cancer cells in test tubes. Further studies are needed to confirm quercetin's benefit in the treatment of prostate cancer.

Quercetin also protects insulin-producing beta cells of the pancreas from free radical damage and enhances insulin secretion. It functions like other bioflavonoids in enhancing the body's collagen network (structural integrity) of blood vessels.

Quercetin is an anti-tumour agent that is believed to reduce DNA damage caused by different cancer-causing substances such as aflatoxins. If you are planning to undergo chemotherapy, quercetin would be a useful addition to your program to ensure that you maintain the health of your capillaries and veins, as one of the major side-effects of chemotherapy is damage to the body's veins.

The recommended dosage of quercetin is 200mg three times per day. It is best taken with either bromelain or vitamin C to increase its absorption.

A synthetic derivative of bioflavonoids, flavone aceteic acid (FAA) has been used to enhance the function of the body's immune system. FAA possesses natural killer cell activity and used with interleukin-2 has a positive effect on kidney cancers. (There are known side effects associated with the use of FAA.)

Good sources of bioflavonoids and quercetin are the white pulp of citrus fruits, blackcurrants, blackberries, cherries, grapes, buckwheat, apricots and plums.

Herbal sources are Echinacea, hawthorn, milk thistle and bilberry.

Coenzyme Q10

Coenzyme Q10 is an essential component in the body's respiratory chain, where energy is produced. CoQ10 is necessary for human life to exist and a deficiency can contribute to ill health, rapid ageing and disease. Since its discovery 40 years ago, hundreds of clinical research studies have been done on CoQ10 and it is now abundantly clear that this nutrient is absolutely vital to health.

Coenzyme Q10 is found throughout the body in cell membranes, especially in the mitochondrial membranes and is particularly abundant in the heart, lungs, liver, kidneys, spleen, pancreas and adrenal glands. The total body content of CoQ10 is only about 500–1500mg and decreases with age.

Coenzyme Q10 is necessary for the formation of adenosine triphosphate (ATP), a compound which acts as an energy donor in chemical reactions. Within the mitochondria of a cell (the cell's power plant where 95 per cent of the cell's energy is created) CoQ10 is needed to not only create energy but to prevent the excess production of free radicals caused by insufficient energy production. If too many free radicals are created because of a lack of CoQ10 the DNA and RNA (our genetic material found in the cell) becomes mutated. This can ultimately lead to cancer formation.

Coenzyme Q10's energy production and antioxidant properties helps the body to protect against the formation of free radicals. It also works hand in hand with vitamin E as an antioxidant and as a vital friend in helping to protect vitamin E from damage.

Antioxidants are substances that scavenge free radicals, damaging compounds in the body that alter cell membranes, tamper with DNA and even cause cell death. Free radicals occur naturally in the body, but environmental toxins (including ultraviolet light, radiation, cigarette smoking, and air pollution) can also increase the number of these damaging particles. Free radicals are believed to contribute to the ageing process as well as the development of a number of health problems, including heart disease and cancer. Antioxidants such as CoQ10 can neutralise free radicals and may reduce or even help prevent some of the damage they cause.

As an antioxidant, Coenzyeme Q10 may have a role to play in both cancer prevention and cancer treatment. Coenzyme Q10 has been shown to reduce tumour growth, stimulate the immune system, possibly increase the size of the body's thymus gland (the maestro gland of the immune system) and improve cellular energetics. It appears to be very effective in breast cancer. Even in patients that presently have cancer, CoQ10 is believed to prevent the spread of cancer, improve the quality of one's life, prevent weight loss and reduce pain.

Coenzyme Q10 normalises cancer cell energetics, thereby improving one's chance of beating cancer. One of the most beneficial functions of coenzyme Q10 is its ability to improve oxygenation throughout the body. It enhances the body's immune system by doubling the body's levels of antibodies and is useful for lowering high blood pressure, lowering cholesterol levels, improving the function and condition of the heart and improving general circulation. Coenzyme Q10 is also thought to promote longevity. It is a wonderful nutrient for improving energy levels and increasing the effectiveness of cancer treatments such as radiation therapy and chemotherapy.

The level of CoQ10 in humans peaks around the age of 20 and then declines fairly rapidly. The decrease in CoQ10 concentration in the heart is particularly significant with a person of 77 having only 57 per cent less CoQ10 in the heart muscle than a 20-year-old. Research shows that many people, especially older people and people engaging in vigorous exercise, may be deficient in CoQ10 and may benefit from supplementation.

Good sources of CoQ10 include hazelnuts, walnuts, chestnuts, almonds, pistachio nuts, peanuts, mackerel, salmon, sardines, eel, yellowtail, organ meats, soy beans, rice bran, wheat germ and rapeseed oil. Average amounts of Co Q10 are also found in broccoli, spinach, cauliflower, cabbage, garlic, onion, eggplant and carrot.

Folic Acid

Folic acid is essential for the synthesis of DNA and RNA, the genetic material of cells. It plays a vital role in the growth and reproduction of all body cells, maintaining the genetic code, regulating cell division and transferring inherited characteristics from one cell to another.

Maintaining the health of our genetic material found within cells (DNA and RNA) is essential in preventing dangerous changes in cells that can lead to cancer formation. Unfortunately, folic acid deficiency is rife in most countries around the world and likewise the incidence of cancer is also rising. This is not to say that lack of folic acid is the cause of a higher rate of cancer in the world; more so, that a number of different nutrient deficiencies are reducing our body's ability to cope with an overload of cancer promoters in today's modern world.

Folic acid deficiency is the most common nutritional deficiency in the world. Diets low in vegetables, frequent alcohol and prescription drug use, and the sensitivity of folate to light and heat contribute to this widespread deficiency. When folate intake is inadequate, levels in serum fall, levels in red blood cells also fall, homocystine concentrations rise and finally, changes in the blood cell-producing bone marrow and other rapidly dividing cells occur.

Folic acid increases the body's production of white blood cells and helps to defend against cancer. Cigarette smokers who have a high intake of foods rich in folic acid like dark green leafy vegetables are able to prevent injury to lung tissue and retard the development of lung cancer. Giving 10000mcg of folic acid and 500mcg of vitamin B12 daily may prevent pre-cancerous changes in bronchial tissue for regular tobacco smokers.

A deficiency of folic acid and vitamin B12 makes a person more susceptible to carcinogens. Folic acid protects against birth defects. It also protects against cancerous changes in cervix cells. Low levels of folic causes a woman to be more susceptible to human papilloma virus, which is believed to also cause cervical cancer. This condition tends to improve after being given folic acid. A deficiency of folic acid is associated with cervical dysplasia, a precursor of cancer of the cervix.

Research around the world suggests that there may be a connection between low folate levels and colon cancer. It is thought that men with a high alcohol, low folate and low protein diet are at a higher risk of developing colon cancer than men who consume low amounts of alcohol and who eat a diet rich in folate and protein.

Folic acid is found in most vegetables and fruits.

Inositol

Inositol is an unofficial phtyochemical (a potential cancer-fighting agent found in food) and a powerful antioxidant member of the B vitamin family, derived from high-fibre foods containing phytic acid (legumes, cereal, grains, and citrus fruits). Inositol is found in nearly all body cells and aids the liver in removing excess fat from its tissues, which prevents fat and bile accumulation in the liver. Inositol plays an essential role in transferring signals between cells and the environment and it may be a preventative against large intestine cancer.

Inositol is present in both plants and animals. The best natural sources are lecithin, brewer's yeast, lima beans, peanuts, raisins, wheat germ, cabbage, cantaloupe, grapefruit, molasses, legumes, cereal grains.

Lipoic Acid

Lipoic acid is a B group vitamin which helps to neutralise the effects of free radicals on the body by enhancing the antioxidant functions of vitamin C, E and glutathione. It is the only antioxidant that is both water and fat soluble, which means that it's easily available to all areas of the body. It helps quench free radical damage caused by sugars and it is used by the mitochondria to produce energy. It assures proper functioning of the two key enzymes that convert food into energy.

Lipoic acid stimulates the body's immune system and contains the antioxidant compound sulphur, which is also found abundantly in garlic and onions. Lipoic acid is essential in protecting the body's liver. It can actually restore the liver's most powerful antioxidant, glutathione. A good source of lipoic acid is animal liver.

Vitamin A (Betacarotene)

Vitamin A plays an important role in strengthening the body's immune system. It can protect against cancer formation, suppress the transformation of healthy cells into cancerous cells and is needed for the repair and maintenance of epithelial tissue, of which the skin and mucous membranes are composed.

Shortly after its discovery in 1922, vitamin A was found to be effective in the prevention of cancer. Many studies suggest that high blood levels of vitamin A can help prevent certain forms of cancer. Protein cannot be utilised in the body without vitamin A. It reduces the risk of many types of cancer by improving the structural integrity of mucous membranes that line various organs of the body. Specifically, vitamin A reduces the risk of developing breast, cervical, lung, mouth, pharyngeal, prostate, skin, stomach, testicular and uterine cancer.

Adequate levels of vitamin A protect normal cells from mutating into cancer cells after exposure to carcinogens. Vitamin A minimises the toxic effects of radiation, if taken at 35000 IU – 100000 IU/day.

Vitamin A and Immune Support

Vitamin A is a friend to the body's immune system by increasing efficiency of cells that produce antibodies. It is able to increase the body's resistance to infection by enhancing phagocyte and antibody production and by protecting and strengthening the body's thymus gland, which helps us fight against infectious agents and carcinogens.

Adequate supplementation and absorption of vitamin A can cause the thymus gland to double in size. It likewise enhances the thymus gland to manufacture cancer-fighting T-lymphocytes. During chemotherapy, vitamin A levels are often very low.

Carotenes or Carotenoids or Beta-Carotene

Many studies have suggested that diets high in carotenes can protect against several types of cancer including those of the cervix, ovaries, uterus, mouth, gastrointestinal tract, lung prostate and breast. Other studies have consistently shown that cancer victims have lower carotenoid levels than healthy individuals.

About five hundred carotenes occur in the plant kingdom. Some have vitamin A activity and some do not. Beta-carotene, a precursor of vitamin A, is well studied and is very effective with regard to health benefits. Beta-carotene has some properties unique to itself as well. It is a potent scavenger of toxic oxygen radicals (singlet oxygen), especially those produced by chemicals in the air and those generated by our metabolism.

Beta-carotene has much stronger immune-stimulating and thymic supportive activity than vitamin A, and it is much safer to use. It protects the body's mucous membranes and is effective in guarding against lung cancer and the damages of cigarette smoking on the lungs, and also from ultraviolet-induced skin cancers. In addition, it is an essential nutrient for normal ovarian function. Therefore it is very beneficial to have good amounts of beta-carotene during cancer treatment.

Alpha-carotene can reduce the incidence of liver, lung and skin cancers. It is believed to be 10 times more effective than beta-carotene at preventing various cancers.

Lycopene, the red-pigmented carotenoid, is effective in reducing the risk of prostate, breast, liver and stomach cancer. It also helps to prevent many of the side effects associated with radiation therapy, particularly burning of tissues. Lycopene has strong antioxidant properties and is a very effective quencher of singlet oxygen free radicals (a potentially dangerous cancer-causing agent), two times more effectively than beta-carotene and 100 times more effectively than vitamin E. It is able to retard the damage caused by oxidized LDL cholesterol and protects against cancer of the cervix. Women with high serum lycopene levels have 80 per cent less risk of developing cervical cancer than women with low levels.

Alpha and beta-carotene rich foods include sweet potato, carrots, broccoli, spinach, apricots, pumpkin, cantaloupe (rockmelon) and pink grapefruit. Lycopene-rich foods include tomatoes (fresh, sun-dried and tomato paste), pink grapefruit, red capsicum, watermelon, papaya, apricots and paprika.

Breast Cancer

Breast tissue may be particularly sensitive to the actions of vitamin A. Studies have been conducted where researchers compared the concentrations of various forms of vitamin A in the breast tissue of cancer patients, and patients with benign breast lumps. It was found that there was an increased risk of disease in those with low levels of vitamin A.

Cervical Cancer

Studies suggest that low carotenoid levels, including beta carotene may increase the risk of cervical cancer. Laboratory studies have shown that beta carotene can slow the growth of cervical cancer cells

Colon Cancer

Studies have been conducted that show many patients with colon cancer have significantly lower carotenoid levels.

Leukoplakia

Vitamin A has also been shown to exert protective effects against leukoplakia, a precancerous change in mucous membranes. It often occurs in the mouth and throat and is related to smoking.

Lung Cancer

People suffering from lung cancer can have low levels of vitamin A in their blood. Vitamin A preserves the integrity of red blood cell membranes and skin. Lung cancer due to inhalation of benzo-alpha-pyrene is reduced by vitamin A.

Studies have been done that confirm a high dietary intake of fruit and vegetables and beta carotene supplementation is linked to a decreased risk of lung cancer in both men and women.

Prostate Cancer

High beta carotene intakes may also improve survival in those with prostate cancer, according to some studies.

Good food sources of vitamin A and beta carotene include fish oil, white fish and eggs; green, orange and yellow vegetables such as carrots, kale, broccoli, yams, pumpkin, winter squash, sweet potatoes, apricots, mangos and rockmelon.

Vitamin C

Vitamin C is a powerful water-soluble antioxidant needed for healthy tissue growth and repair and healthy adrenal gland function. It is a valuable vitamin in protecting against many forms of cancer. Vitamin C aids in the production of anti-stress hormones and interferon, an important immune system hormone. It enhances the body's immune system protecting against infection and cancer, and has a vital role in protecting against oxidative damage.

Vitamin C is essential in the rapid healing of wounds and burns. It is one of the best vitamins for detoxifying the body of toxins and chemicals, and it protects against the harmful effects of pollution. It is able to protect against more than 30 common pollutants and enhances their detoxification from the body. In addition, it helps to remove heavy metals such as lead, cadmium, arsenic and mercury from the body.

Low intake of vitamin C appears to be a risk factor for many forms of cancer. Diets high in fruit and vegetables, and therefore high in vitamin C, have been associated with lower risk for cancer of the oral cavity, oesophagus, stomach, colon and lung. Many studies have found a reduced risk of cancer in people who have high vitamin C intakes. The protective effect seems to be strongest for cancers of the oesophagus, larynx, mouth and pancreas. Vitamin C also provides protection against cancers of the cervix, liver, stomach, rectum, breast and lung.

Vitamin C works synergistically with vitamin E. Vitamin E scavenges cancer-causing free radicals in cell membranes and vitamin C attacks cancer-causing free radicals in the body's biologic fluids. It is believed vitamin C enhances longevity, increases the survival time of cancer patients and decreases tumour size.

Vitamin C, vitamin E and other antioxidants inhibit many cancer-causing compounds and may help to prevent cancer of the digestive system. They also have the ability to inhibit many carcinogens in food from causing stomach cancer. Taking 1500 mg of vitamin C a day may also help to prevent the formation of bladder cancer. With lung cancer patients, vitamin C may to increase survival time and improve general well-being.

Vitamin C decreases the toxicity caused from radiation therapy and chemotherapy. It is useful during chemotherapy to help protect sperm from DNA (genetic) damage that can cause inherited disease or cancer in a man's offspring. It is essential in the treatment of cancer by stimulating the production of lymphocytes (cancer-fighting cells) and providing cellular antioxidant defence.

Vitamin C has a protective effect on the lungs and can reduce the cancer-causing and damaging effects of cigarette smoke. It gives strength to all supporting tissues, including those surrounding tumours, and thus can help prevent or delay the spread of tumours. Vitamin C helps to stimulate the activity of white blood cells, inhibiting viruses and bacteria and bringing about a rapid recovery and enhanced wound healing. Its many other health activities include helping in the formation of collagen, giving strength to bones, cartilage and connective tissue, aiding the integrity of blood vessels and helping to slow cellular ageing/destruction and delaying chronic disease. Vitamin C works best in the presence of bioflavonoids.

Breast Cancer
It is believed that women with breast cancer who have a high vitamin C intake have a much lower chance of dying of breast cancer than women with a low vitamin C intake.

Colon Cancer
Studies suggest that higher vitamin C intakes may lead to a decreased risk of colon cancer. Supplemental use of vitamin A and C also showed a protective effect on colon cancer risk.

Lung Cancer
Studies have also shown that vitamin C may have a protective effect against lung cancer. Those with low fruit and vegetable intake and, therefore, low vitamin C intake may face an increased risk of the disease.

Prostate Cancer
Long term studies conducted over a 30 year period have recently suggested that vitamin C improves survival in patients with prostate cancer.

Stomach Cancer
Results of some studies suggest that low vitamin C intake is linked to an increased risk of stomach cancer.

Good sources of vitamin C include acerola, bananas, berries, rosehips, black-currants, cantaloupe, elderberries, grapefruit, guavas, lemons, mangoes, oranges, papaya, persimmons, raspberries, strawberries, tangerines, chillies, parsley, peas (green), soy beans, asparagus, broccoli, brussel sprouts, cabbage (red and green), capsicum, carrot, kale, mustard greens, spinach, tomatoes, turnips, watercress and wheatgrass.

Vitamin D

Vitamin D is more a hormone than a vitamin. It is made (like many hormones) from cholesterol and exposure to sunlight. The healthiest and safest way to procure an adequate supply of vitamin D is through limited exposure to sunlight. Recently, vitamin D has been linked to the prevention of polyps and cancer of the colon and rectum. In smoggy cities where people receive little sunlight there is a high incidence of colon cancer.

Vitamin D is involved in normal cell growth and maturation, and so may play a part in cancer prevention. Laboratory experiments show that vitamin D can inhibit the growth of human prostate cancer and breast cancer cells. Lung cancer and pancreatic cancer cells may also be susceptible to the effects of vitamin D.

Vitamin D is believed to suppress melanoma growth and also to reduce the occurrence of oestrogen-sensitive breast cancers, colorectal cancer and prostatic cancer (deLuca et al., 1998, p 56 (2):S1–S10). An active form of vitamin D, known as vitamin D3 is being considered as a possible treatment to slow the spread and growth of osteosarcoma, melanoma, colon cancer and breast cancer.

Colorectal Cancer and Skin Cancer

Studies are beginning to indicate that people who have a high vitamin D intake are less likely to develop cancer of the colon or rectum than people with a low vitamin D intake. Vitamin D in small amounts is also thought to be protective against skin cancer, particularly malignant melanoma.

Prostate Cancer

Various studies throughout the world indicate that there may be a reduced risk of prostate cancer in men with high vitamin D levels. Vitamin D is found naturally only in fish and fish-liver oils. However, it is also found in milk (vitamin D-fortified). Cooking does not affect the vitamin D in foods. Vitamin D is sometimes called the 'sunshine vitamin' since it is made in your skin when you are exposed to sunlight. If you eat a balanced diet and get outside in the sunshine at least one and a half to two hours a week, you should be getting all the vitamin D you need.

A particular form of vitamin D is believed to inhibit the growth of prostate cancer cells in laboratory tests. Fructose, the sugar found in fruits, stimulates the production of this form of vitamin D. Eating plenty of fruits is generally associated with lower levels of prostate cancer (Brawley, O.W & Parnes, 2000;36 (10): 1312–1315).

Good sources of vitamin D include beef, butter, cheese, cod liver oil, cream, egg yolks, halibut liver oil, kippers, liver, mackerel, milk, salmon, sardines, shrimp, sunflower seeds and tuna.

Vitamin E

Vitamin E is often referred to as the 'fertility vitamin' as it needed by both men and women to maintain healthy reproductive organs and fertility. Vitamin E is a potent, fat-soluble antioxidant that protects cell membranes from environmental pollution. It protects against many toxic metals and chemicals (benzene compounds, carbon tetra-chloride and other chemical oxidants), oxidizing radiation, chemotherapy and radiation therapy. It reduces toxicity and side effects of chemotherapy drugs, particularly Adriamycin, Mitomycin C and 5-Fluorouraril (5-FU).

Vitamin E strengthens the body's immune system with supplementation of 800 IU/day. It prevents undesirable oxidation in many organs of the body. Vitamin E protects against and suppresses cancer, particularly inhibiting the development of breast cancer, lung cancer and mouth cancer.

Vitamin E has the ability to extend the lifespan of red blood cells by protecting against oxidative damage and facilitates the elimination of cellular waste from cells. It has a positive effect on circulation increasing the oxygen carrying capacity of blood.

Vitamin E is useful in combating cancers of the lung, prostate, ovaries, oral, breast, stomach, pancreas, colon and urinary tract. It is used both topically and internally to reduce scar formation and to accelerate the healing of wounds and burns. Vitamin E helps to protect against the cancer-causing damage from cigarette smoke and may play a role in protecting the lungs against damage from cancer-causing substances. Infertility and impotence is a major risk of conventional cancer treatments. Vitamin E helps to guard against these unwanted side effects.

Breast Cancer

Researchers in America found that post menopausal women whose intake of vitamin E was high had around 60 per cent less risk of breast cancer compared to those with low intake.

Lung Cancer

Several epidemiological studies suggest that low vitamin E intake increases the risk of lung cancer. High vitamin E levels may protect against lung cancer.

Prostate Cancer

Some recent studies have reported that taking vitamin E reduces the risk of prostate cancer among men who smoke.

Good sources of vitamin E include dietary oils such as wheat germ, soy bean, cottonseed, safflower, sunflower, palm, peanut and maize oils. Fruits and vegetables such as bananas, blackberries, carrots, tomatoes, watercress, spinach, broccoli, brussel sprouts and kale. Nuts, grains and seeds such as peanuts, brown rice, oatmeal, wheat germ and sunflower seeds. Kelp and shrimps are also good sources of vitamin E.

Vitamin K

Vitamin K exists in three forms, including naturally occurring Vitamin K1, K2 and the synthetic form of Vitamin K3. It is well known for its ability to produce prothrombin, needed for healthy blood clot formation. It is also essential for healthy liver function. Vitamin K is considered an effective anti-cancer agent. It is believed a combination of Vitamin K and the drug warfarin prevents a number of different types of cancers, including ovarian, breast, colon, stomach, kidneys, lungs, bladder and their metastases. It is also considered to be effective against liver cancer cells.

Vitamin K has an ability to increase the effect and decrease the toxicity of a number of toxic anti-cancer pharmaceuticals. It is thought to enhance the effects of chemotherapy drugs. It may help to prevent the risk of infection in the kidneys and prevent cancers that target the inner linings of the organs. It is believed to be a major vitamin in aiding longevity.

The 'friendly bacteria' in the intestines synthesizes the majority of the body's vitamin K. Good sources of vitamin K include asparagus, broccoli, blackstrap molasses, brussel sprouts, cabbage, cauliflower, green leafy vegetables, egg yolks, oatmeal, oats, rye, soybeans and safflower oil. Herbal sources of vitamin K include alfalfa, green tea, kelp, nettles and oatstraw.

Vitamin L

Vitamin L is also known as the 'Love Vitamin', as coined by humanologist Bethany ArgIsle. One of our most important nutrients for optimum health is a daily dose of love and nurturing. It is necessary for the optimal functioning of people and all their cells, tissues and organs.

A long term deficiency of vitamin L can cause fatigue, muscle tension, increased likelihood of stress conditions, addictions, sexual problems, digestive upsets and weakened immunity. Vitamin L is essential in any psychological disturbance such as depression, sadness, anger, fear, worry, pain and everyday stresses. Emotions such as these would benefit greatly from a daily dose of 'love therapy'.

Vitamin L is referred to as the 'catalytic vitamin for healing'. As cancer can manifest from repressed emotions, vitamin L would prove essential in healing and preventing cancer. 'Love' is found in a great variety of sources but must be developed and nurtured to be available. It is found readily in mums and dads and grandparents. Sisters and brothers, caring lovers and good friends may also be a good source of 'love'. Vitamin L is also found in animals, in flowers and in trees and plants. In food, 'love' is especially found in home cooked meals. It is digested and absorbed easily, and used by the body in its pure state.

The International Hug Association suggests that a minimum of four hugs a day is needed to prevent vitamin L deficiency, six hugs a day for maintenance and 10 hugs a day for growth and happiness.

*For more food sources of vitamins, refer to Part Three of this book.

Chapter 25

MIGHTY MINERALS

Minerals are the active participants in all internal body functions. Every living cell on this planet needs minerals for proper functioning and structure. Minerals are a part of every living cell in the human body. They function as coenzymes or spark plugs, enabling the body to perform its functions efficiently, including energy production, growth, cancer prevention, immune system function and healing. Put simply, the human body is similar to a finely tuned motor engine. Just as an engine requires oil, petrol and water in the correct amounts to 'purr' beautifully, the human body also requires minerals to maintain its delicate chemical balance, and if balanced, the human body can also 'purr' beautifully. All enzyme activities use minerals, making minerals essential for the proper utilization of vitamins and other nutrients. The level of each mineral in the body has an effect on the other minerals. One mineral deficiency can retard the functions of various other minerals. When even one mineral is lacking from the diet, the result is felt by the entire body and the role of certain vitamins will also be inhibited, leading to health problems. Minerals are an essential component in winning our fight against cancer.

Calcium

Calcium is the most abundant mineral in the human body. The total calcium content of the body is entirely renewed over a six year period. Calcium's most famous role is found in advertising campaigns throughout the world stating its essential role in preventing osteoporosis. It is vital for the formation of strong bones and teeth, assists nerves, muscles, blood clotting, heart rhythm and parathyroid function. It also aids in the metabolism of vitamin D. Calcium needs magnesium, phosphorous, vitamins A, C, D and E to carry out its functions.

It is believed that by taking 1500mg – 2000mg of calcium daily a person can decrease the incidence of colon and rectal cancer dramatically. It does this by binding to cancer-causing fats and bile acids in the intestines and normalising the growth of cells in the intestinal wall. Low calcium intake may also increase the risk of breast and cervical cancers. The proper calcium/phosphorous ratio reduces the risk of cancer in the large intestine.

A low intake of vitamin D and calcium may increase the incidence of breast cancer.

Cancer research has shown that cancerous tissues are abnormally low in calcium. Due to a lack of calcium, these cancer cells can spread to other areas of the body. Calcium also has the ability to block the toxicity of harmful fats without damaging the colon. Regular calcium supplementation is believed to decrease tumour size.

Calcium helps to prevent some forms of cancer and prevents pre-cancerous cells from becoming cancerous. It also protects the body from toxic heavy metals, including cadmium, lead and mercury by competing with them for absorption. Magnesium and calcium in combination have the ability to eliminate certain types of toxic radioactive isotopes that may become lodged in bones. Calcium also promotes the elimination of arsenic from the body.

Good food sources of calcium include tahini, Swiss cheese, almonds, asparagus, broccoli, buttermilk, sesame seeds, cabbage, carob, cheese, collards, dandelion greens, goats milk, kale, figs, dulse, tofu, watercress, green leafy vegetables, skim milk and low fat dairy products. Excess intake of chocolate, sugar, alcohol and salt all cause a severe loss of calcium from the body.

Copper

Copper is a trace mineral, with most of the copper content of the body being stored in the muscles, liver and bones. Copper may act to prevent cancer. Animal studies have shown that copper has a protective role and this may be due to its antioxidant properties as part of copper-zinc superoxide dismutase.

Copper is required in combination with manganese for the proper assimilation of iron. Copper-rich foods assist tissue respiration, protect the lungs from infections and improve the function of the body's digestive system. This mineral is a key element in the body's healing process and plays a role in energy production.

Good food sources of copper include raw nuts, purple or red onions, almonds, brazil nuts, cashews, legumes, whole grains and prunes.

Fluoride and Fluorine

Fluorine is a trace mineral that is found throughout every human bone. Organic fluorine helps to increase the number of blood cells in our body and to preserve a youthful complexion. Fluorine is important for growing children, due to the need for bone and teeth development. Generally foods are rich in natural fluorine. However, due to overproduction from soils, the fluorine content in foods can be low. This is the reason why sodium fluoride was originally added to our water system.

Fluoridated water contains sodium fluoride. If this tap water is taken excessively it has a detrimental effect on the body, reducing its ability to absorb calcium. Some evidence suggests that water fluoridation may be linked to some types of cancer.

Good food sources of fluorine include asparagus, oats, garlic, brown rice, cabbage, goat's milk, watercress, rice bran, beetroot, endive, corn, barley, millet, wheat, fresh vegetables and fruits.

Germanium

Germanium is a micromineral found in nature as a mineral salt. Germanium helps to retard the ageing process and possesses strong antioxidant properties. It is useful in decreasing high cholesterol levels and alleviating pain. Organic compounds found in germanium are powerful stimulants of the body's immune system and may therefore suppress and prevent some forms of cancer.

Germanium activates resting macrophages and converts them into cytotoxic (killer) macrophages. It also stimulates natural killer lymphocyte activity and the production of suppressor T cells. These unique qualities enable germanium to act as a powerful immune system stimulator.

Germanium is able to activate the body's utilization of oxygen thereby enriching the body's oxygen supplies. It enhances the removal of toxic substances and stimulates the production of interferon. Germanium is essential in keeping the immune system functioning properly. A daily intake of 100 to 300mg of germanium per day may improve many illnesses including rheumatoid arthritis, food allergies, cancer, chronic viral infections and elevated cholesterol levels.

Good food and herbal sources of germanium include chlorella, shitake mushrooms, aloe vera, ginseng, comfrey, suma, onions and garlic.

Iodine

Iodine is most commonly known for its ability to enhance metabolism and support the function of the body's thyroid gland. Iodine is stored in the thyroid gland and its major purpose is to control the metabolism of the entire body.

Iodine has the ability to excrete arsenic from the body and alleviates radiation sickness, especially when it is caused by iodine-131. Iodine deficiency increases the risk of breast, ovarian and uterus cancer. It is able to kill several forms of detrimental bacteria and fungi and is an important mineral in energy production.

Good food sources of iodine include kelp, dulse, turnip greens, watermelon, cucumber, spinach, asparagus, kale, turnip, okra, blueberry, peanuts and strawberries.

Iron

Iron is present in every cell in the human body. It is essential in the formation of rich red blood cells. A combination of protein and iron are required for the formation of blood haemoglobin (haemoglobin carries and releases oxygen in body tissues). Iron foods improve protein metabolism and protein is essential in building a strong immune system.

Fresh oxygen is required in combination with iron for oxygen transfer throughout the body. It is required for the formation of myoglobin, which is essential for oxygen distribution to all muscular cells. Iron is needed to burn up waste matter in the body and then to build new cells, making it an essential mineral in cancer prevention and treatment. Low levels of iron within the body often leads to a deficiency of the body's immune system.

Laxatives cause a severe loss of iron from the body. Drinking tea and coffee limit the body's absorption of iron. Prolonged bleeding, trauma, surgery, malignant tumours, poor absorption of iron and heavy menstruation may also lead to anaemia or iron deficiency.

Good food sources of iron include apricots, clams, liver, oysters, parsley, pine nuts, soy beans, sunflower seeds, pumpkin seeds, wheat germ, yeast, dulse, kelp, sesame seeds, lima beans, meats and spinach.

Lithium

Lithium is a trace mineral which has received a bad reputation over the years and is classified mainly for its use by psychiatrists. It is commonly used in very large doses to treat mania and depressive states. Lithium is toxic and fatal when given in large amounts. However, in small amounts it provides a variety of beneficial functions to the body.

Lithium is able to enhance the body's immune system and it assists in the prevention of cancer. It is thought to stimulate the production of lymphocytes and depresses the immune systems suppressor T cells. It is also able to prevent heart attacks.

Lithium is a prescription drug, not commonly available as a supplement. Pharmaceutical lithium is sold under the names Lithicarb and Priadel.

Good sources of lithium include sea vegetables, sugar cane, drinking water and some mineral waters.

Magnesium

Magnesium is important for the health of every organ within the body. It activates enzymes, aids energy production and helps to regulate the balance of many cancer-fighting nutrients within the body. It is a cofactor in over 100 enzyme reactions occurring in the body. Recent research has shown that magnesium may prevent cardiovascular disease, osteoporosis and certain types of cancer.

A deficiency of magnesium interferes with the relaying of nerve and muscle impulses, causing irritability, muscular cramps and nervousness. It assists in the uptake of calcium and potassium and helps to maintain the body's proper pH balance. This versatile mineral helps us to excrete arsenic and lead from the body, heavy metals which can lead to the development of cancer.

Magnesium promotes steady nerves, reduces irritability, helps to form strong bones and teeth, assists with the digestion of protein and carbohydrates, enhances memory and helps to prevent heart attacks. This essential mineral also helps to prevent abnormalities in the body's lymph glands. The lymph glands are a key component of the body's immune system.

Magnesium cannot be stored in the body for long periods and therefore it must be obtained regularly from the diet. Excess consumption of milk, coffee, tobacco and alcohol can lead to a magnesium deficiency. Soy milk is a perfect substitute for milk.

Good food sources of magnesium include dark green leafy vegetables, kelp, wheat bran, wheat germ, soy beans, dulse, hazelnuts, lima beans, sesame seeds, walnuts, millet, avocado, almonds, pecans, spinach, lentils, dates, brazil nuts, brown rice, wild rice, buckwheat, cashews, dried figs and apricots, bananas, fish and other seafood, apples, peaches, pumpkin seeds, sea vegetables and sprouts.

Herbal sources of magnesium include chickweed, dandelion, eyebright, fennel seed, fenugreek, lemongrass, licorice, parsley, peppermint, raspberry leaf, red clover and yellow dock.

Manganese

Manganese is essential for proper red blood cell formation and to maintain the health of the body's glands. Manganese-rich foods nourish the nerves and brain and aid in the transport of oxygen from the lungs to all of the cells in the body. It assists with healthy sex-hormone production, making it an essential mineral in helping to prevent hormone-induced cancers.

A form of the antioxidant enzyme, superoxide dismutase, contains manganese. Proper function of this enzyme helps protect against free radical damage, which can cause cancer. Manganese also plays a role in detoxifying alcohol from the body. This may make it a key element in preventing cancers related to excess alcohol intake.

Good sources of manganese include chestnuts, brazil nuts, hazelnuts, almonds, pecans, coconut, walnut, buck wheat, kidney beans, lima beans, pineapple, grapes, beetroot, parsley, lettuce, watercress, apricots, bananas, cherries, green beans, kale, avocado, blackberries, dates, celery, dandelion, figs, lemons, pears, apples.

Molybdenum

Molybdenum is termed an essential trace mineral. Molybdenum possesses strong antioxidant properties and is believed to prevent some forms of cancer. It is able to activate the xanthine oxidase enzyme responsible for the production of the powerful antioxidant, uric acid. Molybdenum enhances kidney function and protects the body from some chemical carcinogens.

Molybdenum has a major influence in protecting the body from the carcinogenic effects of dietary nitrosamines (by preventing the conversion of nitrites to nitrates to nitrosamines in the stomach). Nitrates are found in processed and cured meats and are known to be carcinogenic to the human body. It is believed oesophagus cancer is a symptom of Molybdenum deficiency and a low intake of molybdenum is also associated with mouth and gum disorders and cancer.

Population studies have shown that people living in areas where the soil is molybdenum deficient have been found to have an increased risk of stomach and oesophageal cancers. Molybdenum is currently being studied as a possible mineral in the prevention of breast cancer.

Molybdenum can be obtained from both plant and animal sources. Cauliflower, spinach, fish, liver, peas, beans, legumes, cereal grains, wheatgerm, green peas, brown rice, cottage cheese, lentils, split peas, brewer's yeast, potato, molasses and chicken are all good sources of this trace mineral.

Selenium

The function of selenium is closely related to vitamin E and it is a powerful anti-oxidant. Selenium facilitates the deactivation of certain free radicals and therefore helps to protect against many forms of cancer.

Regular intake of selenium is able to decrease the risk of breast cancer and colon cancer dramatically. Epidemiological studies suggest that the risk of cancer is reduced in areas where the soil is high in selenium. Low serum, dietary and soil selenium levels are particularly associated with lung, gastrointestinal tract and prostate cancers. Selenium deficiency is quite common, as many soils around the world are now selenium deficient.

Selenium is able to protect against several forms of skin cancer and oral or topical supplementation with the L-Selenomethionine form of selenium is effective in retarding some skin cancers induced by exposure to UV light.

Selenium is also a beneficial nutrient to the body's immune system by stimulating the action of phagocytes (cells in the immune system that gobble the 'baddies'), improving the defence response of T-Lymphocytes (immune army cells that attack cancer cells) and causing an increase in the size of the body's thymus gland (the 'maestro' gland of the immune army).

Selenium used in combination with other minerals helps to increase our body's levels of white blood cells. It stimulates B-Lymphocytes to produce more anti-bodies and is able to increase the body's defences by up to 3000 per cent if combined with Vitamin E, as it amplifies the health promoting effects of vitamin E. Selenium is able to detoxify harmful fats, inhibiting their cancer-causing potential. It counteracts the toxic effects of tobacco smoking and it also improves liver function.

Polynuclear aromatic hydrocarbons (PAH) are carcinogens found in tobacco smoke and car exhaust fumes, which cause cancer if ingested or inhaled. Selenium retards the ability of PAH from converting to cancer-causing substances in the liver. Selenium binds (chelates) with many toxic minerals and facilitates their excretion from the body including arsenic, cadmium, lead and methyl forms of mercury via the faeces.

Selenium protects the immune system by preventing the formation of harmful free radicals and prevents the formation of certain types of tumours. It improves the ability of macrophages (immune system cells) to attack and destroy tumour cells. Selenium is also essential to the healthy functioning of the body's reproductive organs in both men and women and an adequate amount of selenium in the body will guard against problems to these organs.

In Australia, Naturopaths are no longer able to prescribe good amounts of selenium, as before. There is no logical reason for this, besides once again, the profit-making capacity of a very effective mineral. Doctors have taken over the role of dispensing selenium, with a prescription only. So if you require selenium, ask for liquid form of sodium selenite from your doctor. Take as directed by your health care practitioner.

Colorectal Cancer

A low selenium intake is thought to increase one's chance of developing colon cancer, compared to people with a high selenium intake. Selenium is a potent antioxidant that is now found in low amounts in the foods that we eat.

Lung Cancer

As mentioned previously, Selenium is a potent antioxidant that helps to retard against damage to cells while removing harmful cancer-causing substances from the body. A person's risk of developing lung cancer is reduced with a higher selenium intake.

Good sources of selenium include wheatgerm, wheatbran, barley, mushrooms, asparagus, garlic, tuna, herring, onions, radish, liver, tomatoes, potatoes, celery, brewers yeast, cabbage and shellfish.

Most soils throughout the world are selenium deficient.

Silica, Silicon

Foods rich in silica are essential for healthy hair, skin and teeth. It is the major beauty mineral required for hair growth, proper eyesight, repair of damaged tissues, efficient cell growth, the formation of red blood cells, good circulation and internal cleansing.

Silica-rich foods are believed to protect the body against the development of cancerous growths.

Silica is part of the 'nutrient team' that helps to remove arsenic from the body. One nasty side-effect of cancer treatment is incontinence. Silica helps to strengthen bladder muscles if used regularly for over three months.

Two of the richest sources of silica are the herbs horsetail and dandelion. Lettuce, parsnips, asparagus, rice bran, spinach, onions, cucumber, strawberry, cabbage, leeks, sunflower seeds, artichoke, pumpkin and celery are also rich in silica.

Sulphur

Sulphur is contained in all tissues in the body and is a component of blood haemoglobin, where it acts as an oxidising agent. Sulphur is able to purify and cleanse the digestive tract, making it an essential cancer preventative. It not only provides oxygen to the blood, it is also required for the healthy formation of blood plasma. Sulphur-rich foods prevent the accumulation of waste body toxins, keeping the body clean and healthy. Sulphur helps to protect against many of the dangerous effects of radiation and pollution making it a valuable cancer-preventative and anti-ageing tool.

This mineral is regularly advertised as 'nature's beauty mineral'. An age-old therapy used around the world is balneotherapy or sulphur mud baths. The sulphur contained in these mud baths is believed to alleviate pain, skin disorders and arthritis.

Good food sources of sulphur include brazil nuts, green vegetables, onions, garlic, kelp, watercress, brussel sprouts, cabbage, kale, snap beans, turnips, cauliflower, kelp.

Zinc

Zinc is involved in approximately 90 enzymatic reactions in the body, including activities of the immune system, liver detoxification, protein synthesis and activities of the prostate, thymus and adrenal glands. It is also involved in the function and maintenance of over 200 enzymes in the body, including enhancing the function of Glutathione, a powerful antioxidant. It helps to fight and prevent the formation of free radicals and is a constituent of many enzyme systems, including the antioxidant enzyme SOD.

Zinc facilitates the elimination of toxic metals from the body including arsenic, copper, cadmium and lead. It enhances the ability of the liver to detoxify alcohols and is helpful for the general health of the body's immune system. It protects the liver from chemical damage and maintains the proper concentration of vitamin E in the blood. It also aids in the healing of wounds, prevents scar formation, and is essential for the health and function of the reproductive organs.

Zinc increases the number of circulating T-lymphocytes (by significantly increasing the body's production of thymulin, responsible for causing the further replication of T-lymphocytes within the thymus). Zinc deficiency can cause the thymus gland to shrink and supplementing with zinc causes regrowth of the thymus gland. Zinc increases the production of antibodies and stimulates the production of interferon. People afflicted with cancer of the oesophagus and cancer of the prostate are often deficient in zinc. Zinc is an essential mineral for healthy prostate and reproductive system function. White flecks on the nails are a sign of zinc deficiency.

Mouth ulcers, appetite loss, loss of taste and smell, fatigue, increased stress and poor immunity are all side-effects of conventional cancer treatment. Zinc helps to ease many of these uncomfortable side-effects.

Zinc must be obtained daily from the diet as the body is unable to make enough

Good food sources of zinc include oysters, pumpkin seeds, hazelnuts, fish, oats, ginger, sunflower seeds, pine nuts, almonds, turnips, pecans and brewer's yeast.

*For more food sources of minerals, refer to Part Three of this book.

Chapter 26

AMINO ACIDS, ENZYMES AND RELATED SUBSTANCES

Carnitine (Acetyl L Carnitine)

Carnitine is a B vitamin found mostly in meat and it can be manufactured by the liver from two amino acids, lysine and methionine, and several other vitamins and minerals. Carnitine is needed for the transport of oxidation of fatty acids within the energy centres of human cells (mitochondria). In fact, the energy metabolism of cells is highly dependent on carnitine. Carnitine also plays a role in the effect of the thymus hormone on the metabolism of cells and their ability to multiply. This is very important with reference to white blood cells, the body's first line of defence against infection and cancer.

Elderly people are virtually devoid of carnitine. It protects older people from damage to white blood cells caused from free radicals (cancer-causing substances). It has the ability to increase white blood cell proliferation (replicate themselves) especially in the elderly. Carnitine counteracts the damage certain fats do to the immune system. Chemotherapy destroys carnitine, expelling it in the urine especially in women, causing a marked loss in energy.

Carnitine and azelaic acid have been used to treat malignant melanoma by enhancing the transport of azelaic acid into cancer cells and facilitating their killing ability.

Carnitine protects against the toxic effects of the toxic cancer drug MGBG. It has been shown that carnitine levels are low in people with cancer. It also helps to maintain extremely high energy levels at all times in our life, especially during cancer treatment.

Good sources of carnitine include beef, liver and milk.

Cysteine

Cysteine is a sulphur-containing amino acid. It has a remarkable ability to scavenge gold, silver, arsenic, mercury aluminium, cadmium, lead and other heavy metals from tissues, which are then combined with glutathione and harmlessly eliminated from the body. Cysteine helps to prevent many forms of cancer. Alliin (a derivative of cysteine) prevents chemically-induced cancers

Cysteine increases the production of glutathione (a powerful cancer-fighting antioxidant) and helps to excrete toxic chemicals, tobacco smoke and environmental pollutants from the body. It is a major factor in two antioxidant systems, gluathione peroxidase and glutathione reductase.

Cysteine deactivates acetaldehyde, a toxic waste product from the liver's metabolism of alcohol (also present in cigarette smoke and smog) and carbon tetrachloride. These harmful substances cause massive cell and liver damage, leading to cancer and death. Cysteine also protects the bronchial tubes from the damage caused by smoking cigarettes. It has an ability to protect against free radicals released during chemotherapy, at a dosage of 500mg, three to four times daily. Cysteine also protects the body against the toxic side effects of radiation damage.

Cysteine has powerful immune-stimulating effects and protects cells (neutrophils, macrophages and lymphocytes) from destruction of their own free radical release, which can lead to chronic infection and cancer. It is also able to enhance T cell counts. T cells are important in the defensive actions of the immune system. Cysteine successfully lowers high cholesterol levels.

This versatile amino acid works more effectively if taken with vitamin E and selenium.

N-Acetyl Cysteine (NAC)

N-acetyl cysteine (NAC) is a form of the simple amino acid cysteine. It is more stable than cysteine, absorbed more easily and is used in a better way by the body. A powerful antioxidant, a premier anti-toxin and immune support substance, it is found naturally in foods. It is a precursor for glutathione, an important antioxidant that protects cells against oxidative stress. In addition to maintaining intracellular glutathione levels, NAC supplementation has been shown to be protective against cell damage caused by chemotherapy and radiation therapy, to be immune enhancing, to protect against toxins and other drugs, as well as mercury, lead, and others heavy metals.

NAC is known and marketed as an 'anti-amalgam' medicine, because it helps remove (chelate) mercury from the body. It also generally improves the body's immune system, making it better able to fight off disease. NAC has neither a sedative or stimulant effect and is a safe substance, showing excellent tolerance in patients.

The most commonly used chemo-preventative agents in the prevention of oral leukoplakia, head and neck cancer and lung cancer are beta-carotene and vitamin A. One of the few natural agents not in this group and presently being used in clinical trials is NAC. Research is beginning to indicate that NAC may help to prevent various types of cancer, including bladder, breast, colorectal, lung and skin cancer. It is a protective agent against harmful chemicals and it may prove to be a useful key in the prevention and spread of many types of cancer.

DHEA

Dehydroepiandrosterone, or DHEA is the most abundant hormone or steroid found in the bloodstream, made by the body's adrenal glands. DHEA is produced in large amounts during youth, with production being its highest at around age 25. By the age of 80, people are thought to have only 10 to 20 per cent of the DHEA that they had at 25 years of age. At 25 years old, 20mg of DHEA is found within the body and by age 80 there is an average of six mg in the body.

DHEA contains many health-promoting functions and anti-ageing properties. It helps to generate the sex hormones oestrogen and testosterone, increases the per centage of muscle mass and decreases the per centage of body fat. It also helps prevent osteoporosis.

As the production of DHEA declines with age, certain structures of the body tend to decline with it. This leaves the body vulnerable to developing various cancers, including cancer of the breast, prostate and bladder as well as nerve degeneration.

It has been proposed in various studies on humans that DHEA can increase life span by as much as 50 per cent. While practising in Thailand, I met an American family of two parents and two children who were injecting DHEA directly into their glands. I believe this to be obsessive and not necessary for good health. This family by no means looked younger or healthier than normal, healthy individuals. Moderation is always the key to good health.

DHEA is believed to be highly beneficial in the treatment and prevention of many types of cancer. Studies have found that DHEA protects against breast, colon, liver, lung, lymphoma and skin cancers. It also protects against many viruses and harmful bacteria. DHEA supplementation is believed to improve alertness, one's sense of well-being, energy levels, sex drive, immunity and stamina.

Indole 3 Carbinol (I3C), Diindolymethane (DIM)

Diets rich in cruciferous vegetables are associated with protection against various cancers, including breast cancer. Indole-3-carbinol (I3C) is an important phytochemical present in cruciferous vegetables. One of its most important actions is to change the way that oestrogen is metabolised. It up-regulates the tumour suppressor gene BRCA1 (breast cancer susceptibility gene) through an oestrogen receptor.

I3C increases BRCA1 and works to block oestrogen from sending any signals that enhance the growth of cancer. It is very similar to putting up a type of road block for oestrogen. Even though it is still present, it can do no harm. Additional benefits of I3C include decreasing the risk of forming hormone-induced cancers, halting cancer cell growth and acting as a powerful antioxidant.

Diindolymethane (DIM) is another type of indole found in cruciferous vegetables. It can help to restore and maintain a healthy balance of oestrogen in men and women. It is believed that diets rich in DIM (broccoli, cauliflower, cabbage, brussel sprouts) may prevent chemically-induced cancers. DIM was first used in 1987 in animals and it is non-toxic, with potential for increasing cancer cell death in humans. In studies, DIM is showing favourable results against many types of hormone-induced cancers and breast cancer.

Overall, the indoles ingested through eating plenty of cruciferous vegetables such as broccoli, cauliflower, bok choy, watercress, cabbage, turnips and brussel sprouts have a beneficial effect against the development of many types of cancers.

Enzyme Therapy

Enzymes are known as the 'sparks of life' as they take part in thousands of biochemical reactions in the body. There are over 20,000 different enzymes, which are essential for digesting food, stimulating brain function, supplying cellular energy and repairing tissues, organs and cells. Enzymes assist the kidneys, liver, lungs, colon and skin in the elimination of toxic wastes from the body.

L-asparaginase, an enzyme which is approved for use by the FDA, is used in the treatment of acute lymphoblastic leukaemia.

Native Americans used the potent digestive enzyme in papaya, papain to treat external skin cancers and ulcerative lesions. The active enzymes in green papaya, mainly papain (100 times richer in enzymes than ripe papaya), are believed essential in the prevention and treatment of all types of cancer, especially stomach, colon and lymphatic cancer.

Salad made from green papaya is believed to prevent colon and stomach cancer. Green papaya leaves are used in the treatment of colon, stomach and lymphatic cancers.

The protein digestive enzyme, brinase, increases T cell counts in the body benefiting the body's immune system and preventing the formation of cancerous growths.

For a good part of the twentieth century, European oncologists have included enzyme therapy as a natural therapy against cancer. Most alternative cancer specialists prescribe food enzymes and concentrated enzyme supplements as a primary or accessory treatment for cancer. Studies on human populations show that those who eat fresh fruits and vegetables that are loaded with life-giving, natural enzymes have dramatically reduced levels of cancer and other illnesses.

Glutamine

Glutamine is an amino acid best known for its function in decreasing alcohol cravings. Glutamine is a versatile amino acid with a variety of functions in fighting cancer. It improves the function of the immune system by stimulating the growth of lymphocytes and phagocytes (the immune army's warriors).

The role of glutamine in tumour cells has been studied extensively. A number of new studies suggest that glutamine may be a potent cancer therapy because it increases levels of the powerful antioxidant glutathione. A study in the Annals of Surgery showed that glutamine may increase the effectiveness of anti-tumour drugs by sensitising cells to chemotherapy. The Journal of Parenteral Enteral Nutrition reported that glutamine decreases the rate of tumour growth by promoting activity of natural killer cells. (Natural killer cells are often low in people with cancer. These cells are able to kill certain types of cancer cells.)

Unlike other cells in our bodies, which require oxygen to live, tumour cells are anaerobic and use glutamine as their fuel. To get the food they need, tumours are equipped with glutamine traps, which literally wait for glutamine to float by so they can grab it. If tumour cells consistently sap our natural stores of glutamine, our body will run out and the tumours will demand more. This causes muscle wasting. An obvious solution is to supplement with glutamine to stop the wasting and stimulate the body's natural killer cells. However, herein lies the controversy: glutamine may actually promote tumour growth, as tumours feed on glutamine among other nutrients. Despite glutamine's potential role in alleviating the growth of tumour cells, the danger of the opposite result leaves scientists wary. Still, the beneficial possibilities warrant further research.

Glutamine is an essential amino acid to take while receiving chemotherapy. Glutamine minimises the damage caused by chemotherapy by:

- enhancing the repair of intestines during chemotherapy;
- repairing the damage chemotherapy does to the immune system;
- preventing many of the side-effects of chemotherapy treatment;
- enhancing the actions of chemotherapy – tumours may decrease in size by 45 per cent if taking glutamine, compared to 25 per cent without glutamine;
- increasing the survival rate of cancer patients receiving chemotherapy;
- soothing and relieving the pain of and quickly healing sores in the mouth (oral mucositis). Patients in a hospital in Boston, USA, receive 5000mg of glutamine six times daily to relieve these painful side effects.

Glutathione

Glutathione is a tripeptide or protein produced in the liver from the amino acids, cysteine, glutamic acid and glycine. It is a powerful antioxidant and inhibits the formation of and protects against the damage from free radicals. Glutathione defends the body against damage from cigarette smoking, exposure to radiation, chemotherapy and toxins such as alcohol. It is able to detoxify heavy metals and drugs, and aids in the treatment of blood and liver diseases.

Glutathione guards against many forms of cancer and is similar in its protective functions to beta-carotene. Glutathione protects cells by neutralising oxygen molecules before they harm cells.

Glutathione has the ability to protect the tissues of the arteries, brain, heart, immune system, kidney, lenses of the eyes, liver, lungs and skin against oxidative damage. Glutathione plays a role in protecting against cancer and the effects of ageing. Older cells contain 20 to 30 per cent less glutathione than younger cells.

Red blood cell integrity and structure is improved with the use of this handy amino acid. Glutathione detoxifies arsenic, aluminium, cadmium, lead and mercury and inhibits the excess production of cytokines. It facilitates the transport of essential nutrients to white blood cells and protects white blood cells from damage.

Glutathione deactivates dangerous free radicals, making them harmless to the body thereby helping to prevent the onset of cancer.

Good sources of glutathione include apples, grapefruit, spinach, tomatoes and carrots.

Laetrile

The use of laetrile as a healing agent is surrounded by controversy. Yet there appears to be much scientific proof of its efficiency. There exists a strong possibility that the pharmaceutical companies have launched a harmful propaganda campaign against laetrile due to their inability to patent it to sell. Laetrile is in the same category as formula's such as essiac, perhaps the ultimate cure for cancer, but subjected to wide misinformation campaigns.

Laetrile is a glucoside also known as vitamin B17, amygladin and nitrilosides. It is claimed to be extremely effective in the treatment of cancer, and may reduce the size of tumours and prevent their further spread. It is believed to reduce the pain associated with cancer.

The enzyme beta-glucosidase releases the tightly bound and unavailable toxins, benzaldehyde and organic cyanide from laetrile and allows them to swiftly wipe out cancerous tissues. Another enzyme, rhodanese, which has the ability to detoxify cyanide, is present in normal tissues but deficient in cancer cells. These two factors combine to cause a selective poisoning of cancer cells by the release of cyanide from laetrile, leaving healthy cells undamaged.

Independent research has proven that a Himalayan tribe known as the Hunza never contract cancer of any kind for as long as they adhere to their native diet. Their native diet is exceptionally high in both apricots and millet. Apricots and millet contain high amounts of laetrile. Once exposed to Western diets they become as vulnerable as other populations to cancer.

The scientist who discovered laetrile believes that cancer results as a direct deficiency of laetrile and carcinogens really just worsen cancer by placing further stress on the body.

Good sources of laetrile include apple (seeds), cherry (stones), peach stones, apricot (kernels), nectarine (stones), pear pips, lime pips, prune seeds, plum stones, elderberries, raspberries, currants, buckwheat, tapioca, millet, boysenberries, wild blackberries, gooseberries, almonds, macadamia nuts, flaxseeds, kidney beans, lima beans, alfalfa sprouts, lentils, chickpeas, mung bean sprouts and black-eyed beans.

L-Arginine

L-Arginine inhibits cellular proliferation (multiplication of cancer cells) and stimulates cancer-fighting T lymphocytes. It also stimulates the release of growth hormone, enhances collagen production, aids healthy fertility and lowers cholesterol levels, decreasing the risk of atherosclerosis.

L-Arginine is believed to block the formation of many forms of cancer. Research indicates it has the ability to stimulate the body's thymus gland and increase the size of the thymus. L-Arginine stimulates the production of T-lymphocytes within the thymus and makes them more active and effective. It retards the growth of tumours and cancer by enhancing immune system function. It also enhances the removal of ammonia from the body and detoxifies the liver.

L-Arginine has the ability to increase the survival time of cancer patients.

Good sources of L-Arginine include alfalfa, cheese, chocolate, leeks, celery, wakame, radish, cucumber, potato, carrot, lettuce, and parsley.

Lentinan

Lentinan is a polysaccharide which boosts the immune system and suppresses the growth and spread (metastasis) of some forms of cancer. Lentinan has the ability to increase the lifespan of breast, stomach and colon cancer patients by preventing the spread of cancer. It stimulates the production of interleukin-1 and interferon's, strong cancer-fighting compounds. Lentinan has an extremely positive effect on the body's immune system. The regular use of lentinan possesses virtually no toxic side effects.

Chemotherapy treatment is enhanced through the added use of lentinan. When taken with chemotherapy, it is believed to enhance the lifespan of breast cancer patients.

Lentinan also prevents chemicals and viruses from triggering cancer and shows strong cancer-fighting properties against stomach cancer. Lentinan is found in high amounts in shitake mushrooms.

Melatonin

Melatonin is a hormone secreted by the pineal gland in the brain and it is important for the regulation of many hormones in the body. Melatonin helps to control the body's circadian rhythm, our internal twenty-four hour timekeeping system that plays a role in when we fall asleep and when we wake up. Melatonin is similar to Coenzyme Q10 and DHEA in the fact that as we age, our levels of these important compounds found in our body decrease. In addition, evidence suggests that melatonin is a vital key in maintaining a strong level of immunity.

Melatonin is an antioxidant that scavenges free radicals, particularly the potent cancer-causing agent, safrole. Low plasma melatonin levels are implicated in endometrial cancer. It is an effective addition to the treatment of kidney cancer and it is thought to inhibit the growth of prostate and breast cancer, and hormone-sensitive and oestrogen-dependent tumours. It is also being considered as a possible preventative agent against melanoma skin cancers.

Melatonin is believed to inhibit the growth of several types of cancer including liver and lung cancer. It has been used successfully with cancer patients who do not respond well to chemotherapy and, in addition, it helps to protect against many of the toxic effects of chemotherapy drugs. Melatonin promotes the release of other pineal gland chemicals, to work hand-in-hand with it in the prevention of cancer.

Melatonin as a Treatment for Breast Cancer/ Prostate Cancer

A number of different studies indicate that melatonin levels may be linked with breast cancer risk. For example, women with breast cancer show lower levels of melatonin than those that do not have this disease. In addition, laboratory studies indicate that low levels of melatonin stimulate the growth of certain breast cancer cells. When melatonin is added to these cells, their growth is halted. For women whose breast cancer is not improving with tamoxifen (a commonly used chemotherapy drug), preliminary studies have shown that the addition of melatonin may actually encourage tumours to regress slightly. However, if you are considering taking melatonin supplements, you should first consult with a healthcare practitioner to design a comprehensive treatment approach suited to your individual needs.

Similar to the findings with breast cancer, studies of men with prostate cancer suggest that melatonin levels are lower, compared to men without this cancer. Laboratory studies have shown that melatonin inhibits the growth of prostate cancer cells. Higher levels of melatonin in prostate cancer patients are associated with longer survival rates.

Meditation helps to raise melatonin levels within the body, showing the benefit of incorporating daily meditation into one's cancer-beating regime.

Two severe side effects of orthodox cancer treatment and cancer are weight loss and malnutrition. Melatonin helps to combat these symptoms.

SOD (Superoxidase Dismutase)

SOD is an enzyme possessing strong antioxidant properties. It rejuvenates cells and decreases the rate of cellular breakdown. SOD neutralises the most common and dangerous free radicals and prevents the formation of cancerous cells.

It has been shown that levels of SOD in the body decrease with age, while the levels of free radicals in the body increase with age. It is therefore considered an important factor in anti-ageing and cancer prevention.

There are two kinds of SOD, Manganese SOD (Mn SOD) and Copper/Zinc SOD (Cu/Zn SOD). Each of these enzymes protects a different part of the cell. Cu/Zn SOD protects the cytoplasm (the jelly-like substance that surrounds the nucleus of the cell), while Mn SOD protects the mitochondria of cells, which contains our DNA and acts as the site of cellular energy production.

SOD may inhibit lung cancer. The susceptibility of breast cells to cancer-causing compounds is lessened by the presence of SOD. SOD levels are higher in healthy people than in patients with cancer of the lung, breast, digestive tract and reproductive system.

SOD is a potent free radical scavenger, absorbing harmful free radicals and converting them into hydrogen peroxide, to be broken down by enzymes into harmless water and oxygen. It decreases the side effects of radiation therapy, particularly with relation to fibrous scar tissue. It also has the ability to decrease the side effects of chemotherapy.

Intramuscular injections of SOD are more effective than the oral form, as SOD can easily be destroyed by acids and digestive enzymes in the stomach. The best way to obtain SOD naturally is by stimulating your body's own production of SOD, by supplying the body with adequate manganese, copper and zinc.

Foods rich in SOD include broccoli, brussel sprouts, cabbage, green barley grass, green leafy vegetables and wheatgrass.

Sulphuric Compounds

Allicin is a sulphuric compound formed when fresh garlic is cut. Heat and ageing destroys allicin. Allicin destroys detrimental bacteria within the body.

Diallyl sulphide is formed in the body from the conversion of allicin found in garlic and garlic oil. It is formed and released on consumption of garlic. Diallyl sulphide may decrease the incidence of colon cancer by up to 75 per cent and provide 100 per cent protection against oesophageal cancer.

Ajoene is also formed in the body from allicin ingested with garlic. It helps in the treatment of Burkitt's lymphoma, a type of lymphatic cancer. Ajoene also prevents abnormal blood clotting.

Sulforaphane inhibits the development of cancer cells, by enhancing the function of enzymes that block cancer-causing carcinogens. Rich sources of sulforaphane include broccoli, cauliflower, kale and brussel sprouts.

Glucosinates act as powerful antioxidants, potentially blocking the development of cancer. It kills the highly carcinogenic aflatoxin. Good sources of glucosinates include mustard seed oil, grapeseed oil, watercress, cabbage, cauliflower, broccoli, brussel sprouts and turnips.

Thymus Extracts

Thymosin is a group of thymus hormones that is now available in supplemental form. It is believed to cure several forms of cancer, when cancer is attributable to thymosin deficiency. Thymosin stimulates the body's immune system gland, the thymus, and enhances the ability of phagocytes to decrease free radical reactions within the body. It is thought thymus extracts may be at least 50 per cent effective in treating some forms of cancer.

Chapter 27

THE ANCIENT MAGIC OF HERBAL REMEDIES

Herbs are the plants of nature – rich in vitamins, chlorophyll, minerals and specific cancer fighting nutrients. Over the centuries, healers and health professionals from around the globe have performed miracles by using plants or herbs.

Today, many cancer drugs, chemotherapy drugs and other pharmaceutical medications are derived originally from plants. Even something as simple and commonly used as aspirin is derived from a plant. Its main ingredient, salicin or salicylic acid, is the main ingredient in a herb called white willow bark, which is used in natural medicine to treat headaches.

The company Bayer artificially synthesised salicin in 1899, to make the world's most widely used drug, aspirin. If a medical claim is made by a company as to the amazing healing properties of a herb, big pharmaceutical companies often find a way of imitating, patenting or synthesizing it for their own profit.

Approximately half of the world's pharmaceutical drugs have been derived from herbs and other plants. The medical field in general likes to disregard nature's medicinal herbs as nonsense in the treatment of cancer. Does that mean that thousands of real-life accounts of people helping heal themselves with herbs is nonsense? I honestly don't believe so! To disregard so many miraculous healing stories through the use of nature's medicinal herbs, is a crime to society. Many people have been told that they would die if they did not have orthodox medical treatment and yet here they are, still alive, healthy and cancer-free. I am a perfect example, as are many of my wonderful clients.

Herbal medicine has been practised for centuries by every civilisation. Animals naturally seek out herbs in self-treatment of their diseases. Watch a dog whenever they have an upset stomach automatically look for the right plant or grass to ease the stomach pains. It is natural to assume that man learnt the skill of herbal medicine from animals and therefore places the origins of herbal medicine back to many thousands of years ago.

The dispensing of Chinese herbs can be traced back to 2500 BC by ancient Chinese herbalists. Their goal was to restore harmony and balance to the whole person through the use of herbs and other traditional Chinese treatments. The Indians have incorporated the use of Ayurvedic herbs since 2500 BC to restore equilibrium to the patient. In fact, most ancient cultures including Egyptian, Islamic, Greek, Roman, North American Indian and European natives have actively used herbs in the treatment of illness and disease throughout history. Nature is truly a miracle in her ability to create such a wondrous array of healing plants and herbs to enhance longevity and to restore the delicate balance of health, so often lost in our fast-paced society.

Herbal Teas

Using herbal teas is a great way to add healing plants to your cancer-prevention or cancer-treatment program. Many people dislike the taste of herbal teas. Certainly some herbal teas do taste 'horrible' or 'bitter' to some people but most herbal teas are delicious, providing a variety of different tastes and unique health benefits.

To begin the addition of herbal teas into your life, firstly try the pleasant tasting teas like chamomile, peppermint, spearmint or licorice. Herbal teas can be drunk either hot or cold. However, to receive the full healing potential of a certain herb, they may need to be prepared in a special way. After all, what could be more refreshing than an iced peppermint tea or an iced lemon balm tea on a hot, steamy day?

For cancer treatment, it is best to use the dried or fresh herbs, or herbal tinctures listed in the following pages from reputable companies, to ensure you are actually getting what you are paying for. Herbal teas will supply an array of health benefits and healing properties and are a simple addition to your diet. Our ancestors knew the benefits of herbal teas incorporating teas as a regular part of their diet. The powerful ingredients in herbs are diluted by water when made into a tea. Mild teas can be used daily as a general health tonic and to prevent illness and disease. To make herbal tea, follow the directions I've provided for each herb in the following pages.

Aloe Vera

Aloe vera is a member of the family of plants known as the 'vulneraries' or 'wound healers'. Aloe vera is found throughout the world in warm, tropical climates. As it originated in these sunny, tropical countries, it is no surprise to learn that aloe vera is one of the most effective treatments for sunburn and for preventing peeling. Aloe vera is widely used today in shampoos, beauty creams, after-sun lotions and gels. There are over 200 different species of this gelatinous plant and it has strong healing properties.

Aloe vera is a great skin healer and moisturiser that softens and soothes wounds, burns, cuts, bruises and welts. The juice is regularly used for cleansing of the colon and intestinal problems. Throughout history, human experience has proven in-depth, the miraculous healing powers contained within the aloe vera plant.

Aloe contains high amounts of the compound emodin, which has strong anti-tumour capabilities. It has an ability to stimulate the scavenging activity of white blood cells in the immune system, giving it remarkable anti-cancer activity. Aloe juice is believed to reduce tumour mass and decrease the frequency of metastases (cancer spread). Another cancer-fighting ingredient found in Aloe is acemannan. Acemannan is believed to inhibit cancerous tumours by boosting helper T cells, white blood cells that act as the immune system's alert watchdogs.

Aloe vera is also able to protect individuals with weakened immunity against infection, as it is immune-enhancing. It is extremely protective on the skin against x-rays and can be used both topically and internally. It soothes burned areas and fibrous skin after radiation treatment.

Why is aloe vera such a miraculous plant for healing wounds? Firstly, it contains large amounts of water, which keeps wounds sterile by starving bacteria of the air they need to grow. Additionally, it contains large amounts of magnesium compounds, which act as effective 'pain-killers'. Finally, it contains several essential vitamins and a substance called allatonin, which has been proven to soothe tissues and speed tissue repair.

Aloe vera has strong liver-protecting qualities, particularly against alcohol. In addition, it helps to alleviate the side effects of constipation and diarrhoea caused from radiation damage and chemotherapy.

What is the best way to use Aloe Vera?
- Internal use – take 0.1 to 0.3 grams of the fresh juice. If you have constipation or a stomach upset, take 1 teaspoon of aloe vera juice after meals. For healing purposes, take 1 tablespoon 3 times daily.
- External use – If you have a fresh plant – pull off one of the leaves, open and apply the fresh gel from the leaves to the affected area. If you have a burn, bandage the open leaf onto the affected area and leave on for 24 hours. The fresh gel can be used for any burn, wound, fungal infection or dry skin area.

CAUTION!
As aloe stimulates uterine contractions, it should be avoided during pregnancy and breastfeeding.

Angelica Root (Angelica archangelica)

If you've ever tasted the liqueurs Benedictine, Chartreuse or Gin, you will have tasted the flavour of angelica. The candied stalks and roots were traditionally taken as a tonic to combat infections and improve energy levels. Angelica is believed to have strong anti-inflammatory properties and immune strengthening actions. Folk healers have used Angelica to treat stomach cancer and tumours, and the leaves have been known to treat indolent tumours.

Two nasty side effects of orthodox cancer treatment are bladder infections and appetite loss. Angelica root is a useful digestive aid for appetite stimulation and it contains antiseptic properties and is a mild diuretic, thus flushing out harmful bacteria. It is reputed to be an excellent urinary antiseptic.

What is the best way to use angelica?
- Decoction or herbal tea – put 1 teaspoon of the cut root in a cup of water, bring to the boil and simmer for 2 minutes. Take off the heat and let this sit for 15 minutes. Take 1 cup 3 times daily.
- Tincture – take 2 to 5 ml of the tincture three times daily.

Astragalus (Huang qi)

Astragalus is an incredible immune system stimulant, possessing strong immune-restorative qualities due to its powerful carbohydrate, Astragalan B. It benefits the immune system by increasing the production of interferon and enhancing natural killer cell function. Natural killer cells are vital in fighting cancer and cancer patients often present with low levels of these cells. Astragalan B found in Astragalus protects against several forms of bacteria and tends to stimulate the body's immune system.

Astragalus is believed to protect against distant metastases (spread) of melanoma (a deadly form of cancer) to the lungs. It is also thought to inhibit primary lung cancer. It protects against the toxic side effects of chemotherapy and may protect the bone marrow of patients undergoing chemotherapy.

In China, astragalus is reputed to be a popular and effective 'spleen tonic. It is very effective in increasing wound healing and increasing adrenal gland function, thereby helping to improve energy levels. It increases stamina and the body's production of energy and would be useful in treating fatigue, a major side effect of chemotherapy, surgery and radiation treatment.

Astragalus protects the liver against the toxic effects of the common cleaning fluid, carbon tetrachloride and in persons receiving chemotherapy. It is considered a valuable immune system tonic that nourishes and fortifies a person's constitution, especially in chronic immune deficiency states such as cancer.

What is the best way to use astragalus?
- Infusion – pour 1 cup of boiling water over 1 to 2 teaspoons of Astragalus. Let sit for 10 minutes. Drink 3 cups a day.
- Dried root – take in dosages of 1 to 4 grams per day.
- Capsules or tablets – take as directed by your herbalist, naturopath or health practitioner.

Bedstraw (Galium Aparine, Galium verum or Galium mollugo)

Bedstraw is commonly referred to as goosegrass, clivers or cleavers. All three varieties of bedstraw carry similar medicinal properties. Bedstraw tea is most famous as a remover of toxic wastes, enhancing detoxification through the liver, kidneys, pancreas, spleen and most importantly, the body's lymphatic system. A healthy lymphatic system is an integral key to maintaining strong immunity.

It has been noted that rinsing with and drinking bedstraw tea may be an excellent remedy for cancer of the tongue, just as the freshly pressed juice mixed with butter can be a remedy for cancerous growth and cancer-like skin disorders. In Maria Treben's famous book, *Health Through God's Pharmacy*, numerous real-life accounts of people healing themselves of cancer of the tongue and tumours in the larynx are offered.

The fresh juice of bedstraw and calendula ointment has been used successfully in folklore medicine, in the healing of malignant skin disorders.

Often bedstraw is combined with other blood-cleansing herbs such as yarrow, stinging nettle, calendula and dandelion.

What is the best way to use bedstraw?

- Infusion – 250ml of boiling water is poured over 1 heaped teaspoon of bedstraw, and infused for a short time OR pour a cup of boiling water onto 2 teaspoons of bedstraw, leave to infuse for 10 minutes. Drink 3 times a day.
- Tincture – take 2 to 4ml of the tincture 3 times a day.
- Fresh juice – fresh bedstraw should be washed and put through a juice extractor while still wet.
- Ointment – sufficient fresh juice is stirred into butter (room temperature) to provide an ointment. Place in the refrigerator.

Burdock Root (Arcticum Lappa)

Burdock root, also known as bardana, hardock, lappa, thorny burr or beggar's buttons, is an ancient herb which has been widely used throughout Europe as a common vegetable, and also as a cleansing remedy. Burdock wine was an ancient folk brew popularly used for indigestion and blood purification. Burdock rids the body of long term toxic material and is an antidote for acute poisoning. It cleanses the lymphatic system, blood, liver and kidneys.

If regularly used, burdock may help to prevent tumours, as it neutralises poisons in the body and is a great accessory treatment for cancer. It has been used extensively by natural healers as a treatment for skin cancer. Burdock contains inulin, the major ingredient found in other powerful immune-stimulatory herbs such as echinacea and dandelion. One of its major functions is to act as an immune system stimulant by promoting chemotaxis of neutrophils and monocytes. Its rich berberine contact is also believed to suppress some forms of cancer cells.

Burdock root is a major ingredient in the famous 'cancer herbal formula – Essiac' rediscovered by a French nurse, Jene Caisse. It also has good anti-bacterial properties, is beneficial in restoring gallbladder and liver function and alleviates pain.

What is the best way to use burdock?

- Infusion – put 1 teaspoon of burdock root into 1 cup of boiling water, bring to the boil and let this sit for 10 minutes. Drink 2 to 3 cups per day.
- As a poultice on the skin – apply to affected area.

Calamus, Sweet Flag (Acorus calamus)

Calamus is an aquatic plant often referred to as sweet rush, myrtle grass or sweet myrtle. It is a reputable herb that is able to cleanse and purify the entire internal body system. A 50-year-old man reported to his doctor that he cured himself of lung cancer by eating calamus roots and drinking yarrow tea. Calamus roots are believed to heal disorders of the stomach and intestines, even if they prove to be stubborn or malignant in origin (Treben, 2001, p 10–11).

There have been various reports that calamus, if taken in the incorrect dosages, may lead to duodenal cancer. Caution should be used when taking this herb – always consult with a qualified herbalist first.

What is the best way to use calamus?
- Infusion – this is prepared only as a cold infusion. 1 teaspoon of calamus roots is soaked in ¼ litre of cold water overnight, lightly warmed in the morning and strained. Before using, warm the tea in a water bath.
- Fresh juice – fresh roots are cleaned and placed through a juice extractor.

Calendula (Calendula Officinalis)

Calendula is probably best known for its wonderful use in healing skin conditions and soothing cuts, burns, wounds and sores. After surgery, calendula is able to cleanse the body, stimulate circulation and improve the healing of wounds. Well known physicians and natural healers around the world believe that calendula is a successful natural remedy for malignant growths.

Freshly pressed calendula juice has been used for skin cancers and also for the removal of liver spots, strawberry spots, pigment spots and other cancer-like skin patches (apply the juice several times daily for a prolonged period). Cancer-like growths and ulcers and malignant non-healing wounds have been treated successfully with an infusion of equal parts of calendula and horsetail. The area is washed twice daily.

What is the best way to use calendula?
- Herbal tea – 1 heaped teaspoon of calendula to ¼ litre of water. Pour boiling water over and let sit for 10 minutes. Drink 3 cups per day.
- Washings – 1 heaped tablespoon of herbs to ½ litre of water
- Fresh Juice – leaves, stems and flowers are washed and while still wet, put through a juice extractor.

Cat's Claw

Cat's claw is a mysterious herb that comes from the Amazon. It is actually a climbing vine that has been toted as a 'cure-all' by many natural healers the world over. It is believed to enhance immune system function and is also thought to possess anti-tumour properties. Usually the inner bark or roots of cat's claw are used. The active ingredients within cat's claw are plant steroles, polyphenols, proanthocyanidins, oxindole alkaloids, triterpenes and glycosides.

Cat's claw is able to cleanse the intestinal tract and enhances the function of white blood cells, which are necessary in fighting disease and cancer. Cat's claw is a powerful anti-oxidant, wiping out free radicals and acting as an anti-inflammatory. It is an excellent remedy for intestinal problems and viral infections.

Cat's claw is believed to reduce the severity and side effects associated with chemotherapy and radiation therapy.

What is the best way to use cat's claw?
- Take only as directed – consult with your health practitioner, naturopath or herbalist.
- Capsule Form – Take two to three 1000mg capsules (containing at least 7.5mg of oxindole alkaloids). Generally cat's claw is safe for children; however it should only by taken in 500mg dosages.

CAUTION!
- Do not take during pregnancy.

Chaparral (Larrea divaricate)

Chaparral contains a potent anti-oxidant, nor-dihydroguaiaretic acid (NDGA). NDGA has been found to have anti-tumour activity and life-extension properties. Being a potent antioxidant, chaparral is able to scavenge free radicals and toxins that contribute to cancer formation. People around the world who have used chaparral tea have claimed to have regressed malignant melanomas, lymphosarcomas and other types of cancer.

The oil obtained from the resin of chaparral decreases inflammation of the respiratory and intestinal tract. It has strong anti-bacterial properties and is very effective in the treatment of wounds. It has the ability to enhance energy levels by increasing vitamin C levels in the adrenal glands and it stops the production of LDL cholesterol, the 'bad guy' in fats. It stimulates respiration in the mitochondria of body cells and protects against the toxic effects of radiation. It also protects against skin cancer and improves liver and lung function.

Chaparral has been used for centuries as an anti-cancer remedy in Mexico. When combined with red clover, it is believed effective at removing cancerous growths and tumours by purifying the bloodstream. However, in rare cases it may stimulate tumours, particularly lymphomas. Use of chaparral in cancer treatment should only be pursued by qualified, experienced practitioners.

The major ingredient of chaparral, dihydronorguaiaretic acid has antioxidant properties and is useful for detoxification. It is also useful in the treatment of acne, warts, arthritis, backache, increasing hair growth, improving eyesight, kidney infections, weight reduction and as a laxative.

What is the best way to use chaparral?
- Take only as directed – consult with your health practitioner, naturopath or herbalist.

Chlorella

Chlorella is a single-celled, freshwater green algae that grows in shallow ponds. The name chlorella comes from the fact that it contains the highest amount of chlorophyll of any known plant. There is approximately 100 times more chlorophyll in chlorella than there is in green leafy vegetables. Chlorella stimulates the production of interferon and macrophage activity. The active ingredient, chorellan, is responsible for this and has strong immune-stimulating properties.

Chlorella has anti-tumour properties and it is believed to prevent or inhibit cancer. Many papers have been written on the photodynamic qualities of chlorophyll (found in high quantities in chlorella) against cancerous tumours. Chlorella is also an excellent detoxifier, removing wastes from the body. It is particularly useful in detoxifying heavy metals including uranium, mercury, cadmium, copper and lead. It helps to remove pesticides, insecticides and polychloridebiphenyl (PCB) from the human body.

Chlorella is useful in the treatment of liver toxicity, alcohol hangover prevention, bowel toxicity, pancreatitis, constipation, ulcers, skin problems, allergies, high cholesterol levels and heart problems. Chlorella also contains high amounts of protein (approximately 58 per cent), B vitamins, carbohydrates, vitamin C, vitamin E, vitamin A, amino acids and rare trace minerals. It contains higher amounts of vitamin B12 than liver, plus considerable amounts of beta-carotene. The high chlorophyll content in chlorella enhances blood cleansing.

In addition, chlorella helps to protect against the effects of ultraviolet radiation and orthodox radiation therapy.

What is the best way to use chlorella?
Chlorella normally comes in liquid form. Take as directed by your health care professional.

Dandelion (Taraxacum officinale)

Dandelion root obtained its unique name from a 15th century surgeon, who compared the leaves to the shape of a lion's tooth. Dandelion root is an excellent blood cleanser, specifically for the liver, as well as a mild laxative. Dandelion contains high amounts of inulin, the main immune-stimulatory ingredient found also in Echinacea. Inulin not only strengthens the kidneys, but also stimulates the body's immune system and aids with the function of the pancreas. Dandelion encourages the production of macrophages (the chameleons of the immune system; these cells can function as phagocytes by gobbling up all of the bad guys) and exhibits strong tumour-fighting properties.

The Chinese have used dandelion for the treatment of breast cancer for thousands of years. It increases the production of bile and is a strong diuretic, due to the high potassium content found in the leaves. This is useful when undertaking chemotherapy, as the body tends to retain high amounts of fluid. One cup of dandelion tea after chemotherapy is a natural way to eliminate fluid from swollen knees, ankles, hips and stomach.

Dandelion is useful at improving the function of the body's spleen, kidney, liver, pancreas and stomach. It may aid in the prevention of breast cancer and is beneficial in treating age spots, boils, anaemia, cirrhosis of the liver, jaundice, rheumatism and abscesses. Dandelion is rich in bioflavonoids, biotin, calcium, choline, folic acid, fluten, gum, inositol, inulin, iron, linolenic acid, magnesium, niacin, PABA, phosphorous, proteins, resin, sulphur, zinc, vitamins A, B1, B2, B6, B12, C and E.

What is the best way to use dandelion?

- Herbal tea – put 2 to 3 teaspoons of the root into 1 cup of water, bring to the boil and gently simmer for 10 to 15 minutes. Drink 3 times a day.
- Salads – adding a few dandelion leaves to a salad during cancer treatment is a good way of stimulating the appetite and providing the body with a rich array of beneficial nutrients.
- Juice – the leaves can also be juiced.
- Tincture – 5 to 10 ml of the tincture 3 times per day.

Echinacea (Echinacea Augustifolia)

Echinacea has gained its well-deserved reputation as a successful remedy and is used throughout the world for treating colds, flu's and viruses. The North American Indians used Echinacea as a cure for snakebites and as an effective antiseptic. Echinacea is also known as coneflower, purple coneflower, black sampsom and snakeroot.

Echinacea's use in the treatment of cancer is due to its incredible ability in enhancing the body's immune system. One of its major components, inulin, promotes chemotaxis of neutrophils, monocytes and eosinophils (cancer-fighting cells) and solubization of viruses and bacteria. Other polysaccharides in Echinacea enhance the immune system by stimulating T-lymphocytes (white blood cells used to fight disease), the production of interferon and the secretion of lymphokines. One common side effect of chemotherapy and radiation therapy is the reduction of white blood cells. Echinacea is a useful herb for increasing white blood cell levels as is Ginseng.

Echinacea is a powerful anti-inflammatory with strong anti-viral properties.

Not only does it support the body's immune system, it also helps to cleanse the lymphatic system. Its active ingredients are many and varied, including arabinose, betaine, copper, echinacen, echinacin B, echinacoside, echinolone, enzymes, fructose, fatty acids, galactose, glucose, glucuronic acid, inulin, inuloid, iron, polysaccharides, potassium, protein, resin, rhamnose, sucrose, sulphur, tannins and vitamins A, C and E. Echinacea is truly a miraculous, nutrient-packed plant.

What is the best way to use Echinacea?

- Herbal tea – place 1 to 2 teaspoons of the root in one cup of water and bring it slowly to the boil. Let it simmer for 10 to 15 minutes. Try to drink at least 3 times per day.
- Tincture – take 1 to 4 ml of the tincture 3 times per day.
- Can also be obtained from a health food store in capsule, tablet or liquid form.

Essiac

Essiac is a combination of herbs that activates the body's natural defences, helps relieve pain and has anti-tumour properties. A Canadian Nurse, Renee Caisse (her last name is essiac spelt backwards), originally introduced it to the Western world. Ms Caisse claimed that the formula had been prescribed to her in 1922 by a patient whose breast cancer had been cured by a traditional Native American shaman in Ontario. Essiac is a combination of burdock root (53%), Indian or turkey rhubarb (3%), sheep sorrel (35%) and slippery elm (9%). Many people with cancer have credited it with extending and improving the quality of their lives.

Vast amounts of anecdotal evidence supporting the incredible health benefits of essiac are available, yet have been suppressed. It is highly probable that this misinformation campaign and the playing down of essiac's healing benefits has been started by those with vested interests (e.g. pharmaceutical companies and the orthodox medical community). This has prevented the facts regarding its efficiency in healing from being acknowledged and accepted.

Essiac is believed to eliminate tumours and cancer. In almost every reported case, essiac significantly diminished the pain and suffering of persons afflicted with cancer and prolonged the life of cancer sufferers.

Essiac stimulates the body's immune system and many people who have used it have reported better levels of health. Essiac is thought to increase energy levels, prevent fatigue and aid in the removal of cancer of the cervix. It is an excellent blood cleanser and liver tonic.

What is the best way to use essiac?

- Herbal tea – essiac can only be obtained through a naturopath, medical practitioner or herbalist. 3 to 6 cups per day is normally recommended.
- Always take only as directed by a qualified health practitioner.

European Mistletoe (Viscum Album)

Mistletoe, also referred to as European mistletoe or birdlime mistletoe, is noted worldwide as being effective in cancer prevention and treatment. It is an ancient herbal remedy noted for its anti-tumour properties. Mistletoe also facilitates the production of red blood cells after radiation therapy and chemotherapy.

Mistletoe supports the body's immune system by increasing the size of the body's thymus gland, to enhance the production of white blood cells for a better immune response. It is believed to possess strong immune-boosting effects. Its active ingredients do this by increasing the body's antibody production, increasing natural killer cell activity and improving the scavenging ability of white blood cells.

Mistletoe is very beneficial in the treatment of cancer and it has been extensively marketed throughout Europe for the accessory treatment of cancerous tumours. In Germany, a combination of fermented mistletoe and homeopathic doses of silver, gold or mercury was marketed and sold for the treatment of cancer. During the 1980s, over 40,000 people throughout the world were using this patented formula.

What is the best way to use mistletoe?

- Cold infusion – a heaped teaspoonful of mistletoe is soaked in a litre of cold water overnight, then the next morning it is slightly warmed and strained. If a larger amount is needed, keep in a dark bottle or thermal flask in the refrigerator and use as desired. Try to drink within 48 hours of making the herbal tea.
- Hot infusion – pour 1 cup of boiling water onto 1 to 2 teaspoons of the dried herb and leave to infuse for 10 to 15 minutes. Drink 3 times daily.
- Tincture – Take 1 to 4ml of tincture 3 times daily.
- Fresh juice – fresh leaves and twigs are washed and, still wet, put into a juice extractor.

Fenugreek

Fenugreek is one of the world's oldest medicinal herbs. It is a common herb, containing plant hormones which some breast cancers may respond to. For hormone-induced breast cancer take fenugreek seed tea with a salt-free semi-vegetarian diet. Folk healers around the world believe that large amounts of fenugreek seed tea in combination with a salt free diet may help to eliminate breast tumours.

Fenugreek also helps to prevent inflammation, especially in the lungs, and it breaks down mucous and catarrh. It has long been used in China for abdominal pain, in Egypt for period pain and stomach cramps and in the Middle East for abdominal cramps.

What is the best way to use fengureek?

- Herbal Tea – pour 1 cup of boiling water over 1 teaspoon of the seeds, let this infuse for 10 minutes. Drink 3 times per day.
- Tincture – take 1 to 2ml of the tincture 3 times daily.
- Poultice – pulverise the seeds to make a poultice.

Garlic

Garlic has been prized for over 5000 years in all parts of the world. This bulbous herb is commonly known throughout the world as 'nature's antibiotic', as it protects against infection by enhancing the body's immune function. Garlic acts in a similar way to penicillin, destroying harmful bacteria. It is a strong immune stimulant and possesses anti-tumour and anti-carcinogenic functions. Garlic also detoxifies the body, lowers blood pressure and improves blood circulation. It has an amazing ability to lower high blood cholesterol levels.

Garlic is a power-packed herb containing allicin, allyl disulfides, calcium, copper, essential oils, germanium, iron, magnesium, manganese, phosphorous, potassium, selenium, sulphur, unsaturated aldehydes, zinc, Vitamin A, B1, B2 and Vitamin C. It is a natural antioxidant with an ability to increase natural killer cell activity and T-Cell activity (infection fighting cells of the immune system). Its ability to enhance the immune system is due to its high levels of selenium, gluatathione and germanium. Garlic is good for virtually any illness or infection.

The abundance of sulphur in garlic simply adds to its amazing healing capabilities. People around the world have been visiting hot springs containing sulfur for many years to cure all kinds of serious ailments. The bulb of the garlic plant is the major part used for medicinal purposes.

In over 30 nutritional studies, doctors found garlic and onions play a large role in decreasing the number of cancer deaths throughout the world. Garlic is believed to protect against radiation damage and breast cancer, stop the effects of skin cancer and slow the growth of tumour cells, while speeding the growth of healthy tissues. In countries where a lot of garlic is used in the diet, the cancer rate is very low. In China, people who regularly consume garlic and onions, have a low incidence of stomach cancer.

Garlic contains allyl sulphides, compounds that help the body to excrete cancer-causing substances before they can do any damage. It not only helps in the treatment of cancer, it is also beneficial in circulatory problems, arthritis, arteriosclerosis, colds, asthma, digestive problems, reduces the risk of heart attacks, insomnia, liver disease, sinusitis, skin infections, ulcers, blood sugar problems and yeast infections.

What is the best way to use garlic?

- Juiced or whole – for cancer treatment, try to eat at least 3 cloves per day. These can also be juiced. One clove of garlic yields about 10mg of alliin and a total alliin potential of 4000mcg.
- Capsules – kyolic garlic oil capsules are available from your health food store.

WARNING!
Toxicity of garlic is rare. However, some reports indicate excessive doses can trigger red blood cell destruction and anaemia. To avoid gastric upset, take garlic with meals. I like to juice garlic with a green vegetable juice or crush garlic and spread on whole-wheat toast with avocado. Heating garlic may destroy some of its healing compounds.

Gingko Biloba

Gingko biloba, also referred to as maidenhair tree, is widely used in the orient to improve memory and slow down the ageing process. The maidenhair tree dates back more than 200 million years, making it the longest living tree species. It has long been extinct in the wild, existing only in Asian oriental gardens. It has only become recognised recently in the west for its amazing healing potential, especially on the brain.

Gingko's active ingredients include ginkgolides, heterosides and quercetin. Gingko biloba's main action is to improve circulation throughout the body, particularly cerebral and peripheral blood flow, thereby improving overall brain function.

Gingko is able to stabilise cell membranes and act as an antioxidant, mopping up and neutralising cancer-causing free radicals. It not only destroys free radicals, it stops their formation and protects against free radical damage to the blood vessels, brain and heart.

Gingko increases oxygenation and is useful for depression, headaches, memory loss, tinnitus, leg cramps, asthma, eczema, heart disorders, kidney disorders and cancer. It has a strong ability to lower high blood pressure, improve memory and brain function, and prevent blood clots in the brain. Truly a miracle herb.

What is3 the best way to use gingko biloba?

- Herbal infusion – 50g of dried leaves with 500 ml of water.
- Tablets or capsules – 40 to 600mg/day in tablet form. Before purchasing Gingko biloba tablets or capsules ensure that they contain at least 24% flavone glycosides and 6% terpene lactones (mainly ginkgolides).

Ginseng

Ginseng is an ancient traditional herb used throughout Asia for centuries. People in Asia, including China, Indonesia, Malaysia, Thailand, Vietnam and Japan, use ginseng every day in tea, fresh herb or tablet form. Asian people believe ginseng improves energy levels, increases longevity and promotes a healthy sexual function. It also improves brain function, increases the body's ability to cope with stress, normalises blood pressure and lowers high cholesterol.

Ginseng is reputed to be useful in the prevention of cancer and acts as a general tonic for overall well-being and health. Shortly before I realised I had cancer, I lived in Thailand for five years, working as a natural health practitioner. I had the pleasure of meeting thousands of beautiful Asian people, and ginseng was without doubt, the most regularly used supplement in their lifestyle. I often asked the age of many Asian people and was shocked when discovering that most of them looked 20 years younger than their actual biological age. Further investigation revealed ginseng and green tea had been a major part of their diet for many years.

Ginseng has strong rejuvenating properties and is available in many different varieties, each exhibiting slightly different actions. It is thought to reduce many of the side effects associated with radiation therapy and chemotherapy.

Panax ginseng, also known as American ginseng, has been shown in experimental studies to return cancerous liver cells to normal. Melanoma cells are believed to be reverted to normal by one of the chemicals in ginseng. American ginseng also aids in lung weakness, stimulates vital organs and helps to relieve fatigue.

Korean or Chinese ginseng strengthens the immune system, decreases fatigue by stimulating the adrenal glands and enhances mental function. It also strengthens the endocrine glands and builds vitality and resistance. The Asians attribute their amazing physical, emotional and mental endurance to the regular use of this variety of ginseng.

What is the best way to use ginseng?

- Chewing – the root of ginseng is often simply chewed.
- Herbal tea – put ½ teaspoon of powdered ginseng in a cup of water, bring to the boil and simmer gently for 10 minutes. Drink 3 times daily.

Green Tea (Camellia Sinensis)

Green tea is an ancient brew, traditionally used throughout Asia as an everyday beverage and health-promoting drink. Most Chinese or Japanese restaurants serve green tea as both a delicacy and cholesterol-lowering digestive aid.

A study conducted by the National Cancer Institute in the United States revealed that people who drank green tea regularly and who were also non-smokers decreased the chance of developing cancer of the oesophagus by 57 per cent in men and 60 per cent in women (Gao et al., 1994: 86:855–58).

The main ingredients in green tea believed to be responsible for its amazing cancer-inhibiting action are polyphenols. In animals, polyphenols are believed to protect against cancer by stopping the production of enzymes that produce cancer-causing substances.

A chemical called epigallocatechin gallate (EGCG) has also been isolated from green tea. It decreases cholesterol levels and is also thought to inhibit cancer growth. In particular, it may inhibit tumour promotion in the skin and the gastrointestinal tract and prevent lung and liver cancer. EGCG is a powerful 'free radical' scavenger that neutralises harmful molecules that attack DNA and trigger cancer. Green tea is also believed to prevent stomach and lung cancer, caused by the known carcinogen, NDEA.

Another active health-promoting ingredient in green tea is theophylline, which works synergistically with the anti-cancer drug Chlorambucil to increase its chemical activity. The tannic acids found in green tea are believed to be effective both topically and internally against cancer.

What is the best way to use green tea?
- Herbal tea – Pour 1 cup of boiling water over 1 heaped teaspoon of Japanese or Chinese Green Tea. Let sit for 10 to 15 minutes. Drink 3 times daily or after meals to break down harmful fats in foods.

Horsetail Tea (Equisetum arvense)

In writings of the famous herbalist and nature cure promoter Abbé Kneipp, it is pointed out that horsetail tea arrests the growth of every tumour and slowly dissolves it. He states that horsetail herb is 'uniquely irreplaceable and invaluable' for bleeding, bladder and kidney disorders, and says, 'For foul wounds, even cancer-like growths and ulcerated legs, horsetail is of great value. It cleanses, clears up and burns away everything bad, so to speak. Often the moist, warm plant is placed into moist cloths and applied to the affected parts'.

So why has such little notice been taken of this miracle herb? Nature, in its abundance and variety of miraculous healing plants, offers us the secrets to optimal health and natural healing. In places such as Guatemala, horsetail tea has long been traditionally used to treat and prevent cancer.

It is believed that horsetail tea used over a long period may inhibit the growth of tumours and possibly enhance their elimination from the body. This would also prove useful for polyps in the abdomen or anus area.

Horsetail tea is one of the richest sources of the mineral silica. Silica is fantastic for strengthening bones, hair, nails and skin. This ancient plant with its rich and diverse mineral content is also capable of enhancing healing of deep-seated lung damage.

What is the best way to use horsetail?

- Herbal tea – ¼ litre of boiling water poured over 1 heaped teaspoon of horsetail herb. Let sit for 10 to 15 minutes. Drink 3 cups per day, depending on your requirements.
- Poultice – a heaped double handful of horsetail herb is placed in a sieve and hung over boiling water. When herbs are hot and soft, place in linen or cheesecloth and apply to affected area. Keep warm.
- Pulp compress – fresh horsetail is washed well and crushed to a pulp on a wooden board, then used as a compress.

Licorice Root (Glycyrrhiza Glabra)

We all know the taste of the delicious black sweet, blackstrap molasses licorice. Licorice in herbal tincture form is wonderful for enhancing energy levels by supporting the body's adrenal glands. It contains glycyrrhizin, a glycoside that is believed to prevent the growth and metastasis of some forms of cancer.

Licorice can protect cell membranes from haemolysis (the rupture of red blood cells). It also boosts the body's immune system by stimulating the production of interferon.

Licorice is a beautiful herb for improving the flavour of other nasty tasting herbal mixtures and counteracts the effects of stress.

What is the best way to take licorice?

- Decoction – put ½ to 1 teaspoon of the root in a cup of water, than bring to the boil and simmer for 10 to 15 minutes. Drink 3 times daily.
- Tincture – take 1 to 3 ml of the tincture 3 times daily.

WARNING!
Taking excess amounts of licorice can be detrimental to health as it causes a loss of potassium from the body. Do not take if you have high blood pressure.

Nettle or Stinging Nettle (Urtica dioica)

The general public has no idea just how valuable this medicinal plant actually is. Apart from its amazing blood cleansing and building properties, it also serves as an excellent cancer preventative, as it strengthens and supports the entire body.

Nettle herb assists with liver, gallbladder and spleen disorders, as well as lung, intestine and stomach congestion. As a blood builder, it is extremely useful for treating anaemia and other blood disorders. Nettle herb is also a mild diuretic that is often used by men to improve prostate problems.

In Maria Treben's book, *Health Through God's Pharmacy,* she notes two cases of people who claimed to have removed cancerous growths in the stomach and in the spleen through regular use of nettle tea. However, science refutes these claims. At present, not enough research study has been performed on nettle tea to allow scientists to understand its unique healing properties.

What is the best way to use stinging nettle?
* Herbal tea – 1 heaped teaspoon per ¼ cup of boiling water, infused for 5 to 10 minutes. Drink as needed.
* Tincture – take 1 to 4 ml of the tincture 3 times daily.

Pau d'Arco

Pau d'arco also known as taheebo, lapacho, ipe roxo, trumpet bush or iperoxo, is made from the inner bark of a tree found in South American rainforests. It has long been used as a folk remedy in the treatment of cancer. In recent years, evidence is emerging that it may be helpful in breast cancer, sarcomas, carcinomas and leukaemias.

According to a Brazilian report, one of the Russian tsars and Mahatma Gandhi both drank pau d'arco. It has strong immune stimulating and anti-inflammatory properties. Pau d'arco is beneficial as an adjunct therapy in the treatment of cancer. The native indians of Brazil have used it in the treatment of cancer of the oesophagus, head, intestines, lung and prostate. It is especially good for limiting the pain connected with cancer.

Pau d'arco is rich in iron, an excellent detoxifier, and it gives the body the energy and defences necessary to defend itself and resist disease.

The inner bark of this wonderful plant has also been used to treat constipation, poor circulation, snakebites, viral infections, Candida albicans respiratory problems, boils, fever and wounds just to name a few ailments.

What is the best way to use pau d'arco?
* Herbal tea – use the bark, which has been standardised to 2 to 4% la pachol content, to ensure you are getting the real thing. Use 1 tablespoon of bark per cup of water and boil for 15 to 20 minutes. Drink 2 to 6 cups per day.
* Fluid extract – take 10-30 drops daily.

Red Clover (Trifolium Pratense)

Red clover, also known as trifolium pratense, has beautiful strawberry-coloured flowers. It was traditionally used as fodder for cattle. Today it is used medicinally in cancer treatment and prevention, due to its potent blood cleansing potential.

Red clover contains many nutrients and active ingredients, and is beneficial in preventing and in many cases removing tumours from the body. Many herbalists believe if you drink one cup of red clover tea a day, there is very little chance you will ever develop cancer or harmful tumours, especially if you combine this with a healthy, chemical free diet. Red Clover is rich in biotin, choline, copper, coumarins, folic acid, glycosides, inositol, isoflavonoids, magnesium, manganese, pantothenic acid, selenium, bioflavonoids, zinc, and vitamins A, B1, B2, B3, B6, B12 and C.

Red clover is a natural antibiotic, appetite suppressant and relaxant.

It is useful in the treatment of bacterial infections, HIV and AIDS, inflamed lungs, inflammatory bowel disorders, kidney problems, liver disease, bronchitis, skin disorders and a weakened immune system. It has also be used effectively by herbalists in preventing and treating breast, prostate, ovarian cancer and lymphatic cancer by increasing haemoglobin content in red blood cells.

Red clover became a popular anti-cancer remedy in the 1930s and has been used locally for cancerous growths. It can be very effective in breaking up growths and tumours when used in combination with chaparral and other cancer-fighting herbs.

What is the best way to use red clover?
- Infusion – pour 1 cup of boiling water over 1 to 3 teaspoons of dried red clover and leave to infuse for 10 to 15 minutes. Drink 3 cups per day.
- Tincture – take 2 to 6 ml of the tincture 2 to 3 times per day.

Suma

Suma, also referred to as Brazilian ginseng, contains cancer-preventing properties. Research in Japan has shown that pfaffic acid, found in suma, is capable of inhibiting certain types of cancer. All parts of the suma plant are used, including bark, berries, leaves and root. Its active ingredients are many and varied, including pfaffosides, vitamins A, B, C, D, E and F, sitosterol, stigmasterol, tannins, germanium, malic acid, essential oils, pfaffic acid, albumin and allantoin.

Suma is used to treat anaemia, fatigue and stress. It is a wonderful immune system booster that helps to prevent and improve cancerous conditions, AIDS, high blood pressure, skin cancer, liver disease and a weakened immune system.

What is the best way to use Suma?
- Herbal tea – Use 1 to 2 teaspoons of the dried root. Pour 1 cup of boiling water over this and let it infuse for 10 to 15 minutes. Drink 3 cups per day.
- Poultice – use in combination with comfrey, pau d'arco and red clover. Skin cancer responds very well to this poultice.

Spice Up Your Life – Turmeric (Curcuma longa) and Cayenne Pepper (Capsicum minimum)

Turmeric is an amazing spice which exhibits strong cancer-preventing properties. Turmeric's active ingredients include curcuminoids, essential oils, turmerone, zingiberene, A-atlantone and curcumin. It is such a simple spice to use and can be added to meals to attain a delicious, powerful flavour. Chop turmeric finely, throw into your cooking and you will be endowed with all of turmeric's incredible healing powers.

Turmeric is blessed with antibiotic properties and anti-inflammatory actions, and is a very powerful antioxidant. It protects our liver against many toxins, inhibits platelet-activating factor (major component of inflammation), strengthens gastric mucosa, prevents gastric lesions and also lowers blood cholesterol.

Turmeric also provides DNA protection against damage by carcinogens and is believed to inhibit the development of skin cancer. It is an anti-carcinogen, which neutralises the cancer-causing compounds in tobacco smoke. Turmeric is the main ingredient in curry powder.

Cayenne, known as bird pepper, capsicum or chilli pepper, is the powder made from ground red chillies (the fruit of the plant). We all know the spicy taste of chilli and its wondrous ability to make us sweat. Cayenne is also a remarkable spice in increasing general body and peripheral circulation, and decreasing blood pressure. It also regulates the blood flow, equalizing and strengthening the heart, arteries, capillaries and nerves.

Cayenne suppresses pain and causes the release of the 'pleasure drugs', endorphins. Large quantities of chilli can stimulate the development of cancer, yet small amounts are very healthy for cancer prevention.

What is the best way to take turmeric?
- Fresh – turmeric is best added fresh to cooking. Chop, dice or grate it and add to your favourite healthy dishes. The rhizoma (underground stem) is the part used for healing.
- Powder – turmeric can also be obtained from a health food store.

What is the best way to take cayenne?
- Infusion – pour 1 cup of boiling water onto ½ to 1 teaspoon of cayenne and leave to infuse for 10 minutes. A tablespoon of this infusion should be mixed with hot water and drunk as needed.
- Tincture – take 0.25ml of the tincture 3 times daily or as needed.

Yarrow (Achillea millefolium)

In old herbal texts yarrow was referred to as 'cure of all ills' and was used in many cases that seemed hopeless. Its potent blood cleansing ability helps to expel toxins from the body, eradicating unwanted illnesses.

Yarrow is an excellent remedy used to stop bleeding in the lungs, as it has astringent properties. Used together with calamus roots, it is believed by many folklore healers to heal lung cancer. The calamus roots should be chewed throughout the day and a cup of yarrow tea is sipped every morning and evening.

Yarrow acts directly on bone marrow, stimulating blood renewal, and can be helpful in bone marrow related disorders.

What is the best way to take yarrow?
- Infusion – pour 1 cup of boiling water over 1 heaped teaspoon of yarrow, infuse for a short time, then drink. Drink 2 to 3 cups per day. If feverish, you should drink hourly.
- Tincture – take 2 to 4ml of the tincture 3 times a day.

Other Medicinal Herbs Used Traditionally and Employed Worldwide for possible Cancer Treatment and Prevention

Agrimony (Agrimonia eupatoria)
The Chinese help prevent colon cancer by mixing an extract of the hairyvein agrimonia (agrimony) plant with ethyl alcohol (drinking alcohol). Agrimony is available in most health food stores.

Barberry (Berberis vulgaris)
Barberry is believed to suppress some forms of cancer, due to its high berberine content.

Cinnamon (Cinnamomum zeylanicum)
Cinnamon is believed to reduce the incidence of cancers caused by a number of synthetic food additives.

Greater Celandine (Chlidonium majus)
This plant is renowned for its blood purifying and stimulating qualities. A combination of greater celandine, stinging nettle and elder shoots has been used in cases of leukaemia. But to be effective, at least 2 litres of this mixture must be drunk daily.

Hops (Humulus lupulus)
Traditionally used to treat cancer due to its blood cleansing properties.

Job's Tears (Coix lacryma jobi)
The Chinese believe this herb may inhibit the growth of cancer cells.

Male Fern (Dryopteris filix-mas)
Traditionally used to treat cancerous tumours and to heal wounds.

Plantain, Ribwort (Plantago lanceolata)
A poultice made from the plantain leaves is believed to encourage the removal of malignant growths. It is also believed beneficial in the treatment of malignant glandular disorders.

Saffron (Crocus sativus)
Saffron has been widely used for treating cancer, but has been outlawed for consumption in non-culinary situations in the United States because of an FDA report saying it can cause cancer in rats.

St John's Wort (Hypericum perforatum)
Tests at the United States National Cancer Institute have shown that this herb has promise in the fight against cancer.

Tansy (Tanacetum vulgare)

Traditionally considered by herbalists as a cancer cure.

Wood Sorrel (Oxalis acetosella)

Wood sorrel is commonly known as sour wood or fairy bells. In popular medicine, wood sorrel juice was recommended for stomach cancer in the early stages, and cancer-like internal and external ulcers and growths.

IMPORTANT NOTE!

Specific herbs may be more suited to individual types of cancer. Before deciding to use herbs for cancer treatment, consult with a qualified herbalist or naturopath as to the most beneficial herbs for your particular type of cancer and for the appropriate dosage amounts, according to your body weight. Certain herbs are contraindicated in a variety of different medical conditions, so always seek professional advice before using.

Chapter 28

BLISS AND HARMONY – MEDITATION, GUIDED IMAGERY AND RELIGION

We all have different beliefs, different gods and different religions. There are thousands of religions throughout the world, and although we pray to different gods, a common bond links all people involved with religion. This bond is faith, admiration and love in our god, whoever or whatever our god may be.

With healing, religion can be a beneficial aid in overcoming the fears and anxiety associated with cancer and also in learning to accept the possibility of death openly. Many people turn to religion when faced with sickness or death. We ask our god, or deity for help in overcoming our illness and beating cancer. For many, religion brings a sense of community and acceptance, and enables similar people bound by a common bond to support your condition and join in your fight to beat cancer.

For many people, religion provides them with a reason to live and fills them with a feeling of acceptance and belonging. Feeling needed or accepted is a desire of most humans and a desire which gives us strength to live and overcome difficult obstacles.

Having cancer can open your heart and mind to change and provide a deeper questioning of why this may have happened. Many people feel religious priests, disciples and monks can provide the clues to unravelling their individual mystery. For some this may be true, for others this may not be true. It is solely dependent on the individual. Religion usually incorporates some form of praying or meditation, which is a highly positive therapy in increasing concentration and attention towards the matter at hand.

Meditation is an ancient art which has been studied and practised for thousands of years as an effective means of treating stress, inducing a state of relaxation and bringing about a sense of calm and peace to the mind and soul. Meditation is effective at controlling anxiety, enhancing the immune system and easing chronic pain and illness.

Many people in this world have the impression that meditation has to involve some mystical state that only shamans, swamis, witch doctors or mystics are able to obtain. In actual fact, meditation comes in many different forms and can be practised in your everyday life. It is simply a way of training yourself to turn your concentration inward, away from your normal pressures in everyday life, while focusing on peaceful, calming thoughts.

There are many different types of meditation techniques used throughout the world, but they basically fall into two categories: concentrative meditation and mindfulness meditation. During concentrative meditation, attention is focused on a single sound, object or one's breath to bring about a calm, peaceful mind.

During mindfulness meditation, the mind becomes aware of but does not react to the wide variety of sensations, feelings and images tied in with the current activity. By sitting quietly and allowing the images of your surroundings to pass by your mind without become involved in them, you can attain a calm state of mind. Many Buddhists describe meditation as reaching a state of 'nothingness'. This means having an empty mind without worries, fears, anxieties or illusions – simply nothing but emptiness.

Most religions throughout the world use some form of meditation. The most famous perhaps is Buddhism, which uses Vipassana meditation and everyday mindfulness of actions. Buddhist monks who live in seaside and mountain temples, practise mindfulness or meditation during their everyday activities, no matter how boring the activity may seem. That is, if a monk is sweeping a path he thinks of nothing else but sweeping the path and all of the bodily actions involved in sweeping a path. If he is walking, all attention and concentration is focused on walking and the action of walking.

Transcendental meditation is a well known meditation which attains a state of the body being completely at rest, yet the mind remains alert.

Meditation can exist in many forms. To reach a meditative or relaxed state it is best to place yourself in quiet, serene and beautiful surroundings. Being in a harmonious and peaceful environment slows down the mind and relaxes the body.

Due to work commitments and pressures in our everyday life it is unrealistic to assume that we can keep our minds empty all of the time. However, in reality most of us can try to put aside 10 to 20 minutes everyday to relax, sit still, breathe deeply and empty out the myriad of crazy thoughts that seem to creep into our heads daily. This simple process in itself is a form of meditation that has positive effects on your body and mind.

All forms of meditation are able to facilitate a deep state of relaxation and reduce stress. Relaxation and a positive state of mind are essential in beating and preventing cancer, and maintaining optimal health and well-being.

Guided Imagery to Beat Cancer

Guided imagery techniques are most successful if you already imagine the situation or event as if it has already occurred. Look at it in the recent past – feel content with the outcome and the resolution of the event. Guided imagery is fantastic at reprogramming the subconscious mind, which proceeds to make changes in the physical body. The mind and body work hand in hand to overcome illness and disease. Following are some wonderful guided imagery exercises for overcoming cancer and maintaining a positive, stress-free state of mind.

Exercise One

Lie down in a quiet and peaceful place. Choose somewhere where you feel completely relaxed and totally at ease. This is usually a place with good vibrations – near the ocean, in your backyard, your own bedroom, in the mountains, close to a waterfall or somewhere special to you. It is usually more relaxing to lie flat on your back, although some people may find it more comfortable to be sitting cross legged or in a lotus position. We are all very different. No one position is more perfect than the other as long as your muscles and mind are comfortable, without any external or internal strains.

Breathe in and out very slowly through your nose and imagine yourself becoming more and more relaxed with each breath. On the out breath, imagine your body and muscles and skin and internal organs relaxing more and more. With each breath, imagine your body falling deeper towards the ground as you become more and more relaxed. You can feel your breath becoming slower as you relax.

With every breath out, your mind and body becomes more relaxed and heavy, falling into the earth in total ease. Release all of your thoughts, empty your mind. On every out breath imagine your thoughts flowing out of you with complete ease and on every in breath imagine a beautiful golden or white light entering your body through your nose. Continue to do this until your mind feels empty and clear.

It may take some time to reach this comfortable and relaxed state. When you do, you can begin imagining the following positive imagery to help eliminate harmful cancer cells from your body:

Visualise your body's cells working like a wonderful army, all in unison, all working hand in hand. Each cell is like a small person or an ant marching around, passing commands on to the next cell (person). All of the army of people (cells) are happy and strong, each content with their own job, each needed by the body. Imagine your white blood cells as an army of white-uniformed people. These are the body's natural defences, walking around with mops, brooms and cleaning utensils, cleaning up any dirty, murky patches in the body, known as cancer cells.

If you know where your cancer is, imagine the white army of white blood cells marching towards the cancer cells and with all of their strength and energy, mopping them up, cleaning them and eliminating them. With every stroke of their brushes the dirty cancer cells disappear, leaving a shiny, healthy surface glowing with white light. The white army of people (white blood cells) are smiling, laughing, content and happy. As you look around, you cannot see any dirty patches anymore – everywhere you look, all you can see is clean, white surfaces. Try to do this as often as possible, even during chemotherapy and radiation treatment. What you imprint on your mind leaves an imprint on your subconscious setting up a beautiful, positive outcome of perfect health and happiness. This is also a great preventative against cancer.

Exercise Two

As for Exercise One, lie down in a quiet and peaceful place. Choose somewhere you feel completely relaxed and totally at ease. This is usually a place with good vibrations – near the ocean, in your backyard, your own bedroom, in the mountains, close to a waterfall or somewhere special to you. It is usually more relaxing to lie flat on your back, although some people may find it more comfortable to be sitting cross legged or in a lotus position. We are all very different. No one position is more perfect than the other, as long as your muscles and mind are comfortable, without any external or internal strains.

Breathe very slowly in and out through your nose and imagine yourself becoming more and more relaxed with each breath. On the out breath, imagine your body and muscles and skin and internal organs relaxing more and more. With each breath, imagine your body falling deeper towards the ground as you become more and more relaxed. You can feel your breath becoming slower as you relax.

With every breath out, your mind and body becomes more relaxed and heavy, falling into the earth in total ease. Release all of your thoughts, empty your mind. On every out breath imagine your thoughts flowing out of you with complete ease and on every in breath imagine a beautiful golden or white light entering your body through your nose. Continue to do this until your mind feels empty and clear.

It may take some time to reach this comfortable and relaxed state. When you do, you can begin imagining the following positive imagery to eliminate harmful cancer cells from your body:

You see yourself exactly as you are, yet miniature, wearing a long red magician's coat. Imagine yourself entering through your mouth and sliding down your throat. Everything is soft and smooth, and you are laughing. You have a bright magician's wand in your hand and it is glowing with a white ball of light on the end. You are sliding and laughing as you are drawn gently along to the area of your body where the cancer is located.

Everything around you is shiny, healthy, pink and smooth. As you reach the cancerous area of your body, you see a black ball. Laughing, you run up to the black ball and swipe at it with your magician's wand with the glowing white ball. With every swipe of your wand, the black ball evaporates in the air with a puff of smoke. You do it again and again, laughing and smiling as more and more puffs of smoke evaporate in front of your eyes. Continue to aim with your magician's wand until the black ball has completely disappeared leaving you with a beautiful, glowing pink colour. You feel very happy, all of the darkness is gone and everything has a beautiful pink, shiny, clean surface.

Your job is done and you are drawn back up the whirling slide, up and up, laughing and laughing, back into your mouth as you realise that you have conquered the black ball. As you reach your mouth, you gently tap yourself over the top of your head with the magician's wand and disappear with a puff of smoke. When you are ready you can slowly open your eyes, feeling completely relaxed and clean and clear within your body.

- The magician's wand creative visualisation is an excellent guided imagery for children to use. I know of one wonderful man who made his little sister, who was only five years old, a magician's wand painted with crystals and beautiful colours. We told her that she is a magician and to tap her head every day with the wand, and to imagine the cancer disappearing in the air with a puff of smoke. This gorgeous girl had a brain tumour and the doctor's gave her only a short time to live. She is still going strong and healing every day – proving that magic can occur every day, even in the smallest ways!

You can also create your own imagery exercises. The best exercise to help eliminate cancer is to imagine yourself destroying the cancer in any way you desire and always feeling content and happy with the outcome. Keep the exercises positive. To enhance immune system function, imagine your white blood cells full of energy and glowing with light. See them fighting the diseased cells and destroying them one by one. Any images you imprint on your subconscious mind create the ultimate result in your physical body.

Amazing Cancer Clearing Exercises

The following cancer clearing exercises were passed on to me by one of the most incredible healers I have ever had the pleasure of knowing. This doctor, who was also a naturopath and homeopath, treated cancer patients successfully every day for over 20 years. He knew that to truly heal and to prevent a cancer from returning, a person had to remove the emotional cause of their cancer or illness. Negative emotions, apart from their detrimental effects on our immune system, create a blockage of energy in the body which can cause a tumour to form. If that tumour is fed more negativity, whether it be through diet or emotions, the tumour will continue to live off this.

As a naturopath I have treated thousands of people all over the world and one thing that I have learnt in my experience is that illness is not purely physical, there is nearly always an emotional connection to cancer and chronic disease. I now realise through my own experience as both a cancer survivor and a naturopath, that most of us have some type of hurt in our lives that we push deep down inside of ourselves so we don't feel the pain. Other people may simply choose to live with this pain, anger or sadness in their lives. At some stage, this emotional trauma needs to be released to allow our life energy to flow clearly again.

Saying the following affirmations and doing the exercises with your own fingers reaches the depths of your subconscious mind, clearing deep-seated problems and pains, and creating new positive long-term changes and beliefs. Many psychologists use these types of techniques as a deep cleansing process for past emotional pain and trauma. Holding onto grief, pain, resentments and anger is a definite recipe for developing cancer and preventing its ultimate cure.

- I am eliminating all of the sadness in all of the roots – and the deepest cause – of all of this problem. (Tap with your index finger above the eyebrow, close to the nose.)
- I am eliminating all of the fear in all of the roots – and the deepest cause – of all of this problem. (Tap with your index finger below the eyebrow, close to the nose.)
- I am eliminating all of the anger in all of the roots – and the deepest cause – of all of this problem. (Tap with your index finger above the other eyebrow, close to the nose.)
- I am eliminating all of the emotional trauma in all of the roots – and the deepest cause – of all of this problem. (Tap the thumb and little finger together at least five times.)

- I forgive myself and I know that I am/was doing the best that I can/could. (Tap the two index fingers together, at least five times.)
- I forgive you (Mum, Dad, Paul, Peter etc.) and I know that you are/were doing the best that you can/could. (Do three circles around the outside of the ear with the index finger.)

Bodywork, Shiatsu, Posture, Reiki and Yoga

Bodywork, good posture, tai chi, chi gung and yoga are wonderful forms of therapy for relaxation, pain relief and immune support.

Bodywork incorporates all types of massage therapies and spinal realignment techniques. Massage involves the manipulation of muscles and other soft tissues. It promotes muscle relaxation, increases lymphatic circulation and improves blood flow through the body's tissues. Massage is not suitable for everyone. In some malignant forms of cancer an increase in lymphatic and blood circulation can cause the tumour or cancer to spread further throughout the body. Avoid massage with lymphatic cancer in particular! Massage may also be harmful with other types of cancers.

Shiatsu originated in China and spread throughout Japan, eventually combining bodywork arts of the east and west to form a beautiful healing therapy. Shiatsu works on the belief that energy flows throughout the body along channel lines that are known as 'meridians'. Similar to acupuncture, there are a number of pressure points along the meridians that relate to specific organs.

Shiatsu can be used to treat a number of different health conditions including insomnia, back aches, headaches and nervous tension problems. A shiatsu therapist locates any blockages in energy flow throughout the body and works to unblock these 'roadblocks' allowing energy to flow evenly along our 'energy channels'. Shiatsu in combination with a healthy lifestyle and nutritious diet can help to bring about a feeling of good health on all levels – physical, emotional and spiritual.

Spinal realignment aims at achieving realignment of the body parts and spine. Through manipulation of connective tissues linking muscles to bones and learnt techniques, the therapist attempts to restore greater movement, resulting in a more balanced body. The spine is interlinked to all body systems, internal organs and brain functions. The nervous system controls and co-ordinates all organs and structures of the human body, which are interlinked to our spine. Misalignments and fixations of the spine may cause irritation to the nervous system that affects the functions of the body's organs, tissues and structures. It is therefore essential in the maintenance of good health to maintain as straight and stress-free a posture as possible. If you have any misalignments, have these readjusted by a qualified and experienced osteopath.

Reiki is an alternative therapy that has re-emerged back into society and healing in a dramatic way in the last few years. In Japanese language, Reiki translates to 'universal life energy'. It works on the basis of transferring 'universal life energy' back into the individual and similar to shiatsu, it helps to unblock any 'energy blocks' within the person.

The Reiki practitioner acts as a 'transferrer of energy', sending the energy into the individual that requires healing. By increasing the energy within an individual, the body renews itself, toxins are removed, emotional blocks are released opening the person to an abundance of healing, life energy. It tends to create a feeling of deep relaxation, allowing the individual to heal much more rapidly.

A qualified and experienced Reiki therapist is essential to deal with more chronic conditions such as cancer. As Reiki works on the basis of transferring 'universal life energy', if a negative Reiki therapist is used, this negative energy is passed onto the person. Always seek a healthy, positive and experienced Reiki therapist to realise the full benefits of this subtle, yet powerful healing modality.

Yoga is an ancient practice combining specific stretching movements working synergistically with breathing and relaxation exercises. Yoga is the primary form of meditation practised by many cultures and religions throughout the world. Its movements and techniques have a variety of healing effects on the body, including toning internal organs, balancing body systems and bringing about a state of total equilibrium in the individual.

Those who practise yoga regularly maintain high levels of health and tend to prevent illness and disease. Yoga is believed to enhance longevity, heal chronic illnesses and spinal deformities through its delicate movements and controlled breathing techniques. While working in Asia, I taught regular yoga classes and was continually in awe at the amazing healing power exemplified by the regular use of yoga in many individuals' lives. Yoga and other ancient arts like tai chi and qui gong, all aim to rebalance the body, spirit and mind in gentle yet effective ways. Try one of these unique healing arts today and feel harmony, peace and spiritual fulfilment drift gently into your life.

Chapter 29

BACK TO BODY BASICS

Dynamic Healing Exercises

These dynamic exercises combine movement and breath control. Concentrate on the feelings of inner energy and work through the different levels of awareness in your body. Many people find it difficult to sustain any negative emotional states, such as aggression, anger and nervousness, while breathing out. So during times of stress or challenge, concentrate on your exhalations. The following dynamic exercises are designed to encourage healing on all levels of existence.

Smiling to the World!

This is a beautiful exercise that can be performed anywhere, at any time of the day. It only takes a few minutes and will leave you with a lively and dynamic feeling throughout your body. Concentrate on smiling! Smile at the world – just look around and smile! Smile at the birds, the trees, the grass; at everything surrounding your aura. As you do this, vigorously shake your hand, arms, legs, hips, legs and feet. Allow yourself a few seconds relaxation in between each shake. But continue to smile, and breathe slowly and gently.

This simple exercise can be done standing, sitting or lying down. Repeat as many times as desired! It uplifts the body and mind and brings about a peaceful, yet energetic state.

Humming Bee

Sit in a comfortable position with your back completely straight, yet relaxed. Close your eyes and place your index fingers in your ears. Block out all sounds. Breathe in gently and slowly, through the nose. Hold your breath for a count of three. Keep your lips gently together, yet slightly parted in the middle. As you breathe out through the mouth, let your lips relax and vibrate as you make the humming sound of a bee. Feel your lips vibrate and listen to the sound of a bee emanate through your mind. Repeat as many times as you like.

This exercise releases built up anxiety and tension, and enables you to laugh at yourself and those around you.

Vibrating Hum

This is a simple exercise. People naturally hum when they are contented and happy, totally absorbed and at one with the situation. Mothers hum to their children to calm them down and place them in a state of deep relaxation. Try humming to yourself.

With your lips closed, begin humming 'mmmmmmm'. You can continue to do this for a few minutes, then change the sound to 'mmmmmaaaah' or 'mmmmmm-meeeeh' or 'mmmmmmmoooo'. If you feel like dancing or swaying to your humming sounds, don't hesitate. Feel the healing vibrations through your body and mind.

Silence Exercise

Have you ever immersed yourself in real silence? In this noise-polluted world of appliances humming, trucks roaring, planes soaring and heavy machinery, it is becoming more difficult to find the silence. Yet it is still possible.

Try to find at least five minutes of silence every day. You may find this a challenge at first. Silence is refreshing, relaxing and universally healing. Episodes of silence will reinvigorate your soul and give your body a chance to repair damage and heal.

Unique Techniques to Remove Pain and Emotional Trauma

Releasing the Past with Passion

Approach this exercise with an open heart, full of love and a blameless, non-judgmental attitude to yourself and others. Choose an event in your life that may have caused you pain or made you feel uneasy. This event may have triggered the development of your cancer without you fully being aware of it. It could have been an argument, a lie, a secret that was disclosed, or a hurt done to you by someone else.

Go back into your memory and recreate the experience. Recapture the sensory impressions of the event, the sounds, sights and smells. Re-live how you felt, and your thoughts and emotions, and strive for a re-run of the experience with a new and open compassion and understanding.

Now sing out loud to your memory. Sing your thoughts and feelings. Sing what you would have done and said at the time, knowing what you know now. Appreciate that life's experiences are your teachers and that everyone else associated with this event was learning too. No one is perfect. Learn from your mistakes and release the past, sing it out.

Don't remain in regret. Go through the event as you would have liked it to progress. Imagine it playing like a video tape in your mind. Sing out loud and dedicate your words and tunes to strength, wisdom, forgiveness and love with which you can overcome the situation. Singing through this event will allay your fears and clear your past. Conclude this exercise by bringing your awareness and love firmly back to the present.

Giggle-a-thon

Sit in a comfortable position. It is best to be in a place where you feel totally uninhibited, free from distractions and judgement. Breathing gently and slowly, try to imagine a prominent time in your life which caused you pain or hurt you. Imagine this clearly in your mind. Imagine vividly the people involved, the way you felt and what made you feel so upset. Now turning everything around, imagine yourself laughing at those people and the situation.

You are full of giggles, you can see yourself smiling and laughing, and your laugh makes those around you laugh. You are not laughing vindictively, you are laughing with passion and complete understanding at the stupidity and silliness of it all. Feel the laughter releasing from your heart and chest. Let it vibrate your body and flow from your mouth. Release that infectious giggle! Continue as long as possible.

If you practise this exercise, laughing at yourself and others, it will be impossible to hold onto past hurts with resentment and bitterness. Laughter is the best medicine to heal the body and soul and to clear old wounds! If you can laugh at yourself and life's silly situations, you will be able to release any negative emotions that led to your cancer.

Oxygen Therapy

All human tissues and organs need oxygen in order to function efficiently. Cancerous cells breed in an oxygen-deprived environment. Tumours and cancer cannot survive in an oxygen-saturated environment and nutrients and healing methods that carry oxygen to the cancerous tissues are very effective in fighting cancer.

As a human being we can live without water for five to seven days, we can exist without food for weeks, but we are unable to live without oxygen for a matter of minutes. Every vital process that occurs in our body's cells needs oxygen to allow us to survive. It cleanses our body and removes harmful toxins that can lead to disease.

Oxygen therapy can be given in a number of ways. Simply using liquid oxygen supplements saturates the body's cells with life-giving oxygen. Breathing deeply in oxygen-rich environments or being administered oxygen at high atmospheric pressure are other successful methods of enhancing the body's supply and efficiency of oxygen.

Hyperbaric oxygen therapy (HBOT) saturates the body with oxygen by placing the individual in a chamber that delivers pure oxygen at three times the normal atmospheric pressure. It is most commonly used in cases of trauma, including burns, wounds and the death of tissues from radiation therapy. HBOT increases the rate of healing and speed of recovery after surgery.

Taking walks in the country, being in mountains, walking on the beach and visiting the ocean all enhances the body's supply of life-giving oxygen and helps to remove carbon dioxide and harmful toxins from the lungs. Beautiful environments rich in negative ions help to maintain normal blood oxygen levels. Certain nutrients and herbs also improve the body's utilisation of oxygen and increase oxygen transport throughout the body. These include germanium, coenzyme Q10, vitamin B2, potassium, iron, magnesium, sulphur, gingko biloba, wheatgrass, chlorella, chlorophyll and ginseng.

The most beneficial way to improve the health of your lungs and absorb oxygen for healing is to undertake deep breathing exercises and relaxation techniques such as yoga, tai chi, qui gong and regular aerobic exercise. All of these natural forms of exercise enhance deep breathing and improve concentration, lung capacity, immunity and health.

Breathing Exercises for Relaxation and Health

Slow Deep Breathing or Simple Yoga Breath

This exercise relaxes your mind and body, increases your oxygen supplies and centres your awareness. Sitting or lying in a comfortable position with your eyes closed, bring in your breath slowly and fully to the pit of your stomach. Breathe in and out through the nose only. Place your hands on your abdomen where you can feel each breath coming in and out. As you breathe in, concentrate on letting your abdomen expand. As you breathe out, concentrate on letting your abdomen slowly pull in. Do not force the breathing or hurry. This is a relaxing, deepening and centering practice. Keep your breathing steady, slow and full. Continue for up to five minutes or more.

Vigorous Deep Breathing or Full Yoga Breath

Sit upright, comfortable and in a relaxed position. You can either sit in a chair, in lotus position or cross legged. Make sure your back is completely upright. Take moderate and deep breaths in and out through the nostrils. First begin by filling the lungs. Breathe in and out through the nostrils, bringing the breath only to the chest area. Continue to do this for a few minutes. On the out breath, do a forceful exhalation through the nostrils.

Next, breathing in and out through the nose, bring your breath down to the diaphragm area. Concentrate on bringing the breath through the chest and down to the diaphragm. Continue to do this for a few minutes – bringing the breath down through the lungs to the diaphragm. On the out breath, do a forceful exhalation through the nostrils. Continue to do this for a few minutes.

Next, concentrate on bringing your breath to the lungs, to the diaphragm and down to the stomach area. Breathe in and out, taking the breath right down to the stomach. On the out breath, do a forceful exhalation through the nostrils. Continue to do this for a few minutes.

Deep Relaxation Exercise

This exercise induces a state of deep relaxation. It also helps to rebalance the emotions, controls cravings and relaxes the body's nervous system. Inhale deeply and quietly through your nose to a count of four. Hold the breath for a count of four. Then exhale through the mouth to a count of eight, making a whooshing sound.

Inhale a second time, hold, and release again to a count of eight with a whooshing sound. This can be done in any position at any time of the day. If you are sitting, remember to always keep your back straight.

Tension Release Exercise

This exercise is great for releasing tension and built up anxiety and stresses.

Standing upright with your back perfectly straight, stretch your arms out straight in front of you with fingers outstretched. Breathe in through the nose very slowly. As you do this, slowly curl your hands into fists and bring them close to your body.

Clench your fists as tight as you can as you hold your breath for a count of four. When you are ready to exhale, breathe out through your mouth with a big 'aaaahhhh' and as you do, throw your hands straight out in front of you, releasing your clenched fists.

Repeat this at least 10 times. Remember, when you clench your fists on the inhale and bring your arms close to your chest, imagine pulling all of your tensions back with this. When you exhale and throw your arms out in front of you releasing your fists, release all of your tensions and stresses with a big 'aaaahhh'.

Oxygenation Exercise

This exercise increases oxygenation throughout the body and increases general lung capacity. Holding your left nostril down with your left finger, breathe in deeply through your right nostril. Hold your breath for three seconds. Change to your right index finger and hold down the right nostril. Breathe out of the left nostril until there is no air left in your stomach.

Next, begin by holding the right nostril down with your right index finger. Breathe in deeply through your left nostril. Hold your breath for three seconds. Change fingers to the left nostril and breathe out of the right nostril, until your stomach and lungs are completely empty. Repeat for 10 breaths. Try to breathe more deeply with each repetition.

The Synergy of Exercise

Interest in health maintenance and preventative medicine has become a phenomenon of unparalleled growth in today's world. We are learning to use the simple tools of health to expand and fully utilise the healing powers contained within our natural processes. One of the greatest and easiest methods to enhance healing and to prevent ill health is regular exercise.

Exercise is available to us in a variety of forms, all benefiting the body in a myriad of positive ways. Some of the best forms of exercise available in the treatment of cancer include aerobic exercise like brisk walking, roller blading, surfing, snowboarding, swimming and cycling and joint mobility exercises such as stretching, yoga, breathing routines, tai chi, qui gong, pilates and the list goes on. How does exercise benefit our body in fighting cancer?

Exercise:
- decreases cholesterol and triglyceride levels;
- increases levels of HDL cholesterol – the 'goody' and lowers levels of LDL cholesterol – the 'baddie';
- decreases resting heart rate;
- strengthens the heart;
- lowers blood pressure;
- increases oxygenation throughout the body;
- increases cardiovascular and respiratory function;
- increases the elimination of wastes and carbon dioxide from the body;
- increases the absorption of nutrients into the cells;

- improves memory and learning function;
- increases blood supply to the muscles;
- aids good digestion and elimination;
- increases immune system function;
- increases energy levels and alleviates fatigue;
- improves calcium deposition in bones and prevents osteoporosis;
- promotes lean body mass while burning fats;
- increases muscle strength;
- increases the flexibility of joints and muscles;
- increases bone, ligament and tendon strength;
- enhances posture, poise, physique and hence confidence;
- increases longevity.

Regular exercise has a powerful effect on the mind by enhancing the release of pain-relieving and mood-elevating substances in the brain called endorphins. Endorphins are similar in their effect to morphine, although much milder.

Endorphins are commonly referred to as the 'happy drugs'. For a natural high, try incorporating regular exercise into your daily life.

Exercise also:
- decreases tension and anxiety;
- provides a natural release of pent up feelings and alleviates anger;
- increases self-esteem and mental outlook;
- relieves moderate depression;
- increases the body's ability to cope with stress;
- stimulates healthy mental function;
- improves sleep, prevents insomnia;
- induces relaxation;
- decreases worries, restlessness and elevates low spirits;
- increases general feelings of well-being;
- increases inner peace and has a positive effect on the moods;
- makes us feel great!

Regular aerobic and relaxation exercises are valuable allies in overcoming cancer and preventing illness. Exercise makes you feel great, keeps your body flexible and supple, and promotes longevity and healing. It must be remembered that too much exercise can be just as dangerous for our health as too little exercise. Over-exercising places excess stress on the body, increases nutritional requirements and speeds up the ageing process.

Try to choose exercises that you enjoy. Whichever exercise you do decide to incorporate into your 'healing routine', always start slowly, listen to your body signals and gently increase the frequency and intensity of your work-outs. Moderation and balance in all areas of our life is a simple solution to good health.

Chapter 30

GOOD VIBRATIONS

From the beginning of time, before the first existence of man, lies the origin of music. Music was the key to communication and connectedness between beings, before humans developed language. It has always been a valuable tool for human beings in helping us to feel more courageous, connecting us with the pulsing universe and rhythmic cycles of the world and providing a way to express the ideas and images that occur inside our minds. And in this experience of union, lies the valuable key to music's healing force.

Music is able to overcome the anxiety and fears of separateness in a world so often filled with hostility. It is the reassurance of harmony and meaning, the order and melody for our eternal universe.

Sound is a form of energy that is caused by the vibrations of objects and particles. When sound is combined with rhythm and harmonies, the result is music. Music is the universal human language – a route to deep healing and spiritual fulfilment. Sound and music therapy are the controlled use of music in the treatment of physical, emotional and mental disorders. The origins of healing by sound and music can be traced into the realms of myth and religion, and into prehistory and beyond, to the ancient memory of the soul.

Harmful Noise

We are slowly becoming more conscious of the foods and beverages we put into our body, realising they have an effect on our health. Likewise, healthy and unhealthy sounds also have an effect on our health emotions, and we should learn to become consciously aware of which sounds are most beneficial to our well-being.

Just as we can decrease our health by regularly consuming unhealthy foods over extended periods, we can also undermine our health by consuming harmful sounds and noises over extended periods. A regular diet of certain kinds of music and sound can help our bodies and mind achieve a greater level of health.

Some people are highly taste-sensitive and can differentiate between subtle flavours. Likewise sound-sensitive people react very strongly to sounds, especially detrimental ones. Sounds are clearly felt in their body and can cause headaches and upset stomachs.

Our body's cells are of a vibratory nature. They act as sound receptors. Even while the mind is asleep, the body's cells are aware of harsh sounds and react to these uncon-sciously. The body converts these irritating sounds into feelings of stress and tension, although we may be unaware of the source.

One of the first sense organs to develop in a baby while in the womb are the ears. This indicates how important sound is to our psychological and physical health, from the first moment of our creation as a living being. While in the womb, babies are aware of sounds and can differentiate between harmonious sounds and detrimental noise. Detrimental noise can produce the following effects:

- raised blood pressure
- stress on the heart leading to abnormal heart rhythms
- circulatory problems
- ulcers, balance disturbances
- fatigue
- irritability, increased stress and anxiety
- disruption of the central nervous system
- delayed healing time
- delayed verbal development in children
- lowered immunity
- disturbed sleep
- poor digestion
- lack of concentration, hyperactivity
- tension, headaches, migraines, nausea, hearing loss.

Noise pollution surrounds us, even quiet noise we cannot hear. The rumble of the refrigerator places people in trance-like states, the humming of fluorescent lights, tele-vision, electric blenders, vacuum cleaners, dishwashers, garbage disposals, ventilation fans and knife sharpeners in the home all produce a state of general body arousal (stress) and generate increased nervous tension. All of these constant noises at home and at work affect our normal sleep patterns and decrease our energy levels.

The ill effects of bad sounds are cumulative. Strong vibrations from excessive noise wears out the sensory cells of the ears, until they no longer respond. It is important to become aware of harmful noises and realise they are dangerous, and may pose a hazard to health and general well-being.

Healing Sounds

Music has been shown throughout time to have a number of therapeutic capabilities. Healing mantras, chants, incantations and the knowledge of rhythms, sounds and words of power have survived centuries of materialism and remain a beneficial tool for healing, both now and for future generations. The Egyptians refer to incantations as cures for infertility and rheumatic pain. In 324 BC, the music of the lyre restored Alexander the Great to sanity. The Old Testament records that David played his harp and lifted King Saul's depression. The healing properties of music are time-tried and tested. Following are the healing benefits of good music and sounds, depending on the type of music being played.

Music can:
- bring about a state of relaxation or excitability – depending on tempo;
- increase or decrease body metabolism – depending on tempo;
- increase or decrease muscular energy increasing muscular endurance;
- reduce or delay physical fatigue and stress;
- produce marked and variable effects on blood volume, pulse and blood pressure;
- lower high blood pressure;
- lower the threshold of sensory stimuli and either reduce or induce visualisation;
- lessen irritability and anxiety;
- improve self-confidence;
- enhance creativity, concentration, meditation and learning;
- regulate respiration and digestive processes;
- alter mood and promote self-healing.

Music has the ability to affect us in a variety of ways both physically, mentally, emotionally and spiritually. Our primary attraction to music is most likely through its power to create moods and to elicit emotional responses within us. Music affects us all very differently and provokes different emotions, feelings and thoughts.

Music has a strong effect on levels of consciousness and spirituality. To explore this, is beyond the scope of this book. However, following is a table of levels of consciousness and how music may affect each level.

States of Consciousness Induced by Music

Table 30.1

Level of Consciousness	Characteristics	Relationship to Music
Daydreaming state	Thoughts which bear little relation to your outside environment	In our culture, this is the major use of music – almost everyone daydreams with music
Expanded state	Usually induced through hypnosis, meditation or in the case of some people – psychedelic drugs	Music can encourage expanded states of consciousness on many levels including – sensory (alters our perception of time and space), analytic (releases thought processes), symbolic (has a symbolic meaning), integral (can induce a religious or mystical experience)
Hyper-alert state	Prolonged increased alertness while one is awake, resulting from activities involving intense concentration	Music could prevent, interfere with or even aid this state, depending on the type of music

Table 30.1 *continued*

Level of Consciousness	Characteristics	Relationship to Music
Lethargic state	Dulled, sluggish mental activity – can be induced by fatigue, despondent moods, health problems or lack of sleep	Music can relax the individual into sleep or when caused by depression, lift the individual out of this state
Meditative states	Minimal mental activity, induced by massage, meditation, deep breathing, floating in water and music etc.	This is the primary use of music in many cultures where music is practised as a spiritual discipline – music can lead to meditative state
Normal state	Logic, rationality, thinking, goal directness, reflective thinking	Music can cause a return to the normal waking state and help a person to remain in a normal state depending on the type of music, intention of the listener and type of circumstances under which it was heard
Sleep state	Some mental activity during sleep	Music can induce sleep, prevent sleep or terminate sleep
Hysteria state	Intense overpowering emotions, usually negative and destructive	Music can calm hysteria
Ecstasy state	Intense overpowering emotion, usually pleasurable and positive	Music can induce or intensify this state
Deep memory state	Memory trances of past events that are not immediately available to the individual, but which exist	Music can release stored memory under certain conditions as part of the environment

Methods of Using Music for Healing

Music and sound therapy can induce a state of healing or self-healing through a number of different methods. Soft music and soothing sounds, used alone or with relaxation techniques, can effectively alleviate stress, relax muscles and evoke a positive mood. Relaxation music enables many people to attain a meditative state much more easily.

Everyone can use this form of music therapy by simply listening to relaxation tapes or CDs. Music shops and department stores sell a variety of relaxation tapes and classical music. As human beings, we are all individually sound sensitive. Therefore, different pieces of music will appeal to each of us and evoke a variety of different emotions and responses. Certain types of music, like classical music, are very therapeutic and promote specific healing properties.

Another simple way of incorporating sound therapy into your life is by visiting a waterfall or a stream and listening to the sound of running water, or by going for a walk through the forest and listening to birds harmonising. These environmental sounds relieve stress and uplift depression. This form of music therapy is easy to do and costs absolutely nothing. Many relaxation and meditation tapes contain the sounds of birds, whales and dolphins, which bring about a sense of calm and relaxation. To record your own relaxation music, take a tape player to a peaceful, harmonious environment such as the rainforest and record the delicate sounds of nature yourself.

The best instrument we have for healing is our own voice. The voice has been used as a vehicle for spiritual uplifting and healing in every culture throughout history. Mothers use lullabies every day. They hum and sing harmonies to their babies to soothe and relax their precious souls. The human voice is a magical tool for transformation. You can sing anywhere at any time. Singing brings about a sense of happiness, confidence and improved health. Group singing is also fun and helps to tone the voice and uplift emotions. Certain keys or tones affect different areas of the body. Try to create your own songs. Different songs can free our 'inner child', ease emotional pain, spread joy, open the heart and uplift the spirit. Take a moment to sing a melody.

Toning is a form of music therapy which involves using sounds that create tones, to enhance healing and harmony in the body. To do toning, stand comfortably erect and let your body sway like a flower on its stalk in the breeze. Relax your jaw and let your teeth be slightly parted. Let sound come up from your feet, not from your mind. Begin with the first vowel sound 'ahh'. Ahh signifies oneness or unity and is believed to radiate a golden colour. It is an earth sound, which opens the heart.

Say the 'ahh' on the out breath and let it give you a feeling of release, of emptying out. Let your body groan and vibrate as long as it likes. Repeat a number of times and then move onto another sound. Make the toning session last from 10 minutes to one hour, or until the body feels cleansed and nourished, and a sigh is released. The sigh lets you know the body-voice is satisfied.

You can also do toning with other sounds. The second powerful vowel sound is 'ooo' (cool). 'Ooo' relates to the throat, is associated with water and is believed to draw energy in. The third sound is 'eee' which is associated with air. 'Eee' is related to the mind and radiates a bright blue-green or turquoise colour.

Beyond these are 'hmmm' (humming) and 'oh' sounds. 'Hmmm' is associated with the top of the head and produces all colours of the rainbow. You can do one sound in a session, or a number of sounds. It is up to you; do what feels right for your soul!

Dancing to music is a wonderful method of keeping the body flexible and the spirit uplifted. Dancing to rhythms of the Middle East and Africa invites the body to move in ways that naturally strengthen and relax the pelvis and thighs. Dancing lowers the body's armour of self-consciousness and inhibitions.

Learning to play a musical instrument is another method of incorporating music into your life. Tribal drums such as congas and bongos produce a very healing tone and tend to reconnect the player and listener with mother earth and nature. Percussion instruments produce music by impact, symbolizing rhythmic vitality and enhancing worship and meditation. They are easy to use and can be taken anywhere.

Go to the top of a mountain or a waterfall and drum to the natural rhythms and sounds of nature! In fact, you can use any instrument as an aid to meditation and healing. Bells and gongs are simple to use and tend to purify the surrounding atmosphere of negative energies and emotional debris. Finding out which instrument brings about this harmonious state in you can only be revealed by experiencing different sounds.

Chants are short and simple lines with little or no harmony and few words. Chants are repeated many times. Chanting is easy to do and very powerful. It is a regular part of many cultures, religions and teachings. One of the most effective chants is 'Om' (Aum). Om is believed to be the original sound of the universe; it is the beginning, the creative sound.

Chant Om in a single, sustained note. Begin with the lips shaping an 'ah' sound. Slowly change to an 'o' sound and end with closed vibrating lips on a 'mm' humming sound. After a relaxed inhalation, repeat the Om chant again. The Om sound is made over and over as many times as you desire. 'Om' centres the being, creates energy and takes one's soul closer to God. Other words used in chanting include love, care, peace, healing, one, God, joy and even your own name. Positive affirmations can also be repeated over and over, as a chant.

Music is inside everyone. It is totally free, with no rules and no harmful side effects. Music and sound are one of the greatest vehicles for transformation, healing and growth! The magic of music healing is that its methods and healing actions are available to everyone. Music does not discriminate between education, age, predetermined talent, sex or culture.

Healing Sound Exercises

The following exercises can induce a state of healing. You can do them at any time and they are also totally free!

Voice Release Exercise

Some people find it difficult to release their voice and give freedom to their vocalisations. Many individuals feel suppressed in some way, either due to inhibitions, hurts or past experiences.

Lying on your back, fold and curl your body into a tight compact knot of arms and legs. Curl yourself into the smallest ball possible. Catch your breathing and vocalising organs at the centre of the mass. Breathe in and out and make the space you are occupying even smaller. Hold the position for a moment and then breathe in. On the out breath, stretch out, quickly and vigorously. Release some of your voice with a powerful 'ugh', using the deepest sound you can find far within your soul. Enjoy the stretch. Rest for a moment. Repeat the exercise up to 10 times. Each time, reach deeper within and project your voice more strongly and further.

Sounds of Nature Exercise

You can either do this by yourself or with someone you love and adore. Listen for the silence! Find a place under some trees, by a river, a mountainside or in a tranquil garden. If you are unable to physically go to one of these peaceful places, enter your own inner landscape, the magical garden planted and cherished by your own creative imagination.

Listen! Listen to the sky, the earth, the water, the rocks, the plants and the animals. Listen to their unique and gentle sounds; let them sing from their hearts into yours. Hear the crackling of grass, the chirping of birds, the rustling of leaves and the trick-ling of water over moss-covered rocks. You can stay in this place for a few minutes, a few hours or even a day. Try to remember these sounds in your mind. Just listen.

You can return to your normal world whenever your heart answers the call. Learning to remember the sounds of nature during demanding times can place the body in a peaceful and meditative state.

Musical Notes and Therapeutic Effects
Table 30.2

Note	Sense	Body parts	Effective Therapy For	Reflexed to
C	Smell	Bones, muscles of the lower back, sciatic nerve, hips, buttocks, lower bowel, legs, ankles, feet, prostate, haemoglobin, corrects egocentricity	Poor circulation, iron deficiency and blood disorders, paralysis, swollen ankles, cold feet, stiff joints, constipation or diarrhoea, urinary difficulties, melancholia	Colon, neck, knees, nose
D	Taste	Body fluids, kidneys, bladder, lymphatic system, reproductive system, fat deposits, skin, links physical and mental energies	Breathing difficulties, cancer of kidneys, bladder and reproductive system, gallstones, obesity, purification, removal of toxins and poisons that cause cancer, lethargy and apathy	Breasts, reproductive organs, feet, tongue
E	Sight	Nerves and muscular energies, liver and intestines, solar plexus, spleen, kidneys, cellular repair, stimulates intellectual activity	Constipation, indigestion, flatulence, liver and GIT disorders, coughs, headaches, poor skin condition, sluggishness, boredom, headaches	Head, eyes, solar-plexus, umbilical area, thighs

Table 30.2 *continued*

Note	Sense	Body parts	Effective Therapy For	Reflexed to
F	Touch	Heart and lungs, shoulders, arms, hands, pituitary, hormone glands, immune system, natural antiseptic and emotionally soothing to all areas	Trauma and shock, exhaustion, sleeplessness, irritability, back pains, high blood pressure, head colds, cancer of the pituitary, allergies	Kidneys, shoulders, chest, colon, calves, ankles
G	Hearing	Throat and neck, blood and circulation, spine and nervous system, metabolism and temperature control, ears, immune system, tissue renewal, stimulates extraversion	Throat infections or cancer of the throat and mouth, headaches, eye problems, skin disorders, vomiting, muscular spasms, fevers, centres attention and calms	Reproductive system, saliva, hair
A	Intuition	All the senses, muscular responses, control and coordination, pain and pain control, blood disorders	All nervous ailments, obsession, balance disorders, excessive bleeding, breathing difficulties, swellings, sedative effects.	Sacrum (base of the spine)
B	All	Blood and fluid balance of potassium and sodium, calcium and phosphorus, iron, iodine and other minerals, aid to meditation	Neuralgia and cramps, inflammatory pain, glandular disturbance, immune deficiency, nervous disorders, restores self-respect	Whole body

Chapter 31

MAGNETIC THERAPIES

Magnets and magnetic fields, although unseen and unheard, are an important part of our everyday life. We use magnetic products in many different ways. Just some of these include: telephones, door alarms, audio and video tapes, computer disks, computers, magnetic strips on credit cards, on Medicare and health cards, bus and train tickets, magnetic cupboard door catches, and many more such items.

More importantly, biologically, every cell in our body is an electromagnetic phenomenon. This is very important to understand, and one day, if not now, your good health may depend upon it.

There are two basic classes of magnets or magnetic fields, and several sub types. Permanent or 'static' magnets have been used since 850 BC, that is, for more than 2850 years. The earth has its own magnetic system. The source is in the molten core that generates earth energies and fields on and above the surface between the Magnetic North and South poles. The density is around 0.5 Gauss and oscillating around 9.6Hz to 10.5Hz. There are also the Schumann resonance field harmonics between the earth and the magnetosphere; the most important biologically oscillate between 7.5Hz and 8 Hz, depending largely upon sun spot flare activity. There are other less important Schumann frequencies.

At intervals over time, various physicians have found that the use of magnetic materials has helped to reduce pain and to improve healing processes. Naturally occurring magnetic ore is called 'magnetite' or 'lodestone' (leading stone'), as it aligns with the North-South magnetic poles of the earth and was used by early mariners to help in navigation. Nowadays we refer to this type of device as a compass.

Permanent magnets can be made out of several types of materials such as ferrous (iron), ceramic with iron particles, combinations of nickel-iron-boron-neodymium, and other 'rare earth' minerals, etc. Generally the newer combination materials have stronger holding powers and are not easily de-magnetised.

These permanent or static magnets are used to assist in the alleviation of many aches and pains, and in some instances can help the body to heal from minor discomforts and may assist peripheral circulation.

Some basic physics is necessary to understand what follows:
When a magnet is moved close to a conductor, such as a wire, or any conductor, such as blood or body fluids or nerves, an electric current is induced in that conductor. Generators and alternators operate on this principle. When an electric current flows along a wire or any conductor, a magnetic field is created around the conductor. Electric motors and many other appliances and devices operate on this principle.

Low power magnets, associated with movement such as the blood circulating or muscles moving under where the magnet is placed, have been shown to induce micro electric currents that can balance body energies and may also stimulate the iron content of the haemoglobin in the blood to transport oxygen more efficiently.

The biggest problem we face concerning permanent-type magnets is the false and misleading claims made by a few in the marketplace, and this makes it confusing for the lay person. It is also a worry because many of these people do not know how magnets work, or what to advise their clients. People should consult a qualified specialist in magnetic therapy so that they can get the best products, advice and help.

Electromagnetic energy is a most important part of biological systems. We are at the cell level, electro-chemical-magnetic beings. The DNA in every cell has its own electromagnetic spin, which maintains its controlling functions and is in turn affected by internal and external electromagnetic fields, both good and potentially damaging.

The two types of magnetic energies referred to above exert influences over the environment and the biological processes of all living things. In humans, the pineal gland at the base of the brain is affected by the magnetic emanations and is responsible for producing melatonin, a master controller of hormones, enzymes, immune function, oxidation and cyclic patterns of sleep-wakefulness. It also governs stress levels and reactions, and the anti-oxidant control of free radicals that can break down cells, and this may lead to allowing for the development of cancer.

Our body's cells are also continuously influenced by strong man-made electrostatic and high frequency electromagnetic fields (EMF), which are well outside what the body is meant to tolerate.

These include: continuous overhead power line currents, house wiring, appliances, CRT television and computer monitors, radio, radar, bedside electric powered alarm clocks, and even electric bed blankets.

The unlimited use of these and other man-made EMF radiation products such as microwave ovens and microwave mobile cell phones, close proximity to fluorescent lighting, and even ultrasonic physiotherapy devices poses a grave risk to health in humans and the environment (Coghill,1991, Vol 22 No 2, p 135).

Research indicates that this potentially damaging high frequency EMF that we take for granted can adversely affect the delicate human biological processes such as nerve function, bone growth, tissue regeneration, body communication systems, white cell activity, and immune system status. Many of these environmental hazards, including ionising x-rays, carcinogenic chemicals in agriculture, in the food chain, in the manufacture of many food items, can interfere with and alter the DNA in the cells. If the DNA is not repaired, the result can eventually be cell mutation and uncontrolled growth (Coghill, 1991, Vol 22 No 2). Many types of high frequency EMF have been implicated in immune system deterioration, and together with other factors and stress, can lead to some forms of cancer over time.

The Western technological society has created a Global EMF pollution of the environment, virtually an electronic jungle. 'Our unwise use of electromagnetic energies has produced environmental changes of unparalleled proportions,' as, stated by Robert Becker, an orthopaedic surgeon, researcher, author and adamant believer in the perils created by man-made EMF pollution.

The figures indicating the link between the dangerous EMF and the plethora of new diseases and proliferation of cancers are alarming. For all the billions of dollars spent on cancer research, the situation is getting worse, not better.

If we wish to live healthy, disease-free lives it is time to address these findings by limiting our own personal exposure, becoming aware of these problems and demanding changes. An informed public taking action can be a powerful influence in global change. We owe this to ourselves and to our precious children (Barsamian, S.T. & S.P., Vol 18).

Electromagnetic Therapy as Medicine

At the other end of the EMF scale is the use of the extremely low frequency, low power, and specific type waveform electromagnetic energy therapy, as in the MERIT® device (Grace, 1996, p 60-75) that has been scientifically proven to be of assistance in pain relief and improved healing of damaged tissue. It is also of great benefit in all neurological conditions, to slow down and arrest the progression, and for the promotion of healing in cancer.

The true essence of energy is vibration. What is now officially known as 'bioenergetic medicine' used to be called 'vibrational medicine' until a few years ago. It is now accepted that at certain very specific selected frequencies, or vibrations, rogue cells including cancer cells can be destroyed while usually leaving normal cells unchanged. This can be accomplished by chemical reaction, ionising radiation, (both of which have certain dangers to adjoining tissue), by electrical currents at precise frequencies and characteristics (under the supervision of a specialist), or by a patented form of Magnetic Energy Resonance Induction Therapy (Grace,1993, p 4–23).

For those who have chosen to submit to chemotherapy and/or radiation treatments, the MERIT® system can enhance the effects, and at the same time reduce the adverse side effects. Healing after operations is also greatly improved. Inhibition from any further cancer cell growth is a major benefit for many.

For the best results, the system should be used before, during, and after any procedures or aggressive treatments, along with a balanced and sensible nutrition program for the individual. Although not usually promoted by orthodox medicine, there is immense healing potential with the appropriate low frequency, low strength electromagnetic energy at the correct level. It has been shown to be completely safe for over 20 years (ibid).

Many hundreds of seriously ill persons facing operations, chemotherapy and/or radiation treatment, who have made the decision themselves to either delay or cancel such procedures, and have used the Magnafield® MERIT® therapy device, along with a carefully selected nutrition program, have recovered and five, 10 or 20 years later are not only clear of any cancer, but are enjoying life to the full.

This however, must be the decision of the individual, after considering all the options, getting 'good quality' advice, dealing positively with the stress from 'well-meaning' relatives, and being comfortable with their informed decision. They should also speak with persons who have proven this form of treatment as many orthodox medical hospitals and physicians do not recognise this drug-free threat to the 'establishment protocols'.

Magnetic Energy Resonance Induction Therapy

- MERIT® magnetic energy influences many enzymatic intracellular and membrane systems, (eg alkaline phosphatase); and influences antigen-antibody relations;
- MERIT® magnetic energy also modifies the permeability of the cellular membrane and therefore the Ionic equilibrium. The sodium/potassium pump balance is stimulated. $SpO2$ is increased.

Magnetic Resonance Imaging (MRI) is now widely used in many hospitals around the world, although it does use much higher levels of magnetic field strength than therapy devices, and is coupled with radio frequencies.

The recent developments in magnetic fields in medicine include:

- MRI   Magnetic Resonance Imaging   (once called nuclear magnetic resonance)
- MEG   Magnetic encephalogram (instead of EEG, electro encephalogram)
- MCG   Magnetic cardiogram (instead of ECG or EKG, electro cardio-gram)
- MBFR   Magnetic blood flow rate meters
- MCI   Magnetically controlled implant
- MERIT®   Magnetic energy resonance induction therapy

The new revolution in medicine is in the area of bio-magnetism and magnetic induction therapy. Both these forms of magnetic medicine are useful in the treatment and prevention of cancer (Becker, 1990, p151–53). The difference between electrotherapy and magnetic induction therapy is that electrotherapy uses contact with or through the skin, whereas magnetic induction therapy does not have to touch the person, making it completely non-invasive (Grace,1992, p 119–34).

Magnetic Therapy Methods
Permanent or Static Magnets

Millions of people around the world use small permanent magnets placed on the skin near affected areas. Some magnets are inserted into thin mattresses or pillows, back belts, knee, shoulder, wrist, or elbow supports, or in small stick-on plasters. Others are used in jewellery or pendants. Many of these do work for some of the people, some of the time, for a few hours until the body accommodates or adapts to the constant energy at or very close to the magnet. These people usually experience some temporary relief of pain, stiff joints, and often an improvement of peripheral blood circulation. The benefits are mainly available when some movement is associated with the magnet. Many swear by them. The placebo effect is very real.

As long as the energy force of the magnetic product is not too high, no harm is caused. It is important to note that 'stronger' is not necessarily better in biological systems. Taking such products off or away from the body for a period of two to four hours and then placing them on again obtains the best results. This avoids the 'accommodation' factor and additional benefits are usually then experienced. It is a symptom alleviator (Rinker, 1997, p 3–113).

Continuous or Pulsed Magnetic Therapy

Continuous electric or magnetic energy is not advisable. Any continuous energy is not beneficial as in nature every energy is vibrating (vibrant) or pulsing, and usually in an oscillating fashion with constantly varying waveforms. A continuous current, especially if in a synthetic sinusoidal (sine) waveform as on the power line supplied to our homes and workplaces, has been shown in many studies to become detrimental to human cell life (Persinger,1988, p 592). It affects the nerves first, and eventually can cause nerve related damage and neurological syndromes.

Pulsed magnetic therapy is far better than continuous, but there are several factors that must be considered in order for the real benefits to be available. Just to pulse at a frequency may or may not be the right method.

Oscillating Magnetic Therapy

This involves an energy field that is oscillating back and forth in positive and negative modes, biased towards more negative. The waveform must be close to that of the human body which is not a sine, sawtooth, or square waveform, as these are not common to the body, but were developed for communications, radio, TV and computers, and are usually filtered to remove the 'hash' or harmonics that interrupt a clear signal. Medical researchers found that the body needs and uses these harmonics (Grace, 1992, p 119–34).

There also must be a correct ON-OFF ratio for each pulse, and there must be a period of time for the treatment followed by at least a similar period of time of rest or 'pause' before the subsequent treatment. Ideally, the treatment using the patented Magnafield system involves placing an applicator pad on the floor under the bed and leaving it operating 24 hours a day, seven days a week. Many have done this without removing or turning it off for more than 15 years. The greatest benefits are received during the sleeping hours. There are no contraindications.

There is a small portable battery powered version of the Magnafield system, known as the Magnatens® that has many of the Magnafield features built in, but is designed for faster pain relief with some healing. The Magnatens® does not provide the same level of cell repair or inhibition of cancer cell mitosis. It is intended more as a supplement or adjunct to the Magnafield for those who can now get around but require maintenance of energy throughout the day. It is also good for those aches and pains that annoy many people who do not want to rely on pharmaceutical drugs with their side effects (Magnacare Pty Ltd, 2002).

Some of the functions and benefits from this therapy include:

- Healthy cells have different EMF characteristics and DNA/RNA spirals from cancer cells. Under the influence of 0.5Hz Magnafield treatments cancerous cells are inhibited from division or 'mitosis', they just unravel and die off, and are dealt with and removed by the body as all other dead cells.
- At 0.5Hz and particularly at 2Hz the Thymus is stimulated to produce more 'T' killer and helper cells, to assist and build up the immune system defences. This is a balancing system, does not over-stimulate.
- Analgesic effects (pain relief) are best at 0.5Hz to 4Hz.
- Tissue healing is initiated first at 0.5Hz, and then at 2Hz or 4Hz, followed by using 8Hz until healed.
- DNA synthesis is enhanced at 5Hz. Also cellular signalling, repair and health.
- Inflammation is reduced at 0.5Hz, swelling and oedema reduced at 3Hz.
- Peripheral circulation is helped initially at 15Hz, but maintained best at 12Hz.
- Joint mobility is improved at 0.5Hz initially, and then at 4Hz, 8Hz, & 12Hz. ('Auto Cyclic' function).
- Liver function assisted at 10Hz. Also a neutralising or energy balancing frequency.
- At all frequencies there is a promotion of nutrient and oxygen transport and uptake into the cells.
- Calcium, potassium and sodium balance may be restored, essential for normal cell function and health.
- Acid/alkaline pH balance assisted, and helps to reduce over acid conditions, and much more (ibid).

Comments

In my practice, many of my clients with cancer and those who have beaten cancer use the Magnafield as part of their cancer-fighting program with great success. Firstly, it seems to have halted the spread of cancer cells. Secondly, it has enhanced the immune system to help fight any remaining cancerous cells. Also, the patient's energy levels have improved dramatically and the oxygen and nutrient acceptance has increased, allowing for a faster healing process. I also continue to use the Magnafield every day and I remain healthy and cancer-free (four years and counting).

With this corrective form of treatment, using the proven frequencies, waveforms, and low intensity magnetic energy resonant induction therapy, inhibition of cancer cells has been noted and proved for over 20 years, but still not accepted in most orthodox establishments (Persinger, 1988, p 592).

Some Like it Hot – Heat Therapy

Heat therapy has long been used throughout history by both doctors and holistic healers. It has shown some promising results in treating brain, breast, head, neck and skin cancer.

Heat therapy is still highly controversial and should not be undertaken without the guidance or direction of a qualified medical practitioner or therapist.

It involves the application of heat to cancerous tissues and cells, by a variety of different methods. The most common method of heat therapy, brought about by the body's natural defence mechanisms, is a fever. This heats up the body's internal environment, making it difficult for cancerous cells to survive. Fever is a spontaneous form of healing, enhancing the body's natural defence proteins.

Most of us try to suppress fevers. By doing this we are suppressing our body's natural healing response. This may cause the bacteria or virus to be suppressed, allowing it to manifest itself later in a more serious condition. The body in all its magnificence has some amazing healing mechanisms designed to restore harmony and balance.

Cancer cells become damaged at 42 degrees Celsius to 43 degrees Celsius. This intense heat may lead to the self-destruction of tumours and may also slow down the growth of malignant cells and their oxygen respiration. Heat goes selectively to cancerous tissue. The major problem with heat therapy is how to gain access to cancerous cells in the body without severely harming other parts of the body. Skin cancers are the easiest to treat, as they are easily accessible on the outside of the body. It becomes difficult to obtain access to internal organs.

Today, practitioners use a modified food-warming oven consisting of a chamber that produces radiant heat up to 40 degrees Celsius. Using heat therapy in conjunction with chemotherapy and radiation therapy may enhance the effectiveness of these orthodox cancer treatments.

Other new heat therapy techniques includes laser light via needles, radio waves, believed to induce tumour regression, scan focused ultrasound systems and interstitial ferromagnetic seed implants.

Chapter 32

RAYS OF LIGHT –
COLOUR THERAPY

How blessed we are to live in such a magical world, overflowing with vibrant and dazzling colours, sounds, smells and beauty. All around us flowers and trees emit vibrations, each uniquely different in colour, aroma and healing properties. Nature is a spectacle of amazing colours and smells, and yet we often get so caught up in our fast-paced existence that we forget to tap into this divine and mystical realm of healing colours sitting right before our eyes!

Colour can be described as light – visible radiant life-enhancing energy of certain wavelengths. Photoreceptors in the retina, called cones, translate this energy into colours. The retina contains three kinds of cones, one for blue, one for green and one for red. We perceive other colours and tones by combining these colours.

Colour has an amazing ability to alter our moods, health, thought patterns and spiritual well-being in a subtle, yet transformative way. It is believed that when the energy of colour enters our body, it stimulates two of our major glands, the pituitary and pineal glands. This in turn affects the production of various hormones, which in turn affects a variety of physiological and metabolic processes. It is no wonder certain colours have such an effect on our moods, thoughts and behaviour.

Colour is such a powerful healer and we are all intuitively attuned to this, even if we don't consciously think we are, as our whole world is coloured. Each colour, in its original essence, has the ability to conjure up a different emotion, feeling, thought and healing vibration. We all have the ability to react to colours in different ways and all possess different preferences for colours. This preference may be due to either cultural, psychological or intuitive selection as to which colour is best suited to our needs.

For instance, we all know how sedating and calming blues are when we look at the expansive sky or endless ocean. Or how uplifting are the sun's golden rays, penetrating our aura on a beautiful clear day. Allow your own intuition to guide you, experiment with different colours and become aware of how each one makes you feel. God's spectrum of healing colours is available to us every day, allowing us to tap into the immense healing power.

The Spectrum of Healing Colours

Clearly the colours we choose for our clothes, home, work environment, healing spaces and surroundings have a profound impact on our physical, emotional and mental well-being. Colours enable us to ease stress, fill us with energy, alleviate pain, elevate moods, enhance healing and increase positivity. *See back for colour phrases.*

Following is a list of just a few colours from the magnificent spectrum that surrounds us. Each of these colours embodies endless shades and tones, some of which you may find more suited to your healing, therapeutic and emotional needs. Colours can be incorporated into your cancer treatment program easily and effortlessly, and will aid in uplifting the spirit and mind, decrease side effects and aid in a rapid recovery. A great combination of colours for cancer therapy is red, green and violet.

Tap into the beauty of colour, become your own nature doctor and let your intuition guide you towards magical colours most ideally suited to your needs.

Yellow – The Colour of Happiness, Intellect and Memory

Yellow is a vibrant, alive and energising colour. It assists with clear thinking, open-mindedness and confidence. It is one of the most memorable colours known. If you wish to remember something, jot it down in yellow. It helps to stimulate the intellect with logical thinking and reasoning powers. Yellow embodies the light of happiness and a heart overflowing with joy. Yellow in its beauty and aliveness has an invigorating effect on the body.

Yellow gently increases pulse rate, blood pressure and respiration. It is great for nervous exhaustion, depression, feelings of hopelessness, despair and despondency. Physically, it helps to generate energy in the muscles, purifies the bloodstream, activates the lymphatic system, liver and intestines. It also increases bile flow and is believed to assist with digestive problems, gallstones, muscle cramps, under-active thyroid and hypoglycaemia.

Avoid Yellow

Yellow should be avoided in cases of acute inflammation, diarrhoea, fever, over-excitement, heart palpitations and delirious states. This vibrant colour is too stimulating for these physical ailments.

Natural Sources of Yellow

Vibrant sun, sunflowers, daffodils, lemons, bananas, grapefruit, squash, pineapples, citrine crystal, birds.

Blue – The Colour of Calmness, Serenity and Inspiration

Serenity, coolness, calm, truth and peace embody the essence of the colour blue. Blue helps to stimulate the intuition, aids with communication and enhances creativity. Blue gently calms the body, brings peace of mind, relaxation and is calmly sedating. It is a contracting colour and is therefore great in easing overexcited states. Blue is a 'major healing colour'. It is also often used in classrooms, to calm down aggressive and hyperactive children.

Physically, blue is able to decrease blood pressure, lower heart rate, decrease respiration and enable people living in hot and humid climates to feel cooler. Blue is great for throat problems, itching, headaches, back problems, inflammatory disorders, rheumatism, measles, excess bleeding, spasms and stings. It is believed to speed up the healing of burns, help fight infections and improve metabolism.

Blue is also one of the best colours for insomnia and shock.

Avoid Blue
Do not use too much blue if you are suffering from cold conditions, gout, paralysis, muscle contractions, low blood pressure, fatigue or depression.

Natural Sources of Blue
Clear blue sky, waterfalls, lakes, flowers, blueberries, ocean, water in all forms, blue Ulysses butterflies and blue birds.

Green – The Colour of Love, Harmony and Renewal
Green is known as the 'balancer' as it is believed to help neutralise disharmony of malignant cancerous cells, making it one of the most healing colours for cancer. It relieves tension and is calming, soothing and relaxing to the body and mind. It is able to balance the heart both physically and emotionally. Soothing greens stimulate feelings of empathy, growth, balance, harmony and love. A great overall body tonic – green stimulates without over-stimulation.

Green gently stimulates the pituitary, aids depression, anxiety, nervous exhaustion and contains disinfectant qualities. Using green is very beneficial in the treatment of shock, illness, fatigue, cancer and negative emotions.

Avoid Green
Do not use green if you are suffering from anaemia or chronic exhaustion.

Natural Sources of Green
Trees, leaves, rolling green fields, grass, mountains, honeydew melon, green vegetables, green plants, seaweed, chlorophyll, green apples, green birds and butterflies.

Red – The Colour of Vitality, Passion and Strength
Red is very stimulating and therefore must be used carefully. It stimulates and vitalises the entire body increasing power, confidence, courage and initiative. Red is the colour of passion and energy, enhancing sexual desire and is therefore great for frigidity and impotence. Red is often associated with sexiness and passion. This passionate colour may conjure up images of attractive red-lipped beauties, sexually active men wearing red socks and beautiful, sexy women in red lingerie – no wonder it is linked to sexuality.

Physically, red activates blood circulation, maintains red blood cells, promotes heat and increases body temperature. It is therefore great for anaemia, chronic chills and colds, bladder infections, low blood pressure, inertia, depression and tiredness. Red releases adrenaline and stimulates sensory and cerebro-spinal nerves. Green or blue should follow after red.

Red also increases heart rate, respiration and brain wave activity. It truly is a great colour for improving energy levels. If you feel tired or run down, try putting on a red top and watch the difference it makes.

Avoid Red

Avoid red if suffering from inflammatory conditions, severe emotional disturbances, poor concentration or high blood pressure. In fact, avoid red in any excess heat-related condition.

Natural Sources of Red

Watermelon, tomatoes, red meat, cherries, red roses, fire, red hair, advertising colours, red-lipped women, aggressive drivers in red cars, sexy red underwear and red apples.

Orange – The Colour of Spirituality, Energy and Abundance

Orange radiates feelings of warmth, intimacy, abundance and tolerance. Orange removes repressions and inhibitions, and opens one's heart to understanding and acceptance. Wearing the colour orange can increase a person's courage and raise both mental and physical energy. Orange broadens our outlook on life and opens one's horizon to new possibilities.

Physically, orange assists with assimilation and circulation. It is one of the best colours for stimulating the appetite. Putting orange place mats or an orange tablecloth on the dinner table is a great way to encourage fussy eaters to indulge. Cancer treatment often diminishes a person's appetite, yet it is extremely important to keep up nutritional levels during this period. Wearing orange or placing orange colours around food may encourage a person to dig in and enjoy. A great colour to uplift a person who is feeling ill.

Orange is also good for gallstones, disturbances of the pancreas, spleen and kidneys and strengthens the lungs. It is helpful with bronchitis, asthma and emphysema. It aids healthy calcium metabolism and is excellent for general weakness and fatigue.

Avoid Orange

Avoid if trying to lose weight. Also steer clear if suffering from high blood pressure and hyperactive conditions.

Natural Sources of Orange

Oranges, cantaloupe, carrots, papaya, mangoes, apricots, peaches, pumpkin, sweet potato, fire, spectacular orange sunsets and sunrises, Hare Krishna clothing colour, Thai and Asian monks' robes are adorned with orange.

Scarlet – The Colour of Arousal and Sexual Stimulation

Like red, scarlet is a powerful sexual stimulant that helps with impotence and frigidity. It increases blood pressure and is great for fluid retention. Scarlet works on stimulating the body's hormones and blood.

Avoid Scarlet

Try to avoid scarlet if pregnant, as it may encourage uterine contractions.

Natural Sources of Scarlet

Plums, grapes, cherries, flowers and roses.

Magenta – The Colour of Universal Love, Divine Understanding and Joy

Believed to be seen in the aura of pregnant women, magenta is a vitalising colour that is particularly good for low energy. It has a stabilising effect on the heart and adrenal glands. Magenta is a tonic and revitaliser to the body's ethereal field.

Avoid Magenta

Avoid magenta when in feverish and excited or hyperactive states.

Natural Sources of Magenta

Flowers, birds, clouds and jacaranda trees.

Violet – The Colour of True Devotion and Spirituality

Violet is believed to halt the growth of tumours. It is very useful in meditation and enhances the development of spiritual intuitive processes. It also has a soothing and tranquilising effect on the body's nervous system. Violet is great for people who are nervous or highly-strung by nature. Surrounding yourself in violet creates a peaceful environment.

Violet maintains the delicate balance between sodium and potassium in the body, thereby preventing fluid retention. Violet is good for rheumatism, cancer, kidney and bladder disorders, scalp problems and migraines. Violet has a subtle effect on the appetite, controlling excess hunger. It is therefore very good for weight loss programs.

This inspirational colour radiates inner wisdom, pure knowing and opens one's heart to spirituality.

Avoid Violet

Avoid violet when suffering melancholic states, depression, chronic fatigue, low vitality, cold and negative conditions.

Natural Sources of Violet

The most enlightened and respected priests and monk's robes are adorned with violet, lavender flowers, grapes, butterflies and flowers.

Gold – The Colour of Divine Wisdom, Forgiveness and Love

Gold is a great colour to use in any healing that requires forgiveness, love and acceptance. The golden rays assist with the deepest healing of the soul itself. This colour, used in conjunction with the breath and words of love and acceptance, can change and heal past mistakes, old patterns, resentments, blocks and fears. Gold connects us to our god within.

Avoid Gold

There is no time when it is necessary to avoid the beautiful colour, gold.

Natural Sources of Gold

Glowing golden light, firelight, golden haired children, gold jewellery, golden Buddhas, gold statues and deities.

White – The Colour of Purity, Innocence and Trust

White is the combination of all other colours. It is a great colour to use if you are confused about which colour is needed. White cleanses and purifies the soul and body. White is the divine, white light can be called upon for any imbalance. This clear colour helps to remove negativity, fear, toxins and mental blocks. It is therefore a purifier on all levels – emotional, spiritual and physical.

Avoid White

There is no time when it is necessary to avoid white.

Natural Sources of White

White clouds, swans, whitewash from waves, stars, the moon, nuns' uniforms (black and white), robes of high priests, white roses (signify friendship), flowers, snow, cauli-flower, parsnips, radish (inside), nuts, milk and seeds.

Pink – The Colour of Unconditional Love

Pink is one of my favourite colours. Surrounding yourself in pink evokes feelings of romance, unconditional love and peace. Pink is a great colour to use in creative imagery and meditation. My favourite imagery techniques involve using pink bubbles.

Pink has a soothing effect on the body and muscles. Pink is often painted on the walls in prisons, juvenile and drug centres to calm and tranquilise aggressive and violent people. It is a great colour for anxiety and withdrawal symptoms. Pink is the colour to open the heart.

Avoid Pink

There is no time when it is necessary to avoid the beautiful colour of pink.

Natural Sources of Pink

Pink flowers, birds, guava fruit, clouds, rose quartz, sunsets and sunrises.

Black – The Colour of Power, Success and Drive

Black increases strength, drive and self-confidence. Think of high powered business people in smart black suits. They seem to give off a powerful and successful aura – exactly what black is representative of. If you want to feel more confident, put on a glamorous little black number and watch the doorways of success open right before your eyes. Black is also a very effective appetite suppressant. Placing black tablecloths on the dinner table will decrease one's desire to eat heartily.

Avoid Black

Avoid black if suffering from underweight problems.

Natural Sources of Black

Night skies, black cats, slinky black dresses, crows and blackberries.

Ways to Use Colour for Healing

There are many different methods of using colour to provoke individual feelings, emotions and healing reactions.

Colour Breathing

Colour breathing can be done anywhere and is particularly useful to do while in hospital. First, lie or sit in a comfortable position. Become totally relaxed, block out distractions and noises. Think of a time where you felt totally happy, content and peaceful. Visualise the colour needed or keep a coloured piece of cotton, material, silk scarf or piece of clothing near you, so you can look at it.

If you are having trouble seeing the colour, place the coloured item over your eyes. Breathe the colour in through your nostrils or the solar plexus (lower chest area). Direct it to the area of the body, which needs the healing. Imagine the colour flowing down to this area and feel its healing essence. Say to yourself that this area is getting better and better every moment, and improving all of the time. Know this and believe this!

Do this exercise for 10 to 15 minutes at any time of the day. It is a great therapy to do in the morning before starting the day, or in the evening before retiring for bed. Imagine the appropriate colour permeating your entire being and always re-affirm greater health and well-being.

Colours on the Body

Another simple method is to place a coloured item (silk scarf, material, coloured cloth or a piece of coloured clothing) over the area of the body that requires the healing. Imagine the colour soaking into your skin and saturating this area with its beautiful healing qualities. Re-affirm its healing potential and feel yourself getting stronger and healthier every moment.

Coloured Clothing

Wearing the right colour in your clothing is very beneficial. Look at your clothes, feel them and let the colours emanate into your aura. Even dying your hair different colours has an effect on your physical and mental health. While going through chemotherapy I wore a pink wig to open my heart to love and calm my mind. It always made me feel peaceful and content.

There are so many wonderful natural vegetable dyes available today. Try colouring your hair to enhance the feeling or emotion you wish to provoke. They say 'blondes have more fun'. In colour therapy this rings true, as yellow is the colour of joy and happiness. They say 'redheads are sexy'. After all, red is the colour of passion and sexual desire!

Coloured Foods

Eating different coloured foods also enhance healing. Red, orange and yellow foods have an alkaline and stimulating effect, similar to the colours. Green foods tend to be neutral and balancing. Blue, indigo and violet foods have an acidic and calming effect.

Coloured Stones

Coloured stones and crystals have a powerful healing effect when held over the appropriate area of the body. Each crystal releases a different vibration through its essence and colour. Crystals radiate their healing vibrations to the area required and assist in rebalancing emotions.

Drinking Colours

Using coloured cellophane paper is useful. Wrap the right colour around a glass of water and leave in the sun for two hours. The water absorbs the vibrations and power from the sun and the colour. Drink the water and you will be absorbing the coloured vibration required.

Green drinks made with wheatgrass, chlorella or spirulina help encourage renewal and balance, as green is the colour of empathy, healing and harmony. Other fresh fruit and vegetable juices, according to their colour, exert many healing effects from their subtle, healing vibrations.

***

Other methods of colour healing include surrounding yourself with coloured flowers and plants, artwork, paintings, using coloured paints, crayons and pencils, coloured make-up, hair ribbons and decorations. Be aware of the colour you decide to paint your home, as this will have either a stimulating or calming effect on yourself and your family.

Table of Healing Colours, Body Areas, Emotions and Crystals

Table 32.1

Colour	Organ, Body Part	Negative Emotion	Positive Outcome	Healing Crystal
White, blue or green	Lungs	Death, grief, sadness, fearful of being judged or rejected	Life, courage, listening to the inner voice, release of sadness	Clear quartz crystals, turquoise, aquamarine, moonstone, carnelian turquoise
Blue or orange	Kidneys	Disappointment, fear, lack of money, unsure in emotional matters	Peace, tranquillity, no problem with sharing emotions	Lapis Lazuli, turquoise, sapphire, carnelian, tourmaline
Golden Yellow or Green	Liver	Anger, resentment	Harmony, love, strength	Jade, emerald, aquamarine, amber, tiger's eye, citrine

Table 32.1 continued

Colour	Organ, Body Part	Negative Emotion	Positive Outcome	Healing Crystal
Pink or green	Heart	Hatred, violence, impatience, looking for rewards, insincere love	Unconditional love, compassion, strength, JOY, peace, understanding	Rose quartz, red/pink tourmaline, bloodstone, jade, emerald
Yellow	Spleen, pancreas, stomach	Worry, anxiety	Joy, lightness	Citrine, amber, tiger eye, carnelian
Orange or bright red	Intestines	Pain, separation	Flowing easily, abundance	Citrine, amber, zircon
Red or orange	Sexual organs	Guilt, struggle	Balanced, grounded	Ruby, garnet, bloodstone moonstone
Blue or orange	Bladder	Anxiety, fear of letting go, something is upsetting you	Powerful, emotional release, positive expression	Jasper, bloodstone, vanadinite
White or bright red	Bones	Feeling unstructured, unbalanced	Grounded, balanced, strong enough on own	Selenite, fluorite, coral
Green or blue	Breasts	Over-nurturing, unable to let go	Balanced nurturing, peace, tranquillity	Hematite, lapis lazuli
Gold, all colours	Cancer	Deep hurt, long-time resentment, deep grief or secret, carrying hate	Peace, tranquillity, forgiveness, happiness, contentment	Sodalite, amethyst, smoky quartz, cobaltite

Chapter 33

SCOPE OF HEALING

The scope of healing is as wide and varied as the peoples of our amazing planet. Below are some more wonderful healing methods that have been tried and tested, but are perhaps yet to be accepted by the orthodox medical world.

Earth Energy – Crystal Healing

People from all over the world have been mesmerised by the beauty of stones and crystals. The power of crystals is said to lie in their ability to focus and transmit energy – particularly thoughtforms. It is believed that crystals can be charged with energy and directed into a chosen object or person. Crystals are often used for healing, on both the physical and the psychological level.

How to Use Crystals

These mystical rocks obtained from the earth's powerful energies of sun, earth, wind and fire, are extremely simple and easy to use. Following are some examples of crystal healing therapy.

- If you wish to heal a particular body area, lie down in a comfortable position, close your eyes and breathe deeply. Place the appropriate crystal over the body area you are treating. When you are relaxed, imagine the energy of the crystal flowing into you. Repeat the words or affirmations in your mind for the positive outcome that you would like to attain.
- Wear the crystals either on a necklace or bracelet, or even place them in your pocket. The energy of the crystals will radiate through your physical and emotional being bringing about your most desired outcome. Let only people with good energy touch your crystal, as crystals tend to retain energy when touched.
- Place your crystals in your house, in your office, beside your hospital bed or treatment area, on your desk or even in your car.
- Try to leave crystals out in the full moon overnight in a tree, at least once a month. The energy of the full moon is able to cleanse the crystal of impurities.

Table of Emotional States and Beneficial Crystals

Table 33.1

Negative State	Positive State	Beneficial Crystals
Authority issues, not facing reality	Success, achievement, grounded and focussed	Ruby, black tourmaline, bloodstone, onyx
Relationship issues	Balance, poise, harmony, resolution	Aventurine, aquamarine, pink topaz, sapphire, red jasper, pink tourmaline, rose quartz
Critical self-analysis, bad dietary habits	Self-acceptance, purification, good health	Garnet, topaz, turquoise, agate
Ego-glorification, power-driven	Expression, pleasure, grounded power, creativity	Gold, ruby, kunzite agate, rose quartz, emerald
Mother issues, emotionally unfulfilled	Nurturing, inner strength, positive expression of emotions	Silver, amazonite, moonstone, rutilated quartz
Issues with security, lacking direction	Prosperity, groundedness, knowing own self-worth	Fluorite, citrine, emerald, brown jasper, black opal
Lacking confidence, aggressive release of emotions	Confidence, improved self image, courage, positive reactions, assertiveness	Amber, bloodstone, haematite, carnelian, onyx, ruby
Idealism, addictions, dependency	Spirituality, meditation, release, tranquillity	Kunzite, pearl, lapis lazuli, blue tourmaline, sapphire, amethyst, topaz, rutilated quartz
Fear of intimacy, afraid to confront	Renewal, regeneration, transformation	Alexandrite, obsidian, quartz, tourmaline, moonstone
Emotional blocks	Release of negativity, enhanced health and well-being	Quartz, smoky quartz, agate, jet
Poor health	Complete mind and body healing and purification	Amazonite, moss agate, rhodocrosite, turquoise

Hydrotherapy

Hydrotherapy is an ancient form of healing dating back to 1500 BC. Sebastien Kneipp, a German physician, instituted health spas throughout Germany and Europe in the 19th century, popularising water therapy even further. No one can ignore the soothing and relaxing qualities of a hot bath or the invigorating, stimulating effects of a cold dip in a lake or waterfall.

The thermal heating and cooling effects of water are responsible for its therapeutic effects in healing. It is great at enhancing circulation and hence removing toxic wastes through the mobilisation of white blood cells.

Hydrotherapy is effectively used in the treatment of circulatory problems, weakened immunity, colds, pneumonia, nervous conditions, pelvic inflammatory disease, insomnia, prostate, uterine and other organ and glandular congestions, oedema, chronic pain, fatigue and detoxification problems. The use of alternate hot and cold water therapy treatments increases white blood cell counts and causes corresponding increases in IgM antibodies, alpha-2 macroglobulin and C-3 complement, greatly affecting the function of the immune system.

Using hot cloths opens blood vessels and attracts blood, enhancing circulation and improving organ function. Hot baths enhance circulation, aid relaxation and by adding oils, Epsom salts and specific herbs different healing properties can be stimulated. Epsom salts added to bath water can help to draw impurities out of the body.

One night recently, I had a wonderful Indonesian meal that tasted great but unfortunately was loaded with tonnes of MSG (monosodium glutamate). The next day I felt fatigued, nauseas and I had a splitting headache that wouldn't go away. I jumped into the spa and poured in half a packet of Epsom salts. After only 20 minutes I felt amazing. As I began to empty the bath water I noticed the colour of the water had a murky, brown tone. The Epsom salts (magnesium sulphate) had actually drawn the impurities out of my kidneys and body and deposited these into the water. Nature often provides us with the most simple and inexpensive tools to restore us back to health and wellness.

Hot Sitz Baths involve sitting in a deep bath so the buttocks and pelvis are immersed. Sitz baths are great for pain or any condition in the uterus, urethra or testes. In Thailand I had the pleasure to work at one of the most beautiful health spas in the world. In my travels I visited health spas all over the world and witnessed some incredible stories of self-healing from the regular use of hydrotherapy. Spa baths, hot and cold water plunge pools, flotation tanks, steam rooms and hydro Jacuzzis are all forms of hydrotherapy that enhance the body's healing potential on both a physical and emotional level.

A simple and effective way to incorporate hydrotherapy into your life is to alternate hot and cold showers, backwards and forwards, ending with the cold water. This simple method increases blood circulation, improves lymphatic circulation, boosts immunity and enhances general well-being and health.

Chelation Therapy

Chelation therapy is a safe, non-invasive therapy designed to rid the body of excess toxins, particularly heavy metals. Over 400,000 people throughout the world have received EDTA chelation treatments over the past 30 years. It has been proven safer than taking aspirin.

There are two methods of dispensing chelation therapy. Firstly, doctors can administer intravenous solutions (through the veins, in a drip). The most common chelating agent is an amino acid called ethylene-diamine-tetra-acetate (EDTA). The molecules of EDTA bond to and chelate (remove) many toxins and heavy metals from the body, via the kidneys. Chelation helps to remove lead, strontium, aluminium, cadmium, mercury and other toxins. Twenty to 30 treatments are recommended per course.

The second method is oral chelation therapy. A number of different chelation agents can be taken orally to remove toxins and heavy metals, which impair body functions and nutrient absorption. These agents include:

- alfalfa, fibre, rutin and selenium
- bentonite clay
- calcium and magnesium chelate with potassium
- charcoal tablets remove poisons
- chromium, garlic, pectin and potassium
- coenzyme Q10
- copper chelate, iron, sea kelp and zinc chelate.
- L-cysteine (removes mercury) and L-methionine
- L-lysine and glutathione (removes toxins and heavy metals)
- miso paste helps to remove nicotine and toxins from the body
- wheatgrass, barley grass, chlorella, chlorophyll, green magma etc.

Chelation therapy is useful in treating any illness or disease caused by toxins or heavy metals. Listed below are conditions chelation therapy is successfully used for:

- removal of calcified, hardened plaque from arterial walls
- circulation problems
- cancer and chemically induced tumours
- angina
- atherosclerosis
- arrhythmias
- intermittent claudication
- Alzheimer's disease
- tinnitus
- vertigo
- and many more.

Colon Cleansing

The bowel or intestines is the body's primary organ of waste elimination. It is also the primary site for nutrient absorption and assimilation. Waste matter tends to accumulate in the bowel area and can collect for many years. Some people may have waste matter in the intestines similar to rubbery, black substances. Many people accumulate toxins in the bowel for 30 years or more.

If the bowel is congested, the rest of the body has difficulty in performing its normal function of detoxification and filtration. Fermentation, putrefaction and encrustation of the bowel are believed by some to be the cause for nearly every ailment known to man.

If the lower bowel is congested with bacteria and toxins, fermented wastes and chemicals, it tends to seep its grime into the bloodstream and lymph system. The blood and lymph take these wastes to every area of the body, synergistically decreasing the absorption of nutrients and increasing the production of mucous and disease. The wastes from the bowel cause a steady self-poisoning of the body.

Symptoms of auto-intoxication from the bowel may be bad breath, body odour, weight gain, headaches, acne, depression, rashes, boils, constant bloating, flatulence, mood swings, fatigue, anxiety, irritation, constipation, diarrhoea, furry tongue, hard stools and a multitude of other health problems and symptoms.

Iridology is a fantastic tool for visually assessing health problems occurring in the body, particularly colon toxicity, digestive problems and chronic conditions that can lead to the onset of disease or cancer. It is one of the best natural tools to use as a preventative as good, professional and experienced iridologists who use high quality computerised iridology equipment, can detect many pre-disposition signs towards illness. Once these are detected, the practitioner uses their nature care skills to provide the appropriate remedies to enhance and restore good health, and to prevent illness from occurring in the future.

The eyes truly are a window to the soul, as through the eyes we can see emotional, physical and psychological well-being from birth through to death.

There are a number of different ways to cleanse the colon. Fasting or detoxification diets are simple and easy to do (Refer to Chapter 21). By simply abstaining from food for one day every week and drinking only water and freshly made juices, you allow your body and bowel a chance to detoxify wastes. Three day cleanses once a month are also very helpful at cleaning the bowel.

Maintaining a good, healthy diet rich in wholegrains, fruits and vegetables, nuts, seeds and legumes will ensure your body stays clean and healthy. There are many natural herbal laxatives and fibres, which can be taken if you experience any problems. It is always best to obtain fibre from your everyday, healthy diet. Try to avoid laxatives, as they are not a 'cure' for bowel congestion and they flush out important nutrients from the body.

Professional colon cleansing techniques are also available. Colonic irrigation is the most popular. There is some controversy over this method. Many practitioners believe the flushing of the colon with large amounts of water causes the good microflora and nutrients to also be flushed out of the body. However, many colonic irrigationists provide these nutrients in ample quantities to ensure the body is reinoculated with good flora. It is best to do your own investigation and see what works best for you. It has also been suggested that colonic irrigation causes the bowel to lose its natural tone (through the flushing of water in the opposite direction through the bowel).

It is imperative to good health that we keep a clean and well-functioning digestive system, as the digestive system is the fuel line that feeds the rest of your body. If your fuel line is congested with muck, it will not only feed small amounts of fuel to the rest of your body, the fuel supply will be dirty and contaminated. This contaminates other areas of your body leading to ill health.

Everyone can perform enemas at home. Natural methods of cleansing the colon include:

- Herbs to give you a good flush out include aloe vera, cascara sagrada, flaxseed, red raspberry, rhubarb and senna.
- Fenugreek, yarrow and elecampane flush mucous from the intestines.
- Marshmallow restores the acid/alkaline balance of the colon, promotes healing and loosens and flushes mucous from the intestines.
- Slippery elm tea soothes inflammation and cleanses excess wastes from the colon.
- Eating only a raw foods diet for 7 days is great for detoxifying and cleansing the bowel and other organs.
- Drinking at least 8 glasses of water every day; upon arising, drink 2 glasses of lukewarm water squeezed with ½ a lemon or lime. Lemon neutralises and detoxifies the bloodstream.
- Every morning, take a brisk walk and drink a fresh vegetable juice, preferably a green juice.
- Colon cleansing drink – 1 tablespoon of bentonite powder, 1 teaspoon of psyllium, ½ cup of apple juice, ¼ cup of aloe vera juice and ½ cup of warm water; drink once a day until the colon is clean and not foul-smelling.
- Avoiding saturated fats, sugar, processed foods, fried foods, dairy products, oils and a heavy meat intake.
- The 'Healthy Breakfast Mix' in the recipes section in Part Three of this book is an excellent, everyday solution to maintain a healthy and clean bowel.
- Exercise on a regular basis. Lack of exercise can cause constipation.

The best form of colon cleansing is 'common sense' with eating. Maintain a good, healthy diet, do not overeat and avoid artificial, processed foods as much as possible. Become aware of signs or symptoms indicating toxicity and perform positive steps, such as those outlined above, to remove these before a health condition begins.

Chapter 34

MY SUCCESSFUL CANCER-FIGHTING PROGRAM

Daily Routine (Including Diet and Supplements)

First Task

To help my healing process I had to remove everything in my life that was causing me emotional stress or trauma. I ended all negative and energy-robbing relationships and let go with love, remembering the good times and the lessons learnt, and decided to keep only positive, beautiful energy in my life. You can do all of the healing therapies you like, but nothing will ever change until you remove the actual cause of your illness, whether it be a physical stress or an emotional burden that you have been carrying. Closing the door of negativity and bad energy in your life will allow a new door to open for you, full of vibrant health, creativity and divine love.

Upon Arising

Two glasses of lukewarm water squeezed with ½ fresh lemon or ½ fresh lime or 1 teaspoon of pure apple cider vinegar.

All Day

Throughout the day I drink 8 to 10 glasses of pure water to flush my system of internal and external body toxins.

Yoga/Exercise

Half an hour of yoga and stretching exercises every morning. In the morning I begin with energising yoga postures, such as Salute to the Sun and the Triangle. If you have never practised yoga or tai chi before, think about joining a class with a qualified instructor or simply purchase an instructional video. I also like to practise 10 minutes of creative imagery, meditation or dynamic healing exercises at the end of every session. Either before or after my yoga/meditation session, I walk briskly on the beach for 30 minutes daily and then take a quick dip in the ocean. If I am in a beautiful place (ocean, mountains) I also practise the deep breathing exercises.

Breakfast

Every morning I consume one freshly squeezed juice. Vegetable juices are rejuvenating and fruit juices are cleansing. My favourite combinations in the morning include carrot/celery/kale/spinach/beetroot and a chunk of ginger or two cloves of garlic. Juices should be watered down 50/50 with spring water.

AND

Special Breakfast Mix (4 parts oatbran, 4 parts psyllium husks, 4 parts L.S.A mix, 4 parts lecithin granules, 2 parts slippery elm and 1 part crushed pumpkin seeds) with ½ cup of soy milk or skim milk, 2 tablespoons of natural acidophilus yogurt and chopped apricots, berries, bananas or figs. If you feel like something sweet, put 1 teaspoon of manuka honey, brown rice syrup or blackstrap molasses on top

OR

Protein/energy shake – refer to the recipes in Part Three of this book.

OR

Yeast-free or sour dough bread – 2 slices toasted and spread with a thin layer of avocado, herb or sea salt, cottage cheese/flaxseed oil mix and a squeeze of lemon juice.

Supplements with Breakfast

Coenzyme Q10	120mg x 1 capsule
Glutathione	100mg x 1 capsule
Vitamin C Powder (with beta-carotene, zinc, quercetin, bioflavonoids)	2000mg of vit C = 2 tsp
Vitamin E tablet or liquid	750 IU x 1 tablet
B Complex tablet	1 tablet
Lipoic acid	100mg x 1 capsule
DHA/EPA – essential fatty acids	1000mg x 2 capsules
Conjugated linoleic acid	1000mg x 2 capsules
Genistein	50mg x 2 capsules
Chlorella/barley grasss/green formula	1 heaped tablespoon
Shark or bovine cartilage/lactoferrin mix	as directed
Medicinal mushroom extract (containing shitake, reishi, ganoderma, cordyceps etc.)	1ml – liquid form

Sodium selenite in one glass of water equivalent to 400mcg/day. This is prescribed by a doctor and can be picked up from a pharmacy. I also added a small amount of liquid oxygen.

Mid-Morning

Either a fresh vegetable or fruit juice (refer to juices in the recipe section in Part Three of this book for different combinations) or a selection of herbal teas. My favourite herbal teas in the morning include essiac, dandelion root tea, echinacea tea, pau d'arco tea, green tea or red clover tea or cancer clear tea (dandelion root, nettle, horsetail, pau d' arco, licorice, red clover – mix herbs together and keep in a glass jar. To make the tea, use only 1 heaped teaspoon. Pour 1 cup of boiling water over the top and let sit for 10 minutes. Sip slowly. Herbs can also be adjusted according to the specific type of cancer you are fighting).

AND

A small handful of my nut and seed mix (pesticide free almonds, walnuts, pecans, brazils, pumpkin seeds and sunflower seeds) and/or a piece of fruit such as apricots, berries, apple, pineapple, kiwifruit or papaya.

OR

Corn or rice thins spread with a thin layer of avocado, rocket or watercresss, cottage cheese and flaxseed oil mix, fresh lemon juice and herb salt.

Supplements in Between Meals

Bromelain	500mg x 3 capsules
Proteolytic/digestive enzymes	6 tablets

Lunch

Try to make one fresh salad every day. Use 6 different coloured vegetables. Choose from grated beetroot, bok choy, sunflower sprouts, fresh broccoli (use stems also), brussel sprouts, cabbage nasturtium leaves, carrot, mixed lettuces, rocket, endive, dandelion leaves, fennel, capsicum, tomato, watercress, celery, spinach, kale, garlic, onions and cucumber. I normally mix in a handful of sun-dried tomatoes and a small amount of goat's cheese or cottage cheese/flaxseed oil mix.

Dressing – 2 tablespoons of organic flaxseed oil, a squeeze of fresh lemon juice or apple cider vinegar to flavour.

AND

A good source of protein such as grilled or steamed fish (salmon, tuna, sardines, mackerel, halibut, herring or cod), organic chicken or turkey breast, grain fed red meat tofu, tempeh, yogurt or nuts and seeds. Try to have at least 2 pieces of healthy protein per day. If you eat red meat, limit to 3 times weekly. For more healthy recipes and salads, refer to recipes in the back of the book.

Supplements with Lunch

Coenzyme Q10	120mg x 1 capsule
Glutathione	100mg x 1 capsule
Vitamin C Powder (with beta-carotene, zinc, quercetin, bioflavonoids)	2000mg of Vit C = 2 tsp
Lipoic acid	100mg x 1 capsule
Chlorella/barley grasss/green formula	1 heaped tablespoon

Mid-Afternoon

One hour brisk walk in a clean, non-polluted environment. It is great to do this with someone you love or with your dog. Dogs are great companions. Often I try to sing or laugh (especially if no one is around) and often I practise cancer-clearing exercises and say positive affirmations out loud while walking.

On returning, I always make a fresh juice. Often in the afternoon I make a combination of fruit juices i.e. strawberries, papaya, apple, lemon, ginger, pineapple, mint, watermelon. Try to buy organic fruits. If you feel like a warm drink, make a fresh herbal tea or make up the cancer clear tea mix. If you feel hungry, grab a piece of fruit or a handful of the delicious nut and seed mix.

OR

Corn or rice thins, spread with a thin layer of either avocado, cottage cheese and flaxseed oil mix, tahini or hummus, sunflower or alfalfa sprouts and fresh lemon juice

The late afternoon is often a peaceful and creative time. The sun is about to settle for the day and the moon is taking its place in the sky to light up our night. This time is perfect for practising meditation, relaxation techniques, yoga, creative imagery and positive affirmations. Use this time wisely to remove any resentment, hurt or anger from your heart and let this rise and disappear into the universe.

Supplements in between meals

Bromelain	500mg x 3 capsules
Proteolytic/digestive enzymes	6 tablets

Dinner

For great dinner recipes, refer to the recipes in Part Three of this book. Try to choose from 5 to 6 different vegetables i.e. broccoli, brussel sprouts, green beans, sweet potato, pumpkin, cabbage, snow peas, kale, zucchini, eggplant, garlic, onions, leeks, cauliflower, radish, carrots and turnips. Try to eat vegetables raw, lightly stir-fried in olive oil or steamed.

AND

One piece of protein such as tempeh, tofu, organic chicken breast or thigh, organic turkey breast, salmon, tuna, mackerel, sardines, halibut, herring or cod (deep water fish is always an excellent option).

OR

Brown or wild rice, legumes or wholegrains.

OR

A beautiful, hearty soup (refer to recipes).

Hydrotherapy

Every night I have a relaxing and healing bath. I place ½ packet of epsom salts in the water and 4 drops of lavender oil (relaxation) or bergamot (uplifting). If you are experiencing fluid retention from cancer treatment, add essential oil of lemon, grapefruit or mandarin to the bath. Before entering the bath, I use a dry skin brush in quick long strokes towards my heart to remove dead skin cells and to stimulate lymphatic circulation.

Supplements with Dinner

Coenzyme Q10	120mg x 1 capsule
Vitamin C Powder (with beta-carotene, zinc, quercetin, bioflavonoids)	1000mg of vit C = 1 tsp
DHA/EPA – essential fatty acids	1000mg x 2 capsules
Conjugated linoleic acid	1000mg x 2 capsules
Genistein	50mg x 2 capsules
Zinc (liquid or tablet)	80mg or as directed
Chlorella/barley grass/green formula	1 heaped tablespoon

Shark or bovine cartilage/lactoferrin mix   as directed
Medicinal mushroom extract (containing   1ml – liquid form
shitake, reish, ganoderma, cordyceps etc.)
1 glass of water with 1 teaspoon of healing digestive formula (may contain slippery elm, fructo-oligosaccharides, glutamnine, aloe vera, guar gum, pectin) – this is normally taken before bedtime.

Meditation

Often at night time, I write down positive affirmations before going to bed. If I feel like a change, I listen to beautiful, uplifting music and inspirational tapes. Sometimes, I find myself dancing or swaying to the rhythms of the music and this makes me smile. I always visualise myself perfectly healthy and full of energy.

If I find my mind wandering throughout the day or drifting into a pattern of endless chatter, I consciously use creative imagery techniques to remove my cancer.

Before falling asleep, I say a prayer to my god and to myself, thanking us both for the wonderful souls I have in my life, for the energy to grow stronger from this lesson and for the magic of creation that I am so blessed to experience.

IMPORTANT POINTS

- Nutritional and vitamin supplements may need to be specifically adjusted for your particular type of cancer. Certain nutrients work better on certain types of cancers. Consult with a qualified and experienced health practitioner as to which program or supplement regime will work best for your needs.
- If using vitamin, mineral and herbal supplements always use a very reputable brand to ensure that you receive the full goodness and healing value from your supplements.
- If possible, try to buy organic produce to ensure that you are not putting more chemicals and pesticides into your body.
- If you are doing chemotherapy or radiation therapy, take all supplements 10 to 12 hours after treatment or six hours before treatment. This ensures that the vitamins do not affect the conventional cancer treatment, but rather enhance the therapy being given.
- The reason so many extra nutrients are given is because the body requires extra nutrition to fight cancer and to boost immune system function. By giving the body what it needs, it is able to take over the process of fighting harmful cells.
- Important Point – In my experience as a naturopath I have witnessed some of the most incredible events of self healing occur. To me it is quite simple. If the body and mind is given exactly what it requires and needs to heal – that is, simple, gentle and natural remedies, the body will restore itself back to a harmonious and healthy state. I am just a normal person, yet I healed myself of a so called 'deadly form of cancer'. If I can do it, anyone can. All you need to do is believe in yourself and get in touch with your fighting spirit and the journey back towards 'ideal health and happiness' is already halfway over. Never give up; the power is present in all of us!

Part 3

RECIPES AND MORE

Chapter 35

THE BEST CANCER-FIGHTING AND HEALING RECIPES

Beverages

Juice Recipes – Vegetable Based Combinations

Cancer Fighting Juice

This juice is action packed with abundant life force and cancer-fighting antioxidants. Juice ¼ red beetroot, 2 carrots, 1 stick celery, radish and a garlic clove. Add potato if you are dealing with liver cancer.

Cleansing Cocktail

A cleansing and refreshing juice made with cucumber, beet, apple and carrot in equal parts. Rejuvenating, energy packed and full of life-giving nutrients.

Green Harmony

Combine 1 stick of celery, 2 leaves of kale, 2 leaves of spinach, 2 leaves of cabbage, 2 green apples and a small chunk of ginger. A great juice to drink every day, as it is rich in chlorophyll, vitamins and minerals.

Green Juices

Watercress, kale, celery, broccoli leaves and parsley. Other combinations include apple/lemon/ginger, carrot/celery/beet/ginger/kale, carrot/spinach/lettuce/cabbage. You can create your own recipes with the above ingredients, to suit your taste. All green juices are rich in antioxidants and chlorophyll. Chlorophyll increases oxygen transport to the body's cells, forcing cancer cells to starve and eventually die.

Liquid Vitamin Pill

Juice spinach, carrot, celery, kale and ginger – this combination is similar to a liquid vitamin pill, providing high amounts of vitamins, minerals, antioxidants and chlorophyll. Combine 2 leaves of spinach, 2 carrots, 1 stick of celery, 2 leaves of kale and a small chunk of ginger to enjoy the benefits of this juice.

Ruby Red

Add 100ml of beetroot juice (raw) to carrot juice, apple juice or some other vegetable juice, and dilute with water. Beetroot is a reputable food used in the prevention and treatment of cancer, the prevention of tumour formation and is an excellent blood cleanser. In fighting cancer, it is recommended to drink beetroot juice on a daily basis.

Wheatgrass juice

This miracle herb is rich in all vitamins, minerals, amino acids and chlorophyll, which is important in fighting cancer. It can be mixed with carrot juice, apple juice or celery juice or simply drink alone. If healing cancer, drink 3 to 6 wheatgrass shots per day.

Juice Recipes – Fruit Based Combinations

Beauty Express

Combine 2 leaves of spinach, 2 carrots and 2 cups of apple juice to make this delicious drink. It is rich in beta-carotene, chlorophyll and cancer-fighting nutrients, and is fantastic for providing a beautiful texture to the skin if drunk on a regular basis.

Fresh Complexion

Another great drink to improve the complexion. Combine 2 cups pineapple juice, 2 cups apple juice and the juice of one cucumber. This juice is rich in enzymes, great for kidney function, fluid retention, digestion and elimination.

Fruit Swirl

A combination of watermelon juice, ginger and fresh papaya. Juice ½ a watermelon and add a chunk of ginger. Then add some fresh pieces of papaya and blend together. Body cleansing, alkalises the body's tissues, aids in detoxification, aids good circulation and benefits the digestive system.

Germ Warfare

This juice helps to boost the body's immune system, acts as a natural antibiotic and contains high amounts of vitamin C and beta-carotene to fight cancer. It also prevents and alleviates symptoms of the common cold. Simply combine 6 oranges, the juice of 1 carrot, 1 lemon and a clove of garlic to make this drink.

Island Mocktail

A delicious combination of oranges, fresh pineapple, banana. First, juice 4 oranges and 1 pineapple. Then put 1 banana in the blender with orange and pineapple juice, mix and serve. Excellent for the skin, digestive system, boosts the immune system and gives a boost to energy levels.

Kiwi Crush

Kiwifruit, green apple and grape juice mixed, roughly in equal parts or according to your taste. All three fruits help to prevent and fight cancer.

Lemon Daiquiri

Combine 1 banana, the juice of 4 lemons, ¼ cup honey and ½ cup natural acidophilus yogurt in a blender, together with some crushed ice. A very refreshing drink that is rich in vitamin C, boosts energy levels and enhances natural immunity.

Lemon or Strawberry Lassi

This juice is excellent for digestion. Blend ½ lemon or 6 strawberries, 1 cup natural acidophilus yogurt, 2 cups apple juice, ¼ cup honey and add crushed ice.

Mint Delight

A simple yet delicious drink made with pineapple and fresh mint (with or without yogurt). First, juice 1 pineapple and 1 handful of mint leaves. Then blend with some crushed ice and if you wish, add ½ cup yogurt. Serve cold. This juice aids healthy digestive function and contains high levels of vitamin C and bioflavonoids to boost immune system function. It also possesses anti-inflammatory actions.

Mint Tang

Add some chunks of papaya to 2 cups orange juice and then add mint leaves to taste. Add some ice if desired and then combine all in a blender. This juice is great for healthy digestive function, boosts immunity and acts as an anti-inflammatory. Also good for healthy skin and eyesight

Petal Cooler or Peppermint Cooler

Make this refreshing drink with any healthy herbal tea, honey, lemon juice and ice. Make herbal tea, let cool. Then blend it with fresh lemon juice to taste, 1 teaspoon of honey and some crushed ice. Cancer-fighting teas include peppermint, dandelion, licorice, pau d' arco, essiac, lemongrass, burdock, red clover and rosehip.

Pink Panther

Juice ½ a watermelon, 4 oranges and 2 chunks of ginger. Serve cold with ice. Increases circulation, aids detoxification and provides high levels of the immune-boosting vitamin C.

Purple Rain

This combination is a rich source of the cancer-fighting antioxidant, manganese. Combine 1 handful of grapes, 3 fresh pears and 1 teaspoon of honey. Juice the grapes and pears. Then add 1 teaspoon of honey and some crushed ice, and blend in a blender.

Siam Sunrise

A sweet, refreshing drink made from papaya and orange juice. Add a large chunk of papaya to the juice of 4 oranges and mix in the blender. Excellent for the skin and healthy digestion. Boosts immune system function.

Strawberry Daiquiri

This juice is high in vitamins A and C, bioflavonoids and other cancer-fighting antioxidants. It is made from fresh strawberries, banana, lemon juice, honey and natural yogurt. Firstly, juice four lemons. Then add 1 banana, ½ punnet fresh strawberries, ½ cup honey and ½ cup natural yogurt. Combine in a blender and then serve cold with ice.

Tropical Fantasy

Strawberry, apple and pineapple juice, in equal parts. This juice is rich in enzymes and phyto-nutrients used to treat and prevent cancer. Strawberries are great for cancer of the oesophagus.

***

The regular addition of juices to a natural, wholesome cancer-fighting diet is a great way to strengthen body functions, prevent illness, maintain healthy skin, digestion and elimination, and enhance longevity. Juices can still be drunk up to six times per day while you are eating other nutritious wholesome foods.

Remember that all juices should be diluted with water. Try to drink more vegetable juices than fruit juices, as too much fruit sugar can rob the body of B vitamins and cause an imbalance in blood sugar levels. Juices do not contain much fibre. If you require a diet rich in fibre, simply add beneficial juices to your normal wholesome diet or add a fibre supplement such as psyllium husk, oatbran or rice-bran to your juices.

Nut Milk

Nut milk is delicious on a hot summer's day. Simply blend 10 to 15 almonds, cashews or another type of nut, with 1 cup of purified water in a blender or food processor. Drink immediately or keep refrigerated.

Protein Energy Drink

1 cup nut milk, soy milk or skim milk
2 tablespoons LSA mix (crushed linseed, sunflower seeds, almonds) or 1 handful almonds, pumpkin seeds and sunflower seeds
1 tablespoon lecithin granules
2 to 4 tablespoons flaxseed oil
1 teaspoon glutamine powder
2 to 4 teaspoons of slippery elm powder
1 banana or ¼ paw paw, 3 to 4 dried apricots or berries
1 teaspoon spirulina, chlorella or barley grass powder or another type of high protein, nutrient packed powder
1 teaspoon of brown rice syrup or honey or 3 drops of stevia to flavour.

Simply place all the ingredients into a blender, blend together and serve.

Cancer-Clear Tea

1 part dandelion root
½ part nettle
1 part horsetail
1 part pau d'arco
½ part licorice root
1 part burdock root
2 parts red clover

Mix herbs together and keep in a glass jar. To make the tea, use 1 heaped teaspoon, pour 1 cup of boiling water over the top and let sit for 10 minutes. Sip slowly.

Herbs can be adjusted according to the specific type of cancer you are fighting. This is also a fantastic cancer-preventative tea.

Better Spreads

Apricot Spread

1 cup pure orange juice
½ cup apple juice concentrate
2 teaspoons agar powder
½ to 1 tablespoon lemon juice
400 grams fresh apricots

Place all ingredients, except for apricots in a saucepan and bring to the boil. Simmer for 5 minutes. Add apricots and simmer for 15 to 20 minutes. Remove from heat. Pour into clean jar. Cool and refrigerate.

Roasted Garlic Butter

Take a whole head of garlic and, without peeling it, wrap it in aluminium foil. Place the garlic in a moderate oven at 180° celsius. Bake for 10 to 15 minutes. Remove the soft flesh from the skin and place in blender. Now you have delicious garlic butter. Stored correctly it will keep for more than 2 weeks in the refrigerator.

Delicious Breakfast Treats

Apple, Date, Apricot and Prune Compote
2 apples
10 prunes, pitted
3 dates
5 apricots
125 ml of water

Wash the apples. Cut each apple into wedges, leaving the skin on. Place the wedges in a saucepan with the water, prunes, dates and apricots. Cover with a lid and place over a medium heat. Bring to the boil and simmer for 3 minutes. Remove the lid and stir the fruits. Cook the fruits until just softened. This recipe can be served either hot or cold (excellent for constipation).

Flaxseed, Fruit and Cottage Cheese Breakfast
2 tablespoons LSA mix (linseed, sunflower, almond)
2 tablespoons cottage cheese (mixed with 1 teaspoon of flaxseed oil)
Your favourite fruit chopped – good choices include berries, papaya, apples, pears, banana, pineapple
3 tablespoons natural acidophilus yogurt
1 teaspoon brown rice syrup or stevia, or manuka honey

Mix the ingredients together in a bowl. Add brown rice syrup, manuka honey or stevia last, for flavouring. Eat fresh.

Fruit Muesli
55 grams oat flakes or 25 grams oats and 25 grams rye flakes
1 serving of fruit – apple, banana, berries, pear
140 grams natural acidophilus yogurt
1 dessert spoon ground flaxseeds and pumpkin seeds
150 ml of skim or soy milk

Soak the oats/rye overnight. Add skim or soy milk. Top with fruit, yogurt and seeds, and serve.

Healthy Breakfast Mix

1 cup oat bran
1 cup LSA mix (crushed linseed, sunflower seeds and almonds)
1 cup lecithin granules (unbleached)
1 cup psyllium husks
½ cup slippery elm
½ cup rice flakes (optional)
½ cup almonds, pecans, sunflower seeds and pumpkin seeds
A handful of dried apple, thinly sliced

Mix all of the ingredients together and keep in a sealed container in the fridge. Serve in a bowl with chopped fruit, fresh juice/soy milk/nut milk or low fat milk. Use manuka honey or brown rice syrup for extra flavouring, if desired.

Curried Mushroom and Tomato Omelette (serves one)

¼ onion, finely chopped
25 ml of vegetable stock
20 grams mushrooms, chopped
1 tomato peeled and diced
¼ capsicum, finely chopped
2 egg whites
2 teaspoons curry powder
2 tablespoons low fat milk
½ teaspoon of olive oil

Place the chopped onion and half of the vegetable stock into a frypan. Simmer until the onions become soft, adding extra stock if necessary. Add the mushrooms and cook until stock has almost evaporated. Dice the tomato and capsicum, and add to the pan. Cook for 1 minute and then set the mixture aside.

Now beat the egg whites and milk together until they are well combined, but not too frothy. Add the curry powder to this mix. Lightly oil the pan with the olive oil. Pour the mixture into the hot pan and cook until almost set. Pile the filling into the centre of the omelette and gently fold over. Turn the omelette out onto a plate and serve immediately.

Natural Antioxidant Muesli

1 green apple
1 teaspoon pecans
1 teaspoon almonds
4 tablespoons oatmeal
1 tablespoon LSA mix
4 chopped apricots
1 tablespoon honey or brown rice syrup
4 tablespoons raisins
125 ml natural acidophilus yogurt

Wash the apple, leave the skin on and cut into fine strips. Place in a bowl with the oatmeal, LSA mix, raisins, apricots, honey and nuts. Add the yogurt to the muesli mixture and leave for 5 minutes. Serve.

Porridge

300 ml water
55 grams porridge oats
1 teaspoon manuka honey
1 dessert spoon ground flaxseeds and pumpkin seeds

Put the water in a saucepan and sprinkle in the oats. Bring to the boil for 5 minutes and keep stirring. When the porridge thickens and is soft, serve with skim milk or soy milk, or fresh juice, seeds and a little honey.

Tofu Omelette

200 grams tofu
2 egg whites
¼ to ½ cup water
1 tomato, chopped
1 garlic clove, chopped
1 small onion, finely chopped
1 tablespoon olive oil
2 spring onions
80 grams mushrooms, chopped

Blend tofu, water and egg whites in a blender. Put olive oil in saucepan and place blended mixture into the saucepan. Then cook over a gentle heat. As the tofu begins to cook, add chopped tomato, garlic, onion, mushrooms and spring onions. Cook until slightly browned. Flavour with sea salt, if desired.

Luscious Soups

Beetroot Soup

1 litre water
3 fresh beetroot, chopped
2 onions, chopped
3 cloves garlic, crushed
1 tablespoon tamari

Boil the water and add chopped beetroot. Cook until the beetroot is soft and water has turned a beautiful pink colour. Add chopped onions, garlic and tamari. Add sea salt for flavour.

Chicken Lime Soup

1 litre vegetable stock
200 grams chicken breasts, skinless
100 grams tomatoes, chopped
100 grams onions, diced
2 chillies to flavour
125 ml fresh lime juice
1 handful green beans
1 handful snow peas

Bring the vegetable stock to the boil and gently poach the chicken breasts in the stock until they are tender. Remove chicken from the stock, allow to cool slightly and then shred it. Add the shredded chicken to the stock, together with diced tomatoes, onions, chillies, lime juice, beans and snow peas. Bring the liquid to the boil and simmer until vegetables are tender. Serve hot.

Chicken Vegetable Soup

800 ml vegetable stock
100 grams organic chicken thighs, skinless and shredded (do not throw away the chicken bones)
6 shitake mushrooms
2 cloves garlic, chopped
2 spring onions, chopped
Pinch sea salt
1 teaspoon tamari
1 teaspoon cornflour
1 zucchini, sliced
1 carrot, chopped
1 handful basil, chopped

Bring the vegetable stock to the boil and add shredded chicken, chicken bones, shitake mushrooms, chopped garlic and chopped spring onions. Season the stock with sea salt (pinch) and tamari, and simmer for 3 minutes. Thicken the soup with cornflour. Add the sliced zucchini and carrot. Cook until the carrot is tender and then remove from the heat. Remove the chicken bones. Garnish with basil and serve. The minerals from the chicken bones will boost your body's immune system and help fight colds and the flu.

Crab, Sweet Corn and Celery Soup

75 grams corn kernels
250 ml vegetable stock
¼ teaspoon sea salt
¼ teaspoon pepper
1 teaspoon Chinese wine
50 grams crab meat
1 stick celery, finely chopped
¼ teaspoon cornflour
1 egg white
Fresh coriander leaves

Place the corn kernels in a blender and blend until coarsely chopped. In a saucepan, bring the stock to the boil with the corn. Add the seasonings, wine and crab meat, and chopped celery. Thicken the mixture slightly with the cornflour and finally, pour in the egg white in a steady stream, and beat. Remove the soup from the heat immediately and garnish with the torn coriander leaves.

Creamy Pumpkin and Soy Milk Soup

1 whole pumpkin
2 litres water
3 cloves garlic, chopped
1 onion, chopped
1 piece ginger
1 cup soy milk
2 tablespoons tamari
Sea salt to flavour

Chop pumpkin and boil in water. When tender, remove pumpkin from water. In a food processor place a small amount of chopped garlic, chopped onion, the ginger and a few chunks of the pumpkin. Add soy milk and blend in the food processor until you have a slightly runny consistency.

Place back in the pan and then blend the rest of the pumpkin. Once all the ingredients have been blended and placed in the pan, add tamari and sea salt, and simmer. Add water if you require less thickness in your soup. Serve with a thick dollop of natural acidophilus yogurt (if desired).

Energy Tonic Soup

8 dried shitake mushrooms
1 slice dried Chinese licorice root
2 cloves garlic, crushed
1 onion, chopped
1 carrot or sweet potato, chopped
1 slice fresh ginger
1 dried hot chilli pepper
1 handful basil leaves
¾ cup pearled barley
6 cups vegetable or chicken stock
1 teaspoon olive oil
2 teaspoons barley miso
Chives, chopped

Soak the mushrooms in hot water until soft. Discard the stems and slice thinly, save the liquid. In a large saucepan, combine ingredients (except olive oil, miso and chives), plus reserved liquid. Bring the soup to the boil, reduce heat and simmer covered, until the vegetables and barley are tender (about 1 hour). Remove from heat and add olive oil. Mix miso with a small amount of water, then add to the soup. Serve hot, sprinkled with chives.

Ginger Pumpkin Soup with Bok Choy

50 grams pumpkin, diced
¼ onion, chopped
3 leaves Bok Choy
½ clove garlic, crushed
¼ teaspoon coriander
¼ teaspoon allspice
1 tablespoon fresh ginger, chopped
350 ml vegetable stock
Pepper
Rye bread

Peel and chop the pumpkin and onion. Shred the Bok Choy. Place the prepared vegetables in a saucepan with the vegetable stock, garlic and spices. Bring to the boil and then simmer until the pumpkin is cooked. Puree to a smooth consistency and adjust seasoning to taste. Serve hot with rye bread.

Hot and Sour Shitake Soup (Immune Booster)

1 litre vegetable stock
Ginger, sliced
3 cm lemongrass
2 tablespoons tamari
½ teaspoon apple juice concentrate
2 tablespoons lemon juice
Pinch of sea salt or herbamere
3 tsp kelp flakes
10 shitake mushrooms
150 grams cherry tomatoes
2 leeks, finely chopped
1 handful basil, chopped

In a large saucepan, bring the stock to the boil. Add lemongrass, tamari, apple juice concentrate and lemon juice. Simmer for 3 minutes. Adjust the taste by adding sea salt and kelp flakes. Bring the stock back to the boil and add shitake mushrooms, cherry tomatoes, leeks and basil. Stir well and garnish with fresh coriander.

Hearty Chicken Soup

You will need:
3 organic diced chicken breasts
8 cups water
1 bay leaf
1 to 2 teaspoons sea salt
½ teaspoon sage
½ teaspoon thyme
3 carrots, chopped
2 onions, chopped
4 sticks celery, chopped
¼ cup parsley
1 handful buckwheat noodles

Bring chicken to the boil in a medium pot with water, bay leaf and salt. Cover and simmer for 30 minutes or until chicken is tender. Leave on medium heat, add chopped vegetables, sage and thyme, and cook until vegetables are slightly tender. Then add parsley and uncooked noodles in the last 10 minutes.

Miso Soup with Kelp

3 cups of water
1 carrot, sliced
1 stalk of celery, chopped
¼ cabbage chopped
3 cloves of garlic, crushed
1 chunk ginger
1 onion
¼ cup of miso paste
2 tsp tamari
½ sheet kelp, shredded

Heat the water. Add carrot slices, chopped garlic, chopped onion, chopped ginger, chopped celery and cabbage. Heat for 10 to 15 minutes until vegetables are slightly cooked. Mix miso with slightly warm water in another cup, until it has a liquid consistency. When vegetables are cooked, bring down heat and simmer. Add miso water, tamari and kelp. Don't boil the miso, as this destroys its valuable digestion-aiding enzymes and micro-organisms. Simmer for a couple of minutes, take off heat and season. Sprinkle sea salt and extra kelp on top.

Vegetable Cleansing Soup

You will need:
2 carrots with tops
2 beets with tops
1 onion
2 stalks celery with leaves
1 potato
1 handful spinach
3 cloves garlic
½ bunch watercress/kale
2 to 3 cups water

Chop all ingredients and add 2 to 3 cups of water. Bring to the boil, reduce heat to simmer and cook about 20 to 30 minutes, until vegetables are soft. Drain off vegetables and use only broth. This recipe can be refrigerated for future use.

Wholesome Country Soup

1 medium onion, chopped
2 cloves of garlic, crushed
2 small organic chicken breasts (cubed)
1 teaspoon of olive oil
500 g chopped fresh seasonal vegetables such as potatoes, swede, celery, leeks, carrots, broccoli, cabbage
225 g tinned tomatoes
1 teaspoon of vegetable stock

Steam fry the onion and garlic in oil with the chicken. Add the vegetables and tomatoes, and enough water to cover, plus vegetable stock or cube. Cover and simmer on low heat until the vegetables are cooked.

Salad Dressings

Antioxidant Dressing
125 ml low-fat acidophilus yogurt
½ teaspoon mustard powder
2 teaspoons apple cider vinegar
2 tablespoons apple concentrate
50 grams cottage cheese
1 tomato
1 small red onion
½ red capsicum
3 cloves garlic
5 ml lime or lemon juice (fresh)
1 pinch of chilli powder
1 teaspoon flaxseed or linseed oil

Combine the yogurt, mustard, vinegar, apple concentrate and cottage cheese in a food processor. Blend until it forms a smooth mayonnaise texture. Peel and de-seed the tomato. Dice the flesh. Dice the onion and capsicum, and crush the garlic. Add all of the ingredients to the yogurt mayonnaise, together with lemon juice and chilli powder. Mix well and serve with salad.

Garlic Dressing
1 cup apple cider vinegar
Juice of 1 lemon
½ cucumber, peeled and seeded
2-3 cloves garlic

Combine all ingredients in a food processor and blend for 1 minute. Place in a sealed jar and store in the refrigerator until needed.

Lemon Tahini Dressing

1 tablespoon tahini
2 teaspoons lemon juice
2 cloves garlic, crushed
Pinch of sea salt
½ teaspoon apple juice or pear juice concentrate

Mix all ingredients together. Pour over salad.

Vitality Dressing

3 tablespoons apple cider vinegar
3 tablespoons olive oil or organic flaxseed oil
1 clove garlic, crushed
If desired, chopped herbs for flavouring
½ lemon, squeezed

Mix all ingredients together in a bowl or food processor. Pour over salad.

Super Salads

Antioxidant Salad

4 stems broccoli
4 stems cauliflower
1 celery stick
4 large lettuce and kale leaves
4 large rocket leaves
1 handful green beans
½ chopped Spanish purple onion
1 stick carrot
½ cucumber
10 cherry tomatoes
1 handful walnuts

Chop and mix all of the ingredients together in a glass bowl. Serve with Antioxidant Dressing.

Apple, Celery and Tuna Salad

80 grams tuna in spring water, drained (not brine)
1 green apple
2 sticks celery, sliced
1 gem lettuce, sliced
1 large handful bean sprouts
75 grams natural live yogurt
2 teaspoons apple cider vinegar
Black pepper to taste
Rye bread
1 avocado

Drain tuna and combine with the other salad ingredients. Blend the yogurt and vinegar into the salad. Season with black pepper. Serve with rye toast, thinly spread with avocado.

Brown Rice Salad

1 cup brown rice
2 stalks celery, chopped
1 handful snow peas
Sweet pepper, chopped
2–3 cloves garlic, crushed
1 small chunk of ginger, crushed
1 tablespoon tamari
1 tablespoon apple juice concentrate
½ lemon, squeezed

Boil the rice and drain. Add the chopped celery and sweet pepper, and the snow peas. Make a dressing from the rest of the ingredients by simply stirring them together. Drizzle dressing over the vegetables and serve.

Brown Rice, Tuna and Bean Sprout Salad

100 grams brown basmati rice
100 grams tuna in spring water, drained (not brine)
1 tablespoon olive oil
1 teaspoon tamari or soy sauce
The juice of half a lemon
100 grams bean sprouts
1 carrot, chopped
1 spring onion, finely sliced

Cook rice and allow to cool. Combine with the other ingredients.

Exotic Bulgar Salad

225 grams bulgar
400 ml boiling water
1 teaspoon salt
2 tablespoons chopped mint and parsley
2 tablespoons sunflower seeds
1 garlic clove, crushed
50 ml olive oil or flaxseed oil
50 ml lemon juice
Freshly ground black pepper
450 grams tomatoes, chopped
1 small cucumber

Mix the bulgar, water and salt. Leave to stand for 15 minutes. Add all but the tomatoes and cucumber, and leave until cold. Stir in the tomatoes and cucumber, and serve. Serves 6.

Thai Style Green Papaya Salad

½ green papaya
2 cloves garlic
2–3 chillies
10 green beans
½ teaspoon apple concentrate
2 tablespoons lime juice
1 tomato, diced
1 handful mung beans
1 teaspoon chopped roasted almonds

Begin by peeling the papaya and place in a food processor. Shred the papaya. With a mortar and pestle, pound the garlic and chillies together. Add the beans (diced) and pound very lightly, just to bruise. Add the apple concentrate, shredded papaya, mung beans, lime juice and tomato. Mix all together. Serve sprinkled with chopped or slivered almonds.

Lentil Chicken Breast Salad

1 tomato
1 green capsicum
100 grams chicken breast, poached
3 spring onions
600 grams green lentils (cooked)
2 teaspoons apple cider vinegar
1 tablespoon apple juice concentrate

Dice tomato and capsicum. Shred the spring onions and chicken meat. Combine with all remaining ingredients and toss well. Season with salt substitute or another delicious dressing for flavour.

Longevity Salad

½ fresh avocado
150 grams goat's cheese chopped (if desired)
1 carrot
A handful of spinach leaves
Mixed lettuce
Snow pea sprouts
2 zucchinis, chopped
½ green or red capsicum, chopped
10 snow peas
5 sun-dried tomatoes, slivered

Chop all ingredients and mix together in a glass bowl. Serve with a garlic dressing.

Mediterranean Tomato and Broccoli Salad

10 to 15 cherry tomatoes, halved
6 medium broccoli florets, chopped
½ a purple or red onion, diced
6 large, fresh basil leaves, roughly torn
1 dessert spoon olive oil or flaxseed oil
2 teaspoons balsamic vinegar
Black pepper to taste

Simply toss all the ingredients together and serve.

Mixed Vegetable Salad

2 tablespoons vegetable stock
2 to 3 chillies
2 tablespoons low-salt tamari
2 tablespoons lemon juice
1 clove garlic, chopped
2 teaspoons chopped almonds
10 green beans
1 small onion
1 stick celery
2 carrots
½ zucchini
2 small cucumbers
3 spring onions
1 tomato
1 handful coriander leaves

Bring stock to the boil and add chillies, tamari and lemon juice. Stir and remove from the heat – this is the dressing. Add chopped garlic and almonds. Cut the beans and shred the onions, celery, carrot and zucchini. Slice the cucumbers and spring onions. Peel and deseed the tomato, cutting into squares. Mix the vegetables with the dressing, garnish with coriander leaves and serve.

Nutty Bean Salad

350 g mixed beans (haricot, kidney etc) soaked and cooked or canned
1 handful walnuts
1 tablespoon fresh parsley, chopped
2 tablespoons olive oil
2 teaspoons tamari or soy sauce
Juice of 1 lemon
100 g fennel, chopped
4 spring onions, finely sliced
½ green apple, peeled and grated

Combine all of the ingredients and serve with a large green salad.

Rainbow Roots Salad

2 medium carrots, grated
¼ purple cabbage, finely chopped
1 small parsnip, grated
1 small beetroot, grated
1 red capsicum, chopped
1 handful of parsley, finely chopped
1 tablespoon olive oil
1 tablespoon lemon juice
Black pepper to taste

Combine all of the ingredients and toss well. Serve with rye toast.

Exotic Eggplant Salad

1 clove garlic
2-3 chillies
1 teaspoon tamari or soy sauce
2 tablespoons lime juice
½ teaspoon honey
4 tomatoes
1 Chinese celery
1 onion
3 small eggplants (cooked and cubed)
200 grams organic chicken breast, poached
15 grams coriander leaves
1 handful fresh lemongrass, chopped

Crush the garlic and chillies together. Add the tamari, lime juice and honey, and combine well, to form a dressing. De-seed tomatoes and slice. Cut celery, shred the onion and chop the eggplant. Tear the cooked chicken strips and mix with celery, eggplant, onion, tomato, coriander leaves, lemongrass and dressing.

Vietnamese Chicken and Cabbage Salad

1 chilli
1 clove garlic, crushed
1 teaspoon of apple juice concentrate
½ teaspoon tamari sauce
3 tablespoons lime juice
1 tablespoon water
1 teaspoon apple cider vinegar
½ small onion, finely chopped
100 grams chicken breast (preferably organic) – poached and finely shredded
220 grams raw cabbage, finely shredded
40 grams carrot, finely shredded
5 grams coriander
1 teaspoon chopped parsley
1 handful raw, organic peanuts (chopped finely)
1 handful fresh mung beans

Combine finely chopped chilli with the garlic, apple concentrate, tamari, lime juice, water, vinegar and onion. Leave to stand for 15 minutes, to help the flavours develop. Add all of the remaining ingredients to the dressing, except the chopped peanuts and mung beans. Mix thoroughly. Then sprinkle the chopped peanuts and mung beans over the top and serve.

Watercress and Goat's Cheese Salad

½ bunch watercress
100 grams diced goat's cheese
1 gem lettuce, sliced
¼ cucumber, sliced
½ green pepper, chopped
1 handful of alfalfa sprouts

Combine all ingredients and toss them with 1 tablespoon of your choice of dressing.

Main Courses

Chicken with Raisins, Pine Nuts and Ginger

20 grams raisins
20 grams pine nuts
1 chunk of ginger, grated
2 tablespoons apple cider vinegar
100 grams chicken breast (preferably organic)
50 grams freshly steamed vegetables
75 grams brown basmati rice, cooked
1 handful black sesame seeds

In a food processor, blend the raisins, pine nuts, ginger and vinegar to a paste. Pour over the chicken breast, coating well, and leave to stand for 1 to 2 hours. Place in a tray and grill, brushing with the marinade as the chicken cooks. Turn and grill the other side, until the meat is cooked through, approximately 8 to 10 minutes. Alternatively, bake in a moderate oven or fry in a frying pan. When cooked, sprinkle the sesame seeds over the chicken. Serve with steamed vegetables (broccoli, bok choy or cauliflower) and brown basmati rice.

Chick Pea Vegetable Curry

100 ml vegetable stock
25 grams diced onion
1 clove garlic
2 teaspoons curry powder
1 teaspoon cumin
1 pinch cayenne pepper
50 grams cauliflower
8 green beans
40 grams tomatoes, roughly chopped
50 ml water
100 grams chickpeas, cooked
50 grams green peas

Simmer 50 ml of the vegetable stock in a saucepan with onion and garlic, until the onion is cooked. Then increase the heat to evaporate the liquid. Add the spices and dry-fry with the onion and garlic. Add a little more vegetable stock. Add the remaining stock, cauliflower, green beans, tomatoes and water. Cover and simmer for 3 to 4 minutes. Add the chickpeas and green peas. Continue to cook until the curry is heated through and the peas are tender. Add sea salt if necessary.

Exotic Fried Wild Rice

1 small onion
½ carrot
½ lemon (squeeze out juice)
1 stick celery
½ green capsicum
75 ml vegetable stock
1 clove garlic, crushed
1 tablespoon tamari or shoyu
150 grams wild rice
Sea salt to taste
1 spring onion, chopped
2 eggs

Finely dice the onion, carrot, celery and capsicum. In a wok or frying pan, add 2 tablespoons of the vegetable stock and heat through until the stock boils (alternatively olive oil can be used). Add the garlic and onion and stir fry. Add the other vegetables progressively, adding a little tamari and lemon juice when necessary. Add the cooked wild rice and mix well. While in the wok, push the rice mix towards the edge of the wok and make a small circle in the centre. Break open the two eggs into this space, let this cook. When cooked, dice with a spatula. Blend in with the rice mix. Season to taste with sea salt. Fold the spring onion through the mixture and serve.

Ginger Snapper Fillets

25 grams asparagus
1 carrot
½ teaspoon ginger root, finely grated
½ teaspoon sherry
½ teaspoon soy sauce
½ teaspoon cornflour
150 grams snapper fillets
50 grams mushrooms
1 teaspoon parsley

Trim the asparagus and cut the carrot into strips. Combine ginger with sherry, soy sauce and cornflour. Set aside. Place fish in a baking dish with the mushrooms and steam or bake in the oven for 5 to 7 minutes, or until done. Meanwhile, steam the prepared vegetables. Drain the juices from the cooked fish and add to the ginger mixture. Bring to the boil (add a little vegetable stock or water if too thick) and spoon a little over the fish – this keeps the heat in the fish when you serve. Arrange the steamed vegetables on the plate with the fish. Spoon the remaining sauce over the fish and serve.

Grilled Pesto Chicken

150 grams skinless organic chicken breasts
1 heaped teaspoon of pesto

Slice the chicken breasts across and spread their insides with half of the pesto.

Spread the remaining pesto on top of the chicken. Grill for 25 minutes or until cooked.

Indian Spiced Chicken

Juice of 1 lemon
1 clove garlic, crushed
½ teaspoon turmeric
½ teaspoon ground cumin
1 teaspoon ground coriander
Dash of cayenne
1 chicken breast (preferably free range)
Steamed broccoli, spinach and cauliflower, or jasmine rice

Blend the lemon juice, garlic and spices. Place the rinsed chicken breast in a dish and toss into the spice blend until it is well coated. Leave to marinate for at least 30 minutes. Place under a hot grill for 25 minutes, or until cooked. Turn it over once, throughout cooking. Serve with steamed broccoli, spinach and cauliflower, or with jasmine rice.

Roast Chicken Breast with a Twist

2 small chicken breasts (with skin)
1 clove garlic, sliced
2 sprigs fresh tarragon
1 dessert spoon olive oil
Juice of ½ a lemon

Place garlic slices and tarragon under chicken skin. Place chicken breasts in a baking dish and drizzle with olive oil and lemon juice. Place in oven. Bake for 20 minutes or until cooked. Remove skin and serve.

Snapper in Apple and Lime Juice

150 grams snapper fillet
30 ml apple juice
½ teaspoon lime juice
½ green apple, peeled
1 tablespoon carrot, finely diced
25 grams cooked pumpkin
2 small potatoes
25 grams green beans
1 teaspoon parsley, chopped

Place the fish fillet in a small baking dish. Pour the apple juice and lime juice over the fish. Slice the apple very thinly and lay on top. Bake in the oven for 8 to 10 minutes or until the apple is soft. Meanwhile, blanch the carrot. Puree the pumpkin and then the blanched carrot. Reheat. Steam the potatoes and beans until tender. Roll the potatoes in the chopped parsley. Put the fish on a plate. Spoon a little of the reduced apple juice over the fish, then surround with hot vegetables and garnish with fresh herbs.

Spicy Mackerel Served with Couscous

2 small mackerel fillets
440 ml boiling water
115 grams couscous
1 teaspoon olive oil and 2 tablespoons water, combined
1 small onion, chopped
2 cloves garlic, crushed
¼ teaspoon chilli powder and 1 teaspoon cumin powder
1 red pepper, chopped
110 grams zucchini, sliced
1 stick celery, finely diced
200 grams tinned tomatoes

Place mackerel fillets in a baking tray, cover and bake for 20 minutes. Pour boiling water over the couscous. Leave it to stand for 15 minutes. Meanwhile, steam-fry the onion, garlic, chilli and cumin powder for 2 minutes, with the olive oil and water. Add red pepper, zucchini, celery and tomatoes, simmer until vegetables are tender. Arrange a fish fillet on the mound of couscous. Top with the vegetables.

Spicy Stuffed Mushrooms

20 large button mushrooms
1 tablespoon low-fat natural yogurt
250 grams smoked tofu (finely chopped and lightly fried)
1½ teaspoons curry powder
2 sticks celery, finely chopped
2 spring onions, finely chopped
4 tablespoons fresh parsley, chopped

Clean mushrooms and remove the stalk. Combine yogurt, tofu, curry powder, mushroom stalks and finely chopped celery and spring onion. Use this mixture to fill the mushroom cups. Garnish with the parsley and serve hot or cold.

Tempting Tofu Burgers with Salad

1 tablespoon soy sauce
1 tablespoon lemon juice
1 clove garlic, crushed
1 slice tofu
1 wholemeal bread roll
⅛ avocado
¼ beetroot, grated
2 tablespoons cottage cheese
½ grated carrot
1 handful shredded lettuce
1 fresh tomato, sliced or 1 tablespoon chopped, sun-dried tomatoes

Mix soy sauce, lemon juice and crushed garlic. Place slice of tofu in this mixture. Let sit for 10 minutes. Cook the tofu in a frying pan until hot. Spread a thin layer of avocado on the bread roll. Add tofu and other salad ingredients. Serve with green salad.

Thai Green Curry

1 small onion, chopped
2 cloves garlic, crushed
1 dessert spoon fish sauce
3 green chillies, finely chopped (if you require extra spice)
2 heaped teaspoons green curry paste
1 teaspoon olive oil
400 grams chicken breasts, cubed or 400 grams of firm tofu cubed
2 tablespoons water
400ml of soy milk
2 kaffir lime leaves
1 large zucchini, chopped
1 handful of fresh basil leaves

Steam fry the onion, garlic, fish sauce, chillies and curry paste in oil for 2 minutes. Add the chicken and fry for a further 5 minutes. Add the milk and kaffir lime leaves. Stir well, cover and leave to simmer for at least 30 minutes. Add the zucchini and basil leaves, and then simmer a further 5 to 10 minutes before serving.

Tuna Served with Grilled Vegetables

3 small potatoes
¼ small pumpkin
2 beetroots, fresh
1 onion
1 zucchini
¼ large eggplant, diced and cooked
½ green capsicum
¼ teaspoon marjoram
¼ teaspoon olive oil
150 grams tuna steak
½ lemon, sliced

Place potatoes, pumpkin and beetroots in a pan with water sufficient to just cover. Boil until soft. Remove from the water and cool. Peel and thickly slice the onion, zucchini and eggplant. Cut the capsicum into slices. Mix the marjoram with the oil and spread a little onto the tuna. Toss all of the vegetables together with the remaining marjoram and oil. Mix well and set aside for 5 minutes. Cut the cooked potatoes, pumpkin and beetroots in half and place cut-side down under a hot grill. Add vegetables and then the tuna. Turn the potatoes, pumpkin and beetroots after 3 to 4 minutes to ensure they are heated enough. Cook the tuna for 5 minutes or until tender. Serve with lemon slices and a sprig of fresh marjoram.

Yummy Sweets

Honey Apricot Oat Bars

90 grams dried apricots
35 grams wholewheat flour or spelt flour
35 grams wheatgerm
½ teaspoon ground cinnamon
75 ml apple juice concentrate
4 tablespoons LSA mix

Chop the apricots and mix with the rest of the ingredients. Pack the mixture into a 20 centimetre square tin and bake in a cool oven at around 100–150° celsius. Cool and cut into bars to serve.

Brown Rice Pudding

1 cup brown rice
½ cup nut milk, soy milk or skim milk
1 handful raisins or currants
1 handful sliced almonds
1 teaspoon vanilla essence
2 teaspoons honey or brown rice malt syrup

Cook the brown rice in boiling water until it is tender. Drain off the water. Then stir the milk through the rice. Add the raisins or currants, vanilla essence and honey, and combine thoroughly. Reheat in a pan on the stove or in the microwave. Can also be served cold.

Apricot and Peach Swirl

110 grams apricots
8 dried peaches, soaked
¼ teaspoon natural vanilla essence
140 grams low-fat yogurt
30 grams cottage cheese
1 egg white

Stew apricots until soft. Blend in a processor, adding the vanilla essence, soaked dried peaches, yogurt and cottage cheese. Whisk the egg white stiffly. Fold into apricot mixture. Place in a bowl or glasses. Chill before serving.

Coconut and Apple Surprise with Apricot, Fig Sauce

25 grams carob
4 green apples, chopped
30 ml honey
15 ml passionfruit juice
25 grams shredded coconut, toasted

SAUCE:
40 grams dried apricots
40 grams of dried figs
water as required

Chop carob and apples into small pieces. Mix this with honey, passionfruit juice and shredded coconut. Press the mixture into a greased tin. Cover this and let it chill in the fridge for 3 hours. To make the topping, cover the apricots and figs with water and bring to the boil. Blend to a watery consistency in the blender. Cool. Serve the coconut and apricot slice on a plate and pour the apricot and fig sauce over the top.

Other Great Recipes

Home-made Vegetable Stock (Cleansing Broth)

4 tomatoes
2 potatoes
¼ small cabbage
2 sticks celery
1 litre water
2 onions
2 carrots
4 spinach leaves

Combine all of the ingredients with skin still on and simmer for one hour. Strain, discarding the vegetables. Store vegetable stock in a glass jar, in the refrigerator.

Salt Substitute

1 teaspoon cayenne pepper
1 teaspoon garlic powder
1 teaspoon dried basil
1 teaspoon dried thyme
1 teaspoon dried parsley flakes
1 teaspoon ground mace
1 teaspoon onion powder
1 teaspoon dried sage

Mix all of the ingredients together.

Yogurt Cheese

100 ml of low-fat yogurt

Line a bowl with muslin cloth. Fill the cloth with yogurt and tie the cloth in a bundle. Suspend the bundle over a sink or bowl for 5 to 6 hours, or until the whey has drained completely. Store and cool.

Vitality Sandwiches for a Snack

Here is a selection of my favourite sandwich fillings. Simply fill two slices of rye bread or pita bread with any of the following combinations. The sandwiches are great with a salad or can be eaten on their own.

- 120 grams cottage cheese with a large handful of alfalfa sprouts.
- 120 grams hummus and a large handful of alfalfa sprouts, together with some refreshing cucumber slices.
- ¼ packet of cooked tofu with lettuce, sprouts and grated carrot.
- 1 sliced tomato and a large handful of watercress.
- 50 grams canned salmon or tuna in brine, cucumber slices and a large handful of watercress.
- 120 grams of cottage cheese, sun-dried tomatoes, rocket leaves
- ¼ packet of cooked tofu, watercress, black sesame seeds
- 1 hard-boiled egg with watercress, tomato and lettuce.

Chapter 36

DANGEROUS FOOD ADDITIVES

A long with the cancer-producing dietary habits we have adopted, we have developed methods of food processing, preserving and packaging that call for the addition of thousands of chemicals to our foods. When these chemicals were first created they were considered a great advance in nutritional technology, making it possible for people to enjoy foods and delicacies from different countries from all over the world.

As with other contributions to industry and technology, what at first appeared to be a breakthrough welcomed by many, has resulted in worries about safety and health issues. Many additives have been banned, yet there are thousands of food contaminants still being used as the profits attained are worth more than the consumer's health. Many of these food additives and preservatives have been linked to serious health conditions and even cancer formation. And we are still asking ourselves why cancer has become so rampant in our society.

I have presented just a few of the most common contaminants in this book. For a more detailed list, you can obtain a food additive chart that provides guidelines as to possible risk factors. Alternatively, a fantastic and well-researched book called *The Chemical Maze* written by Bill Statham provides a comprehensive list of dangerous contaminants found in foods.

Artificial Colourings

Most artificial colourings are synthetic chemicals that do not occur in nature. Colourings are not listed by names on labels. Because colourings are used almost solely in foods of low nutritional value (lollies, soft drinks, gelatine desserts etc.) you should simply avoid all artificially coloured foods. The use of colouring usually indicates that fruit or other natural ingredients have not been used, unless otherwise stated. A small number of dangerous food colourings are listed below, along with code names and other names that may be listed as on the packaging.

Blue No. 1 (Code No. 133, Brilliant Blue FCF)

Found in beverages such as soft drinks, dairy products, gelatine, desserts, cereal, lollies and baked goods. Suggestions of a small cancer risk, allergic reactions in sensitive people, asthma, hyperactivity.

Blue No. 2 (Code No. 132, Indigotine, Indigo carmine)

Found in pet food, biscuits, ice creams, baked goods, beverages and lollies. Reasonable certainty of no harm, however there is some small indication of possible brain tumour formation cancer, asthma, hyperactivity, allergic reactions.

Carbon Blacks (Code No. 153)

Currently banned in America. A black food colouring found in jam, jelly crystals and confectionary. It may be a possible cause of cancer.

Citrus Red No. 2 (Code No. 123, FD & C Red No. 2)

Injected into some oranges, packet cake mix, jelly crystals, soft drinks, cereals, black-currant products. Studies indicate that this additive may cause cancer, asthma, hyperactivity, rashes, malignant tumours.

Red No. 2 G (Code No. 128)

Found in meat products. This additive may cause cancer, asthma, gene damage, skin reactions.

Red No. 3 (Code No. 127, Erythrosine, FD & C Red No. 3)

Artificial colouring used in canned red cherries, snack foods, scotch eggs, packet trifle mix, sweets and baked goods. A possible link to breast and other cancers, hyper-thyroidism, gene damage, thyroid tumours and benign tumours.

Red No. 40 (Code No. 129, Allura Red, FD & C Red No. 40)

The most widely used food dye. The Unites States FDA has admitted to 'problems', but said evidence of harm was not 'consistent' or 'substantial'. It has caused tumours and cancer in mice, hyperactivity and hay fever. Used mostly in junk foods such as soft drinks, lollies, packet cake mix, jelly crystals, chocolate biscuits, sweets, gelatine desserts, sausage and pet foods.

Yellow No. 2G (Code No. 107)

Artificial colouring used in soft drinks. A widely used colouring which causes allergic reactions, primarily in aspirin-sensitive people. May also cause cancer, hyperactivity and asthma. This is labelled on food items.

Yellow No. 5 (Cod No. 102, Tartrazine, FD & C Yellow No. 5)

Used in confectionary, sweet corn, soft drinks, canned peas, cheese crackers, fruit juice cordial, jam, pickles, cereal, lollies, snack foods. It may cause hyperactivity, thyroid tumours, migraines, asthma, insomnia, confusion, blurred vision, cancer.

Yellow No. 6 (Code No. 110, Sunset Yellow FCF, FD & C Yellow No. 6)

This dye may cause tumours in the adrenals and kidneys. It may also cause allergic reactions and is possibly cancer-causing. It is also linked to allergic reactions, asthma, hyperactivity, hay fever and abdominal pains. Found in beverages, fruit juice, cordials, hot chocolate mix, cereals, ice cream, packet soup, snack foods, sausages, baked goods, lollies and gelatine.

Artificial Flavourings and Preservatives

Aspartame
Aspartame, once thought to be the perfect sweetener, is now in serious doubt. People have reported behavioural changes from the use of aspartame and it may pose serious cancer risks. Used as an artificial sweetener in drink mixes, gelatine desserts and other foods.

Brominated Vegetable Oil (BVO)
There is cause for concern with BVO. Gives the cloudy appearance to citrus-flavoured soft drinks and also used as an emulsifier.

Butylated Hydroxyanisole (BHA)
BHA retards rancidity in fats, oils and foods that contain oil. While most studies indicate it is safe, it is known to cause cancer in animals. Safer substitutes are available.

Butylated Hydroxytoluene (BHT)
BHT retards rancidity in oils. May possibly be cancer causing, avoid where possible. Found in cereals, chewing gum, potato chips and oils.

Caffeine
Caffeine occurs naturally in coffee and tea but it is also added to some well-known soft drinks. It may cause miscarriages or birth defects and should be avoided by pregnant women. It also keeps many people from sleeping and may lead to fibrocystic breast disease.

Saccharin
A synthetic sweetener used in diet products. In 1977, the United States FDA proposed that saccharin be banned on evidence that it causes cancer. It was gradually replaced by aspartame.

Sodium Nitrite (Code No. 251) and Potassium Nitrite (Code No. 261)
Sodium and potassium nitrites can lead to the formation of cancer-causing chemicals called nitrosamines, particularly in fried bacon. Has also been linked to asthma, headaches, destruction of red blood cells, breathing problems. Found in preserved and manufactured meats, bacon, ham, frankfurters, luncheon meats, smoked fish and corned beef.

Sulphur Dioxide (Code No. 220) and Sodium Bisulphite (Code No. 221)

Sulphating agents prevent discolouration (dried fruit, shrimp, dried, fried and frozen potatoes, beer, gelatine, cordials, wine etc.). They destroy vitamin B1, vitamin A and may cause headaches, backaches, asthma, hyperactivity, bronchitis, nausea and severe allergic reactions.

Chapter 37

ACID/ALKALINE FOODS

Foods can be either acid forming, balancing or alkaline forming according to the condition that foods create in the body after being ingested. Our body's normal PH is between 6.0 and 6.8 (the human body is naturally mildly acidic). For the body, the values above PH 6.8 are considered to be on the alkaline side, values below PH 6.3 are on the acidic side.

Too much acidity allows parasites, yeast, viruses and rebellious cancer cells to thrive. Symptoms of acidity include frequent sighing, insomnia, water retention, recessed eyes, rheumatoid arthritis, migraines, low blood pressure, dry stools, burning sensation in the anus, burning in mouth or under tongue, sensitivity to vinegar/acidic fruits, bumps on tongue/roof of mouth. Causes of acidity include kidney, liver and adrenal disorders, improper diet, malnutrition, obesity, anger, stress, fear, anorexia, toxaemia, fever and excessive consumption of vitamin C, niacin and aspirin and overwork.

A body system which is too alkaline produces a condition called alkalosis. This causes over-excitability of the nervous system. Symptoms include sore muscles, creaking joints, drowsiness, protruding eyes, hypertension, oedema, allergies, night cramps, chronic indigestion, vomiting, menstrual problems, hard stools, prostatitis, thick skin and calcium build up in the bones.

Causes of alkalosis can be high cholesterol, vomiting, endocrine imbalance, poor diet, diarrhoea, and osteoarthritis.

Acid Forming Foods

Alcohol, artichokes, asparagus tips, aspirin, beans, beef, beer, brussel sprouts, cakes, catsup, cheese, chicken, chick peas, cocoa, coffee, cornflour, cornmeal, cranberries, custards, doughnuts, drugs, eggs, fish, flour, flour products, gelatine, ginger, jams/jellies, legumes, lentils, macaroni, mayonnaise, meat, milk, mustard, noodles, nuts (most), oatmeal, olives, organ meats, pasta, pastries, peanuts, pepper, plums, poultry, prunes, sago, sauerkraut, sesame seeds, shellfish, soft drinks, spaghetti, sugar, tapioca, tea, tobacco, vinegar, whisky and white rice.

Low-level Acid Forming Foods

Butter, canned fruit, cheeses (some), desiccated coconut, dried fruit, fruit treated with sulphur, glazed fruit, grains (most), ice cream and lamb.

Alkaline Forming Foods

Avocados, buttermilk, corn, dates, fresh coconuts, fresh fruits, fresh vegetables, goat's milk, herbs, honey, maple syrup, molasses, raisins, salt, sea vegetables, seeds, soy products, spices, umeboshi plums, whey, wine and yogurt.

Low-level Alkaline Forming Foods

Agar, almonds, amaranth, blackstrap molasses, brazil nuts, buckwheat, chestnuts, lima beans, millet, quinoa and soured dairy foods.

Neutral Foods

All vegetable oils, all sprouts, most dried beans and sunflower seeds.

It is considered optimal for good health, to eat a diet that is composed of approximately 70% alkaline forming foods and 30% acid forming foods.

Chapter 38

MINERAL AND AMINO ACID-RICH FOODS

Minerals

Boron
Apples, carrots, grains, grapes, leafy green vegetables, nuts, and pears.

Calcium
Almonds, apricots, avocado, brazil nuts, broccoli, cabbage, carob powder, chick peas, collard, currants, dates, figs, fish, green leafy vegetables, hazelnuts, kale leaves, kelp, lentils, linseed, molasses, mung beans, okra, olives, parsley, pinto beans, prunes, raisins, rhubarb, sardines, sesame seeds, silverbeet, soybeans, spinach, sunflower seeds, turnip greens, walnuts and white beans.

Copper
Almonds, crab, dry stone fruit, legumes, mushrooms, nuts, organ meats, pecans, perch, seafood (crayfish, prawns, mussel), Spanish onions, sunflower seeds, and whole grains.

Chromium
Asparagus, black pepper, brewer's yeast, clams, grape juice, haddock, lobster, molasses, mushrooms, nuts, oysters, peanuts, prunes, raisins, shrimp and whole grains,

Chlorine
Beans, cabbage, celery, cow's milk, fish, fresh dried figs, kelp, lentils, lettuce, spinach and tomatoes.

Fluorine
Asparagus, cabbage, egg yolk, garlic, goat's milk, mackerel, oats, parsley, rice, sardines and sea salt.

Germanium
Aloe vera, comfrey, garlic, ginseng, onions, shitake mushrooms, and suma.

Iodine
Cucumbers, dairy products, dulse, garlic, iodised salt, Irish moss, kelp, lima beans, mushrooms, saltwater fish, sea salt, seafood, sesame seeds, soybeans, spinach, sunflower seeds, turnip greens and watermelons.

Iron
Apricots, asparagus, barley, broccoli, cabbage, chlorophyll, dates, eggs, figs, fish, kelp, leeks, legumes, lentils, lettuce, oats, onion, organ meats, oysters, parsley, pine nuts, poultry, pumpkin seeds, pumpkin, radish, raisins, red grape juice, red wine, silverbeet, soybeans, spinach, sunflower seeds wheat and wheat germ.

Magnesium
Almonds, beans, beet greens, brewer's yeast, brussel sprouts, cabbage, cashews, corn, dark green vegetables, dates, figs, kelp, molasses, parsley, silverbeet, soybeans, spinach, walnuts and wholegrain cereals.

Manganese
Almonds, avocados, blueberries, buckwheat, coconuts, corn, dried fruits, dried peas, kelp, nuts, olives, pecans, sunflower seeds, walnuts, and wholegrains.

Molybdenum
Buckwheat, dark green leafy vegetables, legumes, lentils, lima beans, liver, oats, peas, soybeans, sunflower seeds, sweet peas and wheatgerm.

Phosphorus
Almonds, asparagus, barley, beans, brussel sprouts, cabbage, cauliflower, chickpeas, corn, cucumbers, egg yolk, fish, garlic, kale, leafy greens, lentils, mushrooms, oats, peas, pumpkin, radish, rhubarb, rice, rye, salmon, soybeans, tuna, walnuts, watercress, wheat and wholegrains.

Potassium
Apricots, avocados, bamboo shoots, bananas, barley, beans, beetroots, broccoli, carrots, cauliflower, celery, citrus fruits, dried fruits, eggplant, garlic, kale, kelp, leafy greens, lettuce, mushrooms, nuts (except macadamias), olives, parsley, peas, potatoes, rhubarb, seeds, silverbeet, soybeans, spinach, sunflower seeds, tomatoes, turnips, watercress, whole wheat and yams.

Selenium
Brazil nuts, brewers yeast, broccoli, brown rice, cashews, chicken, crab, dulse, eggs, garlic, herring, human breast milk, kelp, onions, salmon, seafood, tomatoes, tuna, vegetables and wholegrains.

Silica
Alfalfa, barley, beets, brown rice, dates, dried figs, green leafy vegetables, horsetail plants, oats, root vegetables, soybeans and strawberries.

Sodium

Beans, celery, dates, dried figs, eggs, fish, green olives, kelp, leafy greens, lentils, peas, sardines, silverbeet, spinach, strawberries and tomatoes.

Sulphur

Beans, brussel sprouts, cabbage, carrots, dates, dried figs, eggs, fish, garlic, horseradish, kale, leafy greens, onions, radish, spinach, turnips and watercress.

Zinc

Brewer's yeast, ginger, mushrooms, pumpkin seeds, seafood – especially oysters, soybeans, sunflower seeds and wholegrains.

Amino Acids

Arginine

Alfalfa, almonds, beef, carob, cashews, celery, cheese, coconut, eggs, garlic, ginseng, grains, leeks, lettuce, meats, milk, nuts, peanuts, peas, pecans, soy beans, wakame, walnuts, wheat germ and whole wheat.

Glutamine

Beef, celery, brussel sprouts, cabbage, cottage cheese, dandelion greens, meat, milk, most protein sources, papaya, pork, poultry, raw parsley, raw spinach, ricotta cheese and rolled oats.

Glutathione

Carrots, cysteine supplementation, as glutathione can be made in the body from cysteine, garlic, glutamic acid and glycine, grapefruit, meats, spinach, tomatoes and plant and animal tissue.

Histidine

Bananas, cauliflower, chicken, cottage cheese, egg, fish, meat, pork, rice, rye, wheat and wheatgerm.

Methionine

Bananas, beans, beef, brazil nuts, cottage cheese, chicken, eggs, fish, garlic, legumes, liver, onions, pork, pumpkin seeds, sardines, soybeans and yogurt.

Good Sources of Dietary Fibre

Apple pectin, bran, dates, figs, guar gums, apples, fruits, oatbran, pears, prunes, psyllium seeds or husks, raw salad vegetables and wholegrain cereals.

Chapter 39

FOODS PACKED WITH VITAMINS AND OTHER NUTRIENTS

Biotin
Bean sprouts, brewer's yeast, egg yolks, liver, meat, nuts, oatmeal, pecans, poultry, rice, saltwater fish, soybeans and wholegrains.

Choline
Brewer's yeast, cereals, egg yolks, leafy greens, lecithin, legumes, liver, peanuts, wheat germ and wholegrain cereals.

Coenzyme Q10
Beef, broccoli, cabbage, egg yolks, leafy greens, mackerel, milk, oily fish, organ meats, peanuts, salmon, sardines, sesame oil, soybean oil, spinach, vegetable oils, wholegrains and yogurt.

Inositol
Beans, brewer's yeast, cabbage, cantaloupe, citrus fruits, grapefruit, lecithin, legumes, lima beans, molasses, nuts, raisin, seeds, oats, wheat germ and wholegrains.

Vitamin A (Carotenes)
Apricots, cantaloupe, carrots, dark leafy greens, egg yolks, endive, fish and animal liver, fish oils, lettuce, mangoes, mint, papaya, peaches, prunes, pumpkin, sweet potatoes and yams.

Vitamin B1 (Thiamine)
Beef, brewer's yeast, brown rice, dulse, egg yolks, fish, green vegetables, kelp, lean pork, legumes, liver, milk, nuts, oats, peanuts, peas, rice bran, soybeans, spirulina, torula yeast, wheatgerm and wholegrains.

Vitamin B2 (Riboflavin)

Asparagus, avocadoes, beans, brewer's yeast, broccoli, brussel sprouts cashews and other nuts, fish, leafy greens, legumes, lentils, mushrooms, parsley, spinach, sprouted seeds, wild rice and yogurt.

Vitamin B3 (Niacin)

Almonds, bran, brewer's yeast, broccoli, brown rice, carrots, dandelion greens, fish, leafy greens, legumes, mushrooms, nuts, potatoes, poultry, salmon, sardines, sunflower seeds, tomatoes, wheatgerm and whole wheat products.

Vitamin B5 (Pantothenic Acid)

Avocadoes, brewer's yeast, cashews, cereals, egg yolk, leafy green vegetables, meat, pecans, ricebran, royal jelly, soybeans and wheatbran.

Vitamin B6 (Pyridoxine)

Brewer's yeast, cereals, dried beans, fish, legumes, liver, millet, nuts, oats, organ meats, poultry, salmon, soy beans, tuna, walnuts, wheat germ, wholegrains and yogurt.

Vitamin B9 (Folic Acid)

Almonds, asparagus, avocadoes, beetroot, broccoli, endive, fenugreek, leafy green vegetables, legumes, lettuce, mushrooms, onions, oranges, parsley, soybeans, sprouts, walnuts and wholegrains.

Vitamin B12 (Cyanocobalamin)

Found mostly in meats. Small amounts are found in alfalfa, brewer's yeast, egg yolks, leafy greens, meats, milk, mushrooms, oysters, salmon, sardines, sea vegetables, seafood, soy products, spirulina and yogurt.

Vitamin B15 (Pangamic Acid)

Apricot kernels, brewer's yeast, maize, oats, pumpkin seeds, rice bran and wheat germ.

Vitamin B17 (Bioflavonoids)

Apple seeds, apricot kernels, berries, blueberries, buckwheat, cranberries, grains, legumes, lima beans, linseed, millet, mung beans, nectarines, peaches, plums, prunes, raspberries and young shoots of plants.

Vitamin B Complex

Blackstrap molasses, brewer's yeast, brown rice, dark leafy greens, nuts and seeds, sprouted seeds, wheatgerm and wholegrains.

Vitamin C (Ascorbic Acid)

Apricot kernels, avocado, blackcurrants, broccoli, brown rice, cabbage, cheese, citrus fruits, guavas, nuts, oatbran, parsley, peppers, pineapple, potatoes, rosehips, sesame seeds, strawberries, sunflower seeds and wholegrains.

Vitamin E (D-Alpha Tocopherol)

Avocadoes, barley, cold pressed oils, corn, cotton seed oil, liver, nuts and seeds, oats, soy, sunflower seeds and wheatgerm.

Vitamin F (Essential Fatty Acids)

Cinnamon, cold pressed oils, corn, linseed oil, mustard seed oil, safflower, seaweed, soy, sunflower oil sunflower seeds and tofu.

- **Alpha-Linolenic Acid (ALA, Omega-3)** – canola oil, flaxseed oil, hempseed oil
- **Linoleic Acid (LA, Omega-6)** – evening primrose oil, flaxseed oil, hempseed oil, lard, safflower oil
- **Gamma-Linolenic Acid (GLA, Omega-6)** – blackcurrant seed oil, borage seed oil
- **Eicosapentaenoic Acid/Docosahexaenoic (EPA/DHA)** – cod, haddock, halibut, herring, mackerel, salmon, sardines

Vitamin K (Menadione)

Brewer's yeast, broccoli, brussel sprouts, cauliflower, chickpeas, molasses, seeds soybeans, sprouts (especially alfalfa) and turnip greens.

Vitamin U (Methylmethioninesulfonium Chloride)

Cabbage.

Chapter 40

CYBER INFORMATION

The internet provides a full scope of information on cancer, ranging from conventional medicine to alternative treatments. The best search engines to use include Google, Alta Vista and Lycos. These search engines provide the most detailed sites on cancer. I have listed a few of the best sites here, but there are many others.

Magnacare
www.magnacare.com.
This is the official website of Magnacare Pty. Ltd. and here you will find further information on the Magnafield and other magnetic therapy devices.

Australian Bush Flower Essences
http://www.ausflowers.com.au/
This is the official website for Australian Bush Flower Essences and it is packed with information about these wonderful natural remedies.

American Cancer Society
http://www.cancer.org/
This is a wonderful site for basic information on different types of cancer, as well as some information on alternative and complementary therapies, as given from a conventional or orthodox point of view.

Oncolink
http://www.cancer.med.upenn.edu
This site is provided by the University of Pennsylvania in the United States. It contains some interesting information on cancer including risk factors, screening and treatment options, and personal stories. Oncolink also provides links to other great sites.

Cancer Guide: Steve Dunn's Cancer Information Page
http:///www.cancerguide.org
A wonderful all-round guide about cancer. Steve provides lots of useful information and some great advice on researching the best information.

National Foundation for Cancer Research
http://www.nfcr.org/
Comprehensive site which presents news and reports on the latest strives in cancer research. Also includes an index of treatment and prevention data.

CRFA
http://www.preventcancer.org/
Cancer Research Foundation of America focuses on cancer prevention. Advice on ways to reduce cancer risks and links to other great sites.

Cancer Links
http://www.cancerlinks.edu/
Browse details about the treatment centre and information about clinical trials.

Cancer Care – The American Institute for Cancer Research
http://www.aicr.org/
Practical advice for those undergoing treatment for cancer and their families, and toll-free telephone counselling.

Australian State Cancer Councils
You could also use one of the search engines to look up your local state cancer council. There you will be provided with a great deal of useful and up-to-date information on cancer. If you do not have access to the web, your local cancer council can also be contacted by phone. To get you started, the web address of the Victorian Cancer Council is: www.accv.org.au

MASTER CHART – CAUSES, ORTHODOX AND NATURAL TREATMENTS FOR VARIOUS CANCERS

Master Chart

Type of Cancer	Risk Factors & Major Causes	Orthodox Medical Treatment	Foods to Prevent & Treat	Vitamins & Nutrients	Useful Herbs	Other Alternative Therapies
All Cancers	Alcohol, artificial additives in foods, cigarette smoke, environmental toxins, carcinogens which are many and varied	Generally – surgery, chemotherapy, radiation therapy, immune therapy	Beetroot juice (100 ml/day), broccoli, cherries, cruciferous vegetables, dark green leafy vegetables, garlic, ginger, medicinal mushrooms, onions, turmeric, cabbage	Antioxidants, coenzyme Q10, colostrum, fish oils, GLA, glutathione, lactoferrin, lecithin, lipoic acid, pancreatic enzymes, selenium, omega 3s, shark cartilage	Astragalus, burdock root, essiac tea, medicinal mushrooms – reishi, shitake, ganoderma, maitake, pau d'arco, barley grass, wheat grass	Creative visualisation, detoxification and fasting, magnetic therapy, meditation, NO STRESS, yoga
Bladder	Excess caffeine, low water intake, tobacco use	Surgery, chemotherapy, laser with a cytoscope, radiation therapy, immunotherapy with BCG	Broccoli, brussel sprouts, cauliflower, carrots, celery, garlic, kale, lemon, parsley, plenty of pure water intake. No salt, dairy products, saturated fats, alcohol.	**Alpha-carotene, Beta-carotene, inositol,** DHEA, lactobacilli, selenium, **vitamin** A, vitamin B6, **vitamin C,** vitamin D, vitamin E, vitamin K,	Essiac, **garlic,** medicinal mushrooms	Colon cleansing, positive thinking, pulsed magnetic therapy
Bone (Osteo Sarcoma)	Excess of mould contamination in corn, grains, nuts, peanut butter, bread, cheese, non-inherited errors in DNA, radiation exposure	Surgery, chemotherapy	Broccoli, cruciferous vegetables, dark green leafy vegetables, fruit and vegetable juices, garlic, ginger medicinal mushrooms, onions, turmeric	Antioxidants, carotene, DHA/EPA, digestive enzymes, magnesium, quercetin, vitamin A, vitamin D,	Astragalus, burdock root, essiac tea, green tea, medicinal mushrooms such as shitake	Creative visualisation, detoxification, magnetic therapy, meditation, NO STRESS, yoga

Master Chart continued

Type of Cancer	Risk Factors & Major Causes	Orthodox Medical Treatment	Foods to prevent & Treat	Vitamins & Nutrients	Useful Herbs	Other Alternative Therapies
Brain Tumours	Electromagnetic fields (EMFs) environmental toxins, nitrosamines, polyvinyl chloride, possibly viruses, solvents	Surgery, chemotherapy, injections of chemotherapy drugs into the spine, radiation therapy	Beetroot, broccoli, brussel sprouts, cabbage, carrots, cauliflower, fibre, green tea, kale, mushrooms, spinach	Arginine, beta-carotene, bosweic acid, bromelain, coenzyme Q10, conjugated linoleic acid, curcumin, DHEA, DHA/EPA, essential fatty acids, evening primrose oil, melatonin, quercetin, selenium, taurine, vitamin B6, vitamin D, vitamin K	**Borage oil,** chapharral, essiac, **garlic,** pau d'arco shark cartilage, shark oils	Colon cleansing, light therapy, magnetic therapy, positive visualisation
Breast	**Excess alcohol consumption, excess fat intake, excess intake of sugar, excess oestrogen, fibrocystic breast disease, free** radicals, genetic predisposition, late childbearing age, **long term use of**	surgery, chemotherapy, radiation therapy, tamoxifen, biological therapy	**Broccoli, cabbage,** cherries, citrus peel, fenugreek, **garlic, radish seeds,** garlic, **flaxseed oil and linseed meal,** rice, seaweed, seeds, shitake mushrooms, **soybeans,** soy milk, soy products, tofu, primarily a vegetarian diet	Melatonin may **decrease by 50-70%** Breast dysplasia-give iodine **Beta-Carotene,** bromelain, calcium, coenzyme Q10, conjugated linoleic acid D. glucaric acid, **DHEA, EPA**	Dandelion, essiac, fenugreek, medicinal mushrooms, radish seeds, **red clover, schizandra**	Creative visualisation, magnetic therapies, heat therapy, light therapy, positivity

Site	Causes	Conventional treatments	Foods	Supplements / nutrients	Herbs	Other therapies
	the oral **contraceptive pill**, obesity, physical inactivity, radiation therapy before 30 years of age			genistein, indoles lactobacilli, quercetin, **lentinan**, limonene, lycopene, **selenium**, vitamin A, vitamin B6 **vitamin C**, **vitamin D**, **vitamin E**	Aloe vera, angelica, essiac, **green tea**, medicinal mushrooms – particularly shitake mushrooms, **slippery elm**	Chelation therapy, colonic cleansing, hair analysis to check for heavy metal toxicity, oxygen therapy, positive visualisation, pulsed magnetic therapy
Colon, Stomach, Bowel	**Excess alcohol intake, excess bile,** excess fat, excess intake of foods rich in nitrites, **excess protein (red meats)**, false morel mushrooms, free radicals, **long-term ulcerative colitis,** low intake of fibre, no exercise, pickled foods, polyps, smoking **STOMACH:** Alcohol, foods rich in nitrates and nitrites, helicobacter pylori infection, **low hydrochloric acid,**	Surgery, chemotherapy, radiation therapy, biological or immunotherapy	Barley, berries, broccoli, brown rice, **brussel sprouts, cabbage, cauliflower,** carrots, **celery, chives,** citrus, **garlic,** grapefruit, kale, linseed oil, **rice bran, seeds,** tomatoes, yogurt, soybeans **STOMACH: Capsicum, carrots, cucumber, miso, onions radish, soy – and the foods listed above**	**Beta-carotene, bifidobacteria bifidus, bifidobacteria bulgarius, butyric acid, calcium,** choline, cellulose, conjugated linoleic acid, digestive enzymes, essential fatty acids, fibre, folic acid, genistein, **lactobacillus acidophilus, lentinan lignans,** lycopene melatonin, **modified citrus pectin,** quercitin, selenium, **vitamins A, C, D**		

Master Chart continued

Type of Cancer	Risk Factors & Major Causes	Orthodox Medical Treatment	Foods to prevent & Treat	Vitamins & Nutrients	Useful Herbs	Other Alternative Therapies
Gum, Mouth, Tongue, Oral Leuko-plakia	Excess alcohol intake, nicotine – cigarette smoking	Surgery, radiation therapy	Broccoli, carrots, cauliflower, citrus, garlic, kale, linseed oil, pumpkin, shitake, sweet potatoes	Beta-carotene, carotenes, DHEA, essential fatty acids, folate, glutathione, glutamine, selenium, vitamin C, vitamin E	Essiac, green tea, medicinal mushrooms, pau d'arco, pimpernel tea	Creative and positive visualisation, magnetic therapy, oxygen therapy
Kidneys (renal)	Asbestos, environmental toxins, high blood pressure, long-term dialysis, low water intake, obesity, overuse of pain killers, radiation, smoking, vitamin D deficiency	Hormone treatment, kidney removal in surgery, chemotherapy, radiation therapy , arterial embolisation, immunotherapy	Broccoli, carrots, celery, kale, lemon, parsley, **shitake mushrooms, watermelon, watermelon seeds**	Borage oil, cysteine, DHEA, essential fatty acids, glutathione, melatonin, quercetin, vitamin A, vitamin C, vitamin D, vitamin E	ASTRAGALUS essiac, **green tea,** medicinal mushrooms, watermelon seed tea	Fasting/cleansing, heat therapy, magnetic therapy, positive thinking
Larynx, Oesoph-agus	Excess intake of alcohol on a regular basis, Excess tobacco (the combination of these two can be lethal on the throat membranes)	Surgery, chemotherapy, radiation therapy	Broccoli, brussel sprouts, carrots, citrus, garlic, kale, s strawberries, spinach, shitake mushrooms	Beta-carotene, garlic, genistein, lycopene, molybdenum (for oesophageal), vitamin A, vitamin B2, vitamin C, zinc	Aloe vera, echinacea essiac, **garlic** green tea, medicinal mushrooms, pau d'arco,	Heat therapy, light therapy, magnetic therapy, positive thinking

	Causes	Conventional treatment	Foods	Supplements	Herbs	Other therapies
Leukaemia	Benzene, chemotherapy drugs, exposure to chlordane, genetics, heptachlor, herbicides, irradiated foods, pesticides, radiation, smoking, solvents, viruses	Blood and marrow transplantation, chemotherapy, biological therapy, blood transfusions, Interferon-alpha, prednisone	Broccoli, brussel sprouts, cabbage, cauliflower, medicinal mushrooms – particularly shitake mushrooms, garlic	Antioxidants, **boswellic acid, CLA, coenzyme Q-10, creatine,** genistein, lipoic acid, lycopene, **potassium, quercetin, vitamin** A, vitamin B6, vitamin D, vitamin E **(use caution with folic acid)**	Echinacea, green tea, medicinal mushrooms, pau d'arco, **royal jelly**	Creative visualisation, light therapy, magnetic therapy
Liver	Arsenic exposure, choline deficiency, cirrhosis, **excess alcohol intake, excess intake of peanuts, peanut butter and corn – high in aflotoxins (fungal contaminant),** hepatitis B and C virus, long-term anabolic steroid use, polyvinyl chloride, tamoxifen, thorium dioxide	Surgery, chemotherapy, hormone therapy	Beetroot, broccoli, brussel sprouts, cabbage, carrots, cauliflower, dandelion greens, garlic, green leafy vegetables, kale, lecithin granules, spinach	Alpha-carotene, **beta-carotene,** choline, creatine, curcumin, **glutathione,** lecithin, limonene, **lipoic acid, lycopene,** methionine, quercetin, SAMe, selenium, vitamin C	Dandelion, essiac, **ginseng,** milk thistle, raw potato peel tea (make from the peels of potato), red clover, yellowdock	Blood cleansing, colon cleansing, fasting / cleansing, heat therapy

Master Chart *continued*

Type of Cancer	Risk Factors & Major Causes	Orthodox Medical Treatment	Foods to prevent & Treat	Vitamins & Nutrients	Useful Herbs	Other Alternative Therapies
Lung	Alcohol consumption, asbestos, cadmium, certain chemotherapy drugs, excess caffeine (5 cups or more/day), excess cholesterol consumption, excess fats, excess margarine, nicotine – cigarette smoking, environmental carcinogens like polyvinylchloride, low vegetable intake, petroleum, radon gas, uranium	Surgery, radiation therapy, chemotherapy, photodynamic therapy (PDT)	apricots, beetroot, broccoli, brussel sprouts, cabbage, cauliflower, carrots, kale, pumpkin, shitake mushrooms, squash, sweet potatoes, wakame	alpha-carotene, baicalein from scutellaria, baicalensis, beta-carotene, conjugated linoleic acid, DHEA, EFAs, folic acid, genistein, melatonin, selenium, thymus glandulars, uric acid, vitamin A, vitamin C, vitamin E	Chapharral, Chinese herbs, echinacea, essiac, green tea, lungwort, medicinal mushrooms, mullein, pau d'arco	Breathing exercises, chelation therapy, magnetic therapy, oxygen therapy, positive visualisation, yoga
Lymphomas (Lymphatic cancers)	Aspartame, excess intake of Chapharral (the herb) also found in essiac – use only as prescribed, coeliac disease may increase	Surgical lymphectomy, chemotherapy, radiation therapy, stem cell transplantation, biological therapy	Dark green leafy vegetables, fruit and vegetable juices, lemons, potassium broths, vegetable soups, watermelon	Alpha-carotenes bioflavonoids, bromelain, coenzyme Q10, lycopene, pancreatic enzymes, potassium,	Astragalus, bedstraw or clivers, dandelion root, green tea, lemongrass, medicinal mushrooms	Detoxification diets, fasting – avoid dairy products, salt, sugar, processed foods, magnetic therapy, creative visualisation

	the risk, dilantin, Epstein-Barr virus, exposure to herbicides, history of infections such as HIV or AIDS, pesticides, polyvinyl chloride, solvents			quercetin, vitamin A, vitamin C, vitamin E		Creative visualisation, heat therapy, light therapy, magnetic therapy
Ovarian	Asbestos exposure, **excess fat, excess oestrogen,** fertility drugs, free radicals, herbicide exposure, high intake of butter, milk or red meat, **tobacco smoking**	Surgery – removal of ovaries or tumour, chemotherapy, radiation therapy, biological therapy	Beetroot, broccoli, brussel sprouts, cauliflower, carrots, fibre, garlic, green tea, medicinal mushrooms, seaweed, soybeans	Algae, **bromelain** DHEA, DMSO, enzymes, **essential fatty acids,** genistein, indoles, **iodine,** magnesium, quercetin, **selenium,** SOD, vitamin E, vitamin A	Essiac formula, medicinal mushrooms, **red clover,** garlic	
Pancreas	Cirrhosis, chemicals, excess sugar, **excess alcohol intake (can increase the risk by 100%),** excess animal fat, **excess tea intake,** history of pancreatitis, insecticide exposure, smoking	Surgery, Radiation therapy and chemotherapy in combination, pancreatic enzyme tablets, insulin therapy	Broccoli, brussel sprouts, cabbage, cauliflower, citrus, garlic, grains, kale, linseed oil	**Alpha-carotene,** B vitamins, **beta-carotene,** chromium, DHEA, D – limonine **digestive enzymes,** essential fatty acids, fibre, fish oils, vitamin C	Essiac, green tea, medicinal mushrooms, sage tea	Chelation, colon cleansing, pulsed magnetic therapy

Master Chart continued

Type of Cancer	Risk Factors & Major Causes	Orthodox Medical Treatment	Foods to prevent & Treat	Vitamins & Nutrients	Useful Herbs	Other Alternative Therapies
Prostate	Excess caffeine, excess fat, excess oestrogen production, free radicals, high cholesterol, too much cadmium, use of sunglasses	Surgery, chemotherapy, radiation therapy, hormone treatment, brachytherapy, cryotherapy	Beetroot, broccoli, brown rice, brussel sprouts, carrots, cauliflower, garlic, kale, seeds, tomatoes – including sun-dried tomatoes	Beta-carotene, CLA, DHEA, EFAs, enzymes, essential fatty acids, genistein, indoles, lactoferin, lycopene, melatonin, modified citrus pectin, selenium, vitamin A, vitamin C, vitamin D, vitamin E, zinc	Berries, green tea, medicinal mushrooms, pau d' arco, pygeum, saw palmetto, bovine cartilage, willow herb tea	Colon cleansing, creative visualization, heat therapy, magnetic therapy, oxygen therapy, pulsed magnetic therapy
Rectal	Excess fat, excess refined carbohydrates, free radicals, low intake of fibre, polyps, ulcerative colitis	Surgery, chemotherapy, radiation therapy	Fibre rich foods, garlic, green leafy vegetables, linseed oil, tomatoes, wholegrains, yogurt	DHEA, enzymes, essential fatty acids, fibre, fish oils, lentinan, linseed oil, selenium, vitamin A, vitamin C, vitamin D	Green tea, medicinal mushrooms	Colon cleansing, colonic irrigation, ozone therapy, pulsed magnetic therapy
Skin, Melanoma	Dysplastic nevi, excess alcohol, family history, fair skin, fluorescent lighting, high intake of margarine, microwaves, oral contraceptive pill	Laser removal, surgery, chemotherapy, radiation therapy	Apricots, black-currants, carrots, garlic, grapefruit, grapes, mangoes, onions, papaya, raspberries, shitake mushrooms, sweet potatoes	Alpha-Carotene, azelaic acid, B vitamins, beta-carotene, boswellic acid, CLA, DHEA, EFAs, enzymes, genistein, glycine, lycopene, magnesium,	Aloe vera, astragalus, burdock chapparral, essiac, garlic, green tea, licorice, propolis, raspberry **Rhubarb is believed**	Chelation therapy, colon cleansing, heat therapy, magnetic therapy, positive thoughts

Cancer type	Causes	Treatment	Foods	Nutrients	Other therapies
	for more than 5 years, overexposure to UV sunlight, radiation, severe blistering sunburn, vitiligo, weak immune system			melatonin, N-acetyl cysteine, quercetin, **selenium, vitamin A, vitamin B6, vitamin C, vitamin E**	to retard growth of malignant melanoma — Colonic irrigation, magnetic therapy, oxygen therapy, positive visualisation
Testicular, Penis	Excess fat, free radicals, long term marijuana use	Surgery, radiation therapy, cancer drugs	Broccoli, carrots, cauliflower, garlic, kale, linseed oil, seeds, spinach, wholegrains	**Beta-carotene** DHEA, enzymes, essential fatty acids, flaxseed oil, laetrile	Essiac formula, medicinal mushrooms, green tea, willow herb tea,
Vagina, Cervix, Endometrium and Uterine Sarcomas	**ENDOMETRIUM:** ERT, high dietary fats, high oestrogen levels, irregular ovulation, many sexual partners, not having children, obesity, OHP, tobacco smoking **CERVIX:** Human papilloma virus, long term oral contraceptive use, poor nutrition, STD exposure, tobacco smoking	**ENDO-METRIUM:** Hysterectomy – surgical removal of uterus or endometrium, radiation therapy **CERVIX:** Surgery, radiation therapy, chemotherapy	Beetroot, berries, broccoli, brussel sprouts, carrots, cabbage, cauliflower, celery, figs, flaxseed oil and linseed meal, garlic, kale, shitake mushrooms, spinach, tomato	**Beta-carotene,** coenzyme Q10, digestive enzymes, d-glucarate, **folic acid,** indoles, lipoic acid, **lycopene,** quercetin, iodine, **Vitamin A, Vitamin B6, Vitamin C** injection or infusion **CERVICAL DYSPLASIA:** beta-carotene folic acid, vitamin B6, vitamin C	Astragalus, essiac, green tea, medicinal mushrooms, pau d'arco,
					Colon cleansing, heat therapy, magnetic therapy, positive visualisation

Words that are highlighted indicate extremely important nutrients or points for the individual cancer type specified.
CLA – Conjugated linoleic acid; DHA/EPA – Fish Oils; GLA – Gamma Linoleic Acid; Omega 3s – Omega 3 Fatty Acids; EFA – Essential Fatty Acids

Epilogue

LOOKING BACK ON IT ALL

One morning, I was sitting on the beautiful golden sands of a deserted beach in Thailand and a beautiful tangerine sun glimpsed at me from across the ocean. I sat down and thought to myself, 'Yeah ... I have beaten cancer and defied the odds.'

It hadn't really dawned on me until that moment. I thought to myself, 'God has given me another chance and he is reminding me of the beautiful gifts of nature, friendship and love that I have here all around me. He is giving me another chance to help others through my experience. He has given me the gifts of empathy and understanding.'

At that moment I felt truly blessed and the following words fell from my heart:

Earth's Chorus

As the sun rises,
The magical sounds
Of nature abound;

Echoes in time
Footprints on my heart,
Reflecting its glow
Earth's chorus can start.

The moon casts its spell
Healing the earth,
All creatures in harmony
A magical rebirth;

I take a deep breath
And reflect on this time,
Feeling so loved
As I am part of this rhyme.

Laughter seeps up
From deep in my core,
One of life's rare moments
Reveals a new door.

Thank you universe
For being so kind,
And sharing your treasures
To cleanse my full mind;

Lucky some say
I call it blessed,
To witness a new day
And to know true peace, in rest…

By Katrina Ellis

REFERENCES

Barsamian, S.T. & S.P., *A Morphogenic Process in Low Energy Electromagnetic Fields, Cancer Cells Activity,* Journal of Biological Physics, U.S.A Volume 18.

Becker, R.O., 1990 *Cross Currents- The Promise of Electromedicine, the Perils of Electropollution,* J. P. Tarcher Inc. Los Angeles, U.S.A, p 151-153.

Brawley, O.W., Parnes, H. 2000, *Prostate Cancer Prevention Trials in the USA,* European Journal of Cancer; 36 (10): 1312–1315.

Brock, J. 1995, *Lactoferrin: a multifunctional immunoregulatory protein?* Immunology Today 16, 9, p 417–419.

Coghill, R. 1990, *Electropollution and how to protect yourself against it,* Thorsons, Wellingborough, UK. Reported in *Physiology Journal* Feb 1991, Vol 22 No 2, p135.

Coghill, R. 1991, *DNA Hydrogen bonds and excess EMF energy.* Reported in *Physiology Journal,* Vol 22 No 2).

DeLuca, H.F. et al. 1998, *Mechanisms and function of vitamin D.* Nutr Rev: 56(2): S1-S10, U.S.A.

Feher, J. et al. 1989, *Immunopharmacology & Immunotoxicology,* 11 (1): 55–62, Review of Natural Products, Facts and Comparisons Publishers, St. Louis, U.S.A

Gao, Y.T. et al. 1994, YT Gao, *Reduced Risk of Esophageal Cancer Associated with Green Tea Consumption,* Journal of National Cancer Institute, United States: 86: 855–858.

Geelhoed, G.W., M.D. & Barilla, J., M.S. 1997, *Natural Health Secrets From Around the World,* Keats Publishing, Connecticut, p 44.

Grace, R.J. 1996, *The Role of Biomagnetic Fields in Nutrition Uptake,* 5th Oceania Symposium on Complementary Medicine proceedings, Bio Concepts, Qld. Australia p 60–75.

Grace, R.J. 1993, *Pulse Frequency specificity in magnetic field treatments* Bemic Publishing, Australia, p 4–23.

References

Grace, R.J. 1992, *Health Implications of Magnetic Fields*, 4th Oceania Symposium on Complementary Medicine, Bio Concepts, Queensland, Australia, p 119–134.

Hyperhealth CD Rom, 1995 – 2003, In-Tele-Health, Melbourne, Australia.

Kosaka, A. et al. 1987, *Gan To Kagaku Ryoho*, 14 (2): 516–22. (Japanese Journal of Cancer and Chemotherapy.)

Maekawa, S. et al. 1990, *Gan To Kagaku Ryoho*, 17 (1): 137–40. (Japanese Journal of Cancer and Chemotherapy.)

Magnacare Pty Ltd, 2002, Operator Manual MF2000, Magnacare Pty Ltd, Adelaide, Australia.

Ong TM, et al. 1986, *Chlorophyllin: a potent antimutagen against environmental and dietary complex mixtures.* Mutat research.173:11–5., U.S.A.

Persinger, M.A. 1988 *ELF & VLF Electromagnetic Field effects,* Plenum Press New York, U.S.A., Modern Bioelectricity, Marino, p 592.

Rinker, F. 1997, *The Invisible Force,* Mason Service Publishing, London, Ontario Canada, p 3-113.

Rodrigue, C.M. et al. 2001, *Resveratrol, a Natural Dietary Phytoalexin, Possesses Similar Properties to Hydroxyurea Towards Erythroid Differentiation.* British Journal of Haematology: 113 (2): 500–7, United Kingdom.

Shimizu, Y. et al. 1990, *Nippon Sanka Fujinka Gakkai Zasshi,* 42 (1): 37–44, Japan.

Singleton, P. & Sainsbury, D. 1996, *Dictionary of Microbiology and Molecular Biology,* 2nd ed. Wiley Publishers, U.S.A.

Swart, P.J et al., 1996 Jun 10, *Antiviral effects of milk proteins; Acylation results in polyanionic compounds with potent activity against human immunodeficiency virus types 1 and 2 in vitro.* AIDS Res. Hum. Retroviruses; 12(9), p769–75.

Tagachi, T. 1987, *Cancer Detection and Prevention,* 1 (Suppl): 333–49. U.S.A.

Warner, JR, et al. *Antimutagenicity Studies of Chlorophyllin Using the Salmonella Arabinose-resistant Assay System.* Mutat Res.1991:262:25–30. U.S.A.

BIBLIOGRAPHY

Balch, J., M.D. & Balch, P.A., C.N.C. 1997, *Prescriptions for Nutritional Healing*, Second Edition, Avery Publishing Group, New York, U.S.A.

Berendt, J.E. 1987, *The World is Sound, Nada Brahma*, Destiny Books, Rochester, Vermont, U.S.A.

Bragg, P.C., N.D., Ph.D. & Bragg, P., N.D., Ph.D, 1992, 44th reprint The Miracles of Apple Cider Vinegar, Health Science Publishers, California, U.S.A .

Buchman, D.D., with the Herb Society 1991, *Herbal Medicine, The Natural Way to Stay Well*, Tiger Books International PLC, Random House, Twickenham, U.K.

Chancellor, P.M. 1977, *Handbook of the Bach Flower Remedies*, The C.W.Daniel Company Ltd, U.K.

Cheraskin, E., M.D., D.M.D. 1989, *Health and Happiness*, Bio-Communications Press, Kansas, U.S.A.

Fischer, W.L. 1994, *How to Fight Cancer and Win*, Fischer Publishing Corporation, Ohio, U.S.A.

Gawain, S. 2002, *Creative Visualization: Use the Power of Your Imagination to Create What You Want in Your Life*, New World Library, California, U.S.A.

Golan, R., M.D. 1995, *Optimal Wellness*, Ballantyne Books, a division of Random House, Inc., New York, U.S.A.

Hall, D. 1992, *Dorothy Hall's Herbal Medicine*, Lothian Publishing Company, Melbourne, Victoria, Australia.

Halpern, S., & Savary, L., 1985, *Sound Health. The Music and Sounds That Make Us Whole*, Harper & Row Publishers, Sydney Australia & New York, U.S.A.

Harrison, Dr. J. 1990, *Love Your Disease, It's Keeping You Healthy*, Harper Collins Publishers, Australia.

Haye, L.L., 1984, 1988, You Can Heal Your Life, Specialist Publications, New South Wales, Australia.

Hoffman, D. 1992, *The New Holistic Herbal*, Element Books Ltd for Jacaranda Wiley Ltd, Milton, Brisbane, Queensland, Australia.

Koch, M. U. 1994, *Laugh with Health,* First published by Renaissance & New Age Creations. Revised edition published by Spectrum Access Pty Ltd, Toowong, Queensland, Australia.

Lowen, A., M.D. 1976, *Bioenergetics,* Penguin Books, London, U.K.

Lowenthal, R. 1990, 1996, *CANCER What to Do About It,* Lothian Books, Melbourne, Victoria, Australia.

Lust, J. 1974, *The Herb Book*, Bantam Books, published by arrangement with Benedict Lust Publications, New York, U.S.A.

Moss, R.W., 1996, *Cancer Therapy – the Independent Consumer's Guide to Non-Toxic Treatment and Prevention,* Equinox Press, Inc., New York, U.S.A.

Moule, T. 2000, *CANCER, the Healthy Option,* Kyle Cathie Ltd, London, U.K.

Murray, M., N.D. & Pizzorno, J., N.D. 1997, *Encyclopedia of Natural Medicine,* Revised 2nd Edition, Prima Health, California, USA.

Osiecki, H., B.Sc (Hons.) 1998, *The Physician's Handbook of Clinical Nutrition,* Fifth Edition, Bioconcepts Publishing, Kelvin Grove, Queensland, Australia.

Osiecki, H., B.Sc (Hons.) 2000, *The Nutrient Bible,* Bioconcepts Publishing, Kelvin Grove, Queensland, Australia.

Royal, P.C. 1989, *Herbally Yours,* Sound Nutrition, Utah, U.S.A.

Selbey, J. with Luhmann, M., M.D. 1991, *Conscious Healing, Visualizations to Boost Your Immune System,* Bantam Books, New York, New York, U.S.A.

Simonton, C.O., M.D., Mathews-Simonton, S., Creighton, J.L. 1992, *Getting Well Again,* Bantam Books, New York, New York, U.S.A.

Statham, B. 2002, *The Chemical Maze*, 2nd Edition, possibility.com, Victoria, Australia.

Thorsons Editorial Board 1989, *The Complete Raw Juice Therapy,* Harper Collins Publishers, Hammersmith, London, U.K.

Treben, M., 2001, *Health through God's Pharmacy*, 28th English Edition, Ennsthaler Verlag, A-4402 Steyr, Austria.

White, I. 1998, *Australian Bush Flower Essences*, Bantam Books, Sydney, Australia.

Willner, R.E., M.D., Ph.D. 1994, *The Cancer Solution*, Peltec Publishing Company, Florida, U.S.A.

Small Books and Pamphlets by the Queensland Cancer Fund, Australia.

- Understanding Hair Loss
- Nutrition
- Understanding Emotions
- Understanding Chemotherapy
- The Child with Cancer
- A Guide for the Partners of Women with Gynaecological Cancer

The Queensland Cancer Fund provides a range of support services for people with cancer. It can be contacted at:
www.qld.cancer.com.au

LIST OF TABLES

INDEX

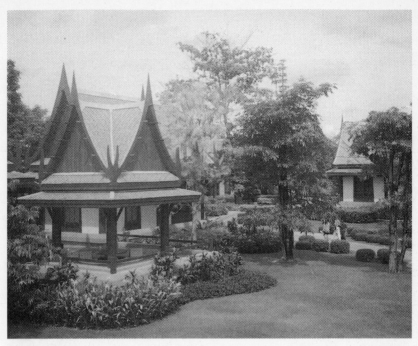

The five star health resort in Hua Hin, Thailand, where Katrina worked as a naturopath, nutritionist and yoga instructor before the onset of cancer.

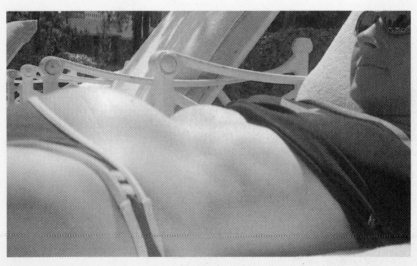

Within one month, Katrina's tumour had grown to 20cm in diameter, causing her stomach to protrude. At this early stage, doctors had diagnosed her condition as an ovarian cyst.

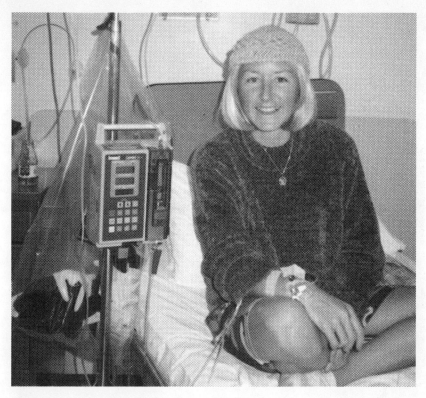

Katrina undergoing chemotherapy. She strongly urges people to remain smiling during this period to help promote a positive outcome.

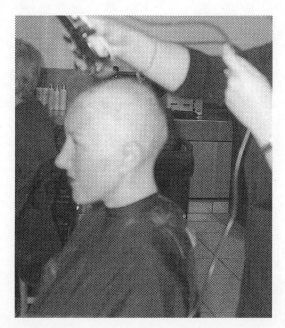

While having her last locks of hair shaved off, Katrina found it hard not to cry.

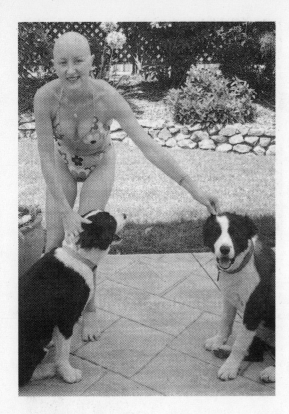

During the chemotherapy period, Katrina used natural medicine to help alleviate symptons. Here she is shown looking relatively healthy playing with her dogs.

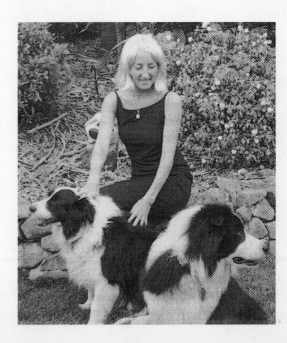

Katrina wearing her favourite wig and playing with her dogs. At this stage she has stopped chemotherapy and is using natural medicine instead.

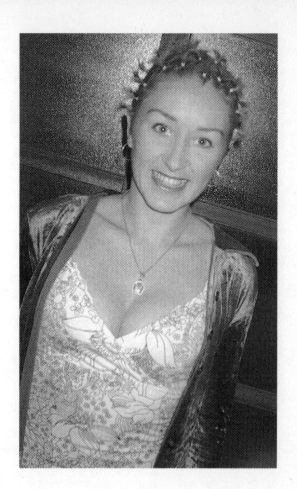

Katrina looking radiant and healthy – with the help of natural therapies, I am cancer-free!

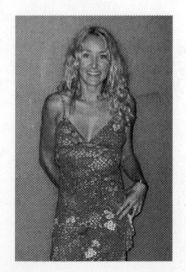

Four years after conquering cancer, Katrina is enjoying a happier and healthier life.

Colours

Famous Phrases

A famous phrase linked to yellow is
'mellow yellow', which means relaxed and happy.

Famous phrases linked to blue are 'feeling blue' and 'baby blue'.

A famous phrase linked to green is 'green with envy'.

A famous phrase linked to red is 'seeing red'.
This phrase embodies the energy of red.

A famous phrase linked to orange is 'orange as a summer sunset'.
This embodies the warmth of this beautiful colour.

A famous phrase linked to scarlet is
'scarlet woman', meaning woman of ill-repute and reminding
us that scarlet can be a powerful sexual stimulant.

A famous phrase associated with magenta is 'magnetic as magenta'.
This phrase embodies the warmth, vitality and attraction of magenta.

Famous phrases linked to violet are 'shrinking violet' and 'sweet violet'.
They may also refer to the violet plant – a plant with beautiful,
delicate flowers with a subtle fragrance that creates a sense of peace
and tranquillity itself.

A famous phrase linked to gold is 'good as gold'.
This embodies the true goodness and healing aspects of gold.

Famous phrases linked to white are 'whiter than new snow on a raven's back',
which signifies the purity of white, and 'white knight', which is often used to refer
to someone who has rescued or saved another, and signifies goodness.

A famous phrase linked to pink is 'pretty in pink', a saying which speaks for itself.

A common phrase linked to black is 'black hearted',
which signifies someone who is lacking in feeling or love,
or is obsessed with success and self-ego enhancement.
This is the colour black expressed negatively.